Pharmaceutical Mathematics with Application to Pharmacy

Pharmaceutical Mathematics with Application to Pharmacy

D.H. Panchaksharappa Gowda
Assistant Professor,
J.S.S. College of Pharmacy,
Sri Shivarathreeshwara Nagar,
Mysore-570 015.

PharmaMed Press
An imprint of Pharma Book Syndicate
A unit of BSP Books Pvt. Ltd.
4-4-309/316, Giriraj Lane,
Sultan Bazar, Hyderabad - 500 095.

Pharmaceutical Mathematics with Application to Pharmacy-

by D.H. Panchaksharappa Gowda

Published by

PharmaMed Press

An imprint of Pharma Book Syndicate

A unit of BSP Books Pvt. Ltd.

4-4-309/316, Giriraj Lane, Sultan Bazar, Hyderabad - 500 095.

Phone: 040-23445605, 23445688; Fax: 91+40-23445611

E-mail: info@pharmamedpress.com

ISBN : 978-93-85433-78-8 (HB)

Foreword

It gives me immense pleasure in introducing this book on **"Pharmaceutical Mathematics with Application to Pharmacy"** authored by Mr. Panchaksharappa Gowda D.H. This book describes the fundamental aspects of Pharmaceutical Mathematics a core subject, Industrial Pharmacy and Pharmacokinetics application in a very easy to read and understandable language with number of pharmaceutical examples. This book not only deals with Pharmaceutical Mathematics but also with related aspects such as Factorial design problems (formulations), Pharmacokinetics and Physical pharmaceutics, etc.

The book is not just theoretical, but based on the practical application by the author over the years. As far as I know there has been no attempts earlier by an Indian author to write a textbook in this area specially related to Pharmacy course.

The author of this book is known for his expertise in teaching for more than twenty seven years, a dedicated, student caring teacher was instrumental in introducing Pharmaceutical Mathematics at B.Pharm and Pharm D level. He worked very hard in restructuring the JSS University, Mysore syllabus of Pharmaceutical Mathematics and Biostatistics and Computer application in Pharmacy. He has conducted workshops on Design of experiments (DOE) and Biostatistics and its application for M.Pharm and Doctoral students.

I am sure this book will be highly informative and interesting reading material for the students of B.Pharm, Pharm D and M.Pharm and other related course in the field of Pharmaceutical Sciences.

It is my great pleasure to commend this textbook, as it will strengthen and support in learning the related Pharmacy subjects.

I wish every success to Mr. Panchaksharappa Gowda D. H. for all such endeavors.

Dr. B. Suresh

President, Pharmacy Council of India
Vice chancellor, JSS University,
JSS Medical Institutions campus,
Mysore-570 015.

Preface

Mathematics has been given an important place in pharmacy course to solve various equations in pharmacokinetics. No students of these discipline can afford without the knowledge of those topics which are explained in this book. The present text is designed to introduce students about the methods and applications of Mathematics in Industrial Pharmacy and Pharmacokinetics.

This book covers theoretical, Practical and applied aspects of mathematics in a clear and exhaustive way. The author has attempted to give as many illustrations as possible in order to make the students to understand various methods in solving or deriving the Pharmacokinetics Problems. I claim no originality for the matter presented in the text, however, the methods of presentation and arrangement of the subject-matter is my own, which reflects an approach for mathematical methods to solve kinetic equation and also understandability based on the long teaching experience of degree (B.Pharm, Pharm.D) and Post-graduate classes.

I hope that the book will be found more useful by the students. I invite suggestions from students as well as my teacher-friends for any improvement (addition or deletion) of the book in future. I would like to thank my colleagues for their encourage and suggestions.

The author accepts full responsibility for any typographical or subject-matter errors, which may be there in the book of this dimension and subject.

- Author

Contents

Chapter – 5

Introduction to Functions

Chapter – 6

Differentiation

CHAPTER 1

PARTIAL FRACTIONS

1.1 INTRODUCTION

We know the method of combining number of fractions into a single by taking LCM (least common multiple) of denominators of the fractions. Now, here we have to learn, converse problem, that is splitting up of a given fraction into a number of simpler fractions called **Partial Fractions**.

In this Chapter, we study the method of resolving a given fraction into Partial fractions.

1.1.1 Polynomial

An algebraic expression of the form $f(x) = a_0x^n + a_1x^{n-1} + \dots + a_n$ is called a polynomial in x, where $a_0 \neq 0$, a_1, a_2, ... a_n are real constants and x is an unknown variable. The highest power of x that exists in the expression is called the degree of the polynomial.

Ex: $f(x) = x^5 + 4x^4 + 3x^3 + 4x^2 + x + 1$

$a_0 = 1$ $a_1 = 4$ $a_2 = 3$ $a_3 = 4$ $a_5 = 1$

$a_6 = 1$ are real constants and degree is 5, because the highest power of x is 5

1.1.2 Rational Fraction

The quotient $\dfrac{P(x)}{Q(x)}$ of two polynomials P(x) and $Q(x) \neq 0$ is called a rational fraction.

Ex: $P(x) = x^2 + 3x + 5$

$Q(x) = 3x^3 + 4x^2 + 5x + 1$

$$\frac{P(x)}{Q(x)} = \frac{x^2+3x+5}{3x^3+4x^2+5x+1}$$

1.1.3 Proper and Improper Fractions

The rational fraction $\frac{P(x)}{Q(x)}$ is a proper fraction, if the degree of the numerator P(x) is less than the degree of the denominator Q(x).

Ex: $\frac{x+1}{x^2+2x+1} = \frac{P(x)}{Q(x)}$

$P(x) = x + 1$ – Degree = 1

$Q(x) = x^2 + 2x + 1$ – Degree = 2

The rational fraction $\frac{P(x)}{Q(x)}$ is a improper fraction, if the degree of numerator P(x) is greater than or equal to the degree of the denominator Q(x).

Ex: 1. $\frac{P(x)}{Q(x)} = \frac{x^2+2x+1}{x^2+3x+1}$

P(x) – degree = 2

Q(x) – degree = 2

2. $\frac{P(x)}{Q(x)} = \frac{x^3+2x^2+3x+1}{x^2+3x+2}$

P(x) – degree = 3

Q(x) – degree = 2

3. $\dfrac{x^3+2x^2+3x-4}{x^2+x+3}$

$$
\begin{array}{r|l}
x^2+x+3 & \;\; x+1 \\ \hline
 & x^3+2x^2+3x-4 \\
 & x^3+x^2+3x \\ \hline
 & \quad x^2+0-4 \\
 & \quad x^2+x+3 \\ \hline
 & \quad -x-7
\end{array}
$$

$$\therefore \quad \frac{x^3+2x^2+3x-4}{x^2+x+3} = x+1+\frac{-x-7}{x^2+x+3}$$

1.2 PARTIAL FRACTION

Consider

$$\frac{1}{x+1}+\frac{2}{x+2}=\frac{x+2+2(x+1)}{(x+1)(x+2)}$$

$$\frac{1}{x+1}+\frac{2}{x+2}=\frac{3x+3}{(x+1)(x+2)}$$

How to resolve $\dfrac{3x+3}{(x+1)(x+2)}$ into $\dfrac{1}{x+1}+\dfrac{2}{x+2}$

1.2.1 Rules to Resolve into Partial Fraction

1. Denominator containing linear distinct factors

$$\frac{p(x)}{q(x)r(x)}=\frac{A}{q(x)}+\frac{B}{r(x)}$$

A and B are constants to be determined

$$\frac{3x+3}{(x+1)(x+2)}=\frac{A}{x+1}+\frac{B}{x+2} \qquad \text{..... (1)}$$

Take LCM for RHS – side equation

$$\frac{3x+3}{(x+1)(x+2)}=\frac{A(x+2)+B(x+1)}{(x+1)(x+2)}$$

Cancel the denominator of LHS and RHS

$$3x + 1 = A(x + 2) + B(x + 1) \quad \text{..... (2)}$$

Put $x + 1 = 0 \rightarrow x = -1$

Substitute $x = -1$ in equation (2)

$$3(-1) + 1 = A(-1 + 2) + B.0$$

$$-3 + 1 = A.1 + 0$$

$$-2 = A, A = -2$$

$$A = -2$$

Put $x + 2 = 0 \rightarrow x = -2$

Substitute $x = -2$ in equation (2)

$$3x + 1 = A(x + 2) + B(x + 1)$$

$$(-2) + 1 = A.0 + B(-2 + 1)$$

$$-6 + 1 = 0 + B(-1)$$

$$-5 = -B \rightarrow B = 5$$

$$B = 5$$

Take equation (1), substitute A and B

$$\frac{3x+3}{(x+1)(x+2)} = \frac{A}{x+1} + \frac{B}{x+2}$$

$$\frac{3x+3}{(x+1)(x+2)} = \frac{-2}{x+1} + \frac{5}{x+2}$$

2. Denominator containing linear repeated factors:

If $$\frac{p(x)}{q(x)} = \frac{x+1}{(x+a)^3}$$

The fraction should be resolve as

$$\frac{x+1}{(x+a)^3} = \frac{A}{x+a} + \frac{B}{(x+a)^2} + \frac{C}{(x+a)^3}$$

Then the values of A, B, C are to be determined

Ex: $$\frac{x+1}{(x+2)^3} = \frac{A}{x+2} + \frac{B}{(x+2)^2} + \frac{C}{(x+2)^3} \qquad .....(1)$$

Take terms LCM and add the RHS side

$$\frac{x+1}{(x+2)^3} = \frac{A(x+2)^2 + B(x+2) + C}{(x+2)^3}$$

$$x + 1 = A(x + 2)^2 + B(x + 2) + C \qquad .....(2)$$

Put $x + 2 = 0$

$x = -2$

Substitute $x = -2$ in equation (2)

$-2 + 1 = 0 + 0 + C$

$-1 = C$

$C = -1$

$x + 1 = A(x + 2)^2 + B\ (x + 2) + C$

$x = 1 = A(x^2 + 4x + 4) + B(x + 2) + C$

$x + 1 = Ax^2 + 4Ax + 4A + Bx + 2B + C$

$x + 1 = Ax^2 + 4Ax + 4A + Bx + 2B + C$

Equate coefficient of x

$$1 = 4A + B \qquad .....(3)$$

Equate coefficient of x^2

$0 = A$

$A = 0$

Take (3)

$1 = 4.A + B$

$1 = 4.0 + B$

$B = 1$

Substitute A, B and C in (1)

$$\frac{x+1}{(x+2)^3} = \frac{A}{x+2} + \frac{B}{(x+2)^2} + \frac{C}{(x+2)^3}$$

$$= \frac{0}{x+2} + \frac{1}{(x+2)^2} + \frac{-1}{(x+2)^3}$$

$$\frac{x+1}{(x+2)^3} = \frac{1}{(x+2)^2} - \frac{1}{(x+2)^3}$$

3. Denominator containing non-repeated non-factorizable factor. To each non-repeated, non-factorizable quadratic factor of the type $(ax^2 + bx + c)$ of the denominator,

Ex: $$\frac{x^2-1}{(x^2+3)(x+1)} = \frac{Ax+B}{x^2+3} + \frac{C}{x+1} \quad \text{..... (1)}$$

Take L.C.M

$$\frac{x^2-1}{(x^2+3)(x+1)} = \frac{(Ax+B)(x+1)+C(x^2+3)}{(x^2+3)(x+1)}$$

$$x^2 - 1 = (Ax + B)(x + 1) + C(x^2 + 3) \quad \text{.....(2)}$$

Put $x + 1 = 0 \rightarrow x = -1$

Substitute $x = -1$ in (2)

$$x^2 - 1 = (Ax + B)(x + 1) + C(x^2 + 3)$$

$$(-1)^2 - 1 = 0 + ((-1)^2 + 3)\, C$$

$$0 = (1 + 3)\, C$$

$$0 = 4.C \qquad C = 0$$

To find $A \propto B$

Equate coefficient x in the equation

$$x^2 - 1 = (Ax + B)(x + 1) + C(x^2 + 3)$$

$$0 = A + B$$

$$A + B = 0 \qquad A = -B$$

Compare coefficient of x^2

$$1 = A + C$$

$$1 = A + 0$$

$$A = 1$$

But

$$A = -B$$

$$B = -A$$

$\therefore \quad B = -1$

$$\frac{x^2-1}{(x^2+3)(x+1)} = \frac{Ax+B}{x^2+3} + \frac{C}{x+1}$$

Substitute A = 1, b = –1, c = 0 in equation (1)

$$\frac{x^2-1}{(x^2+3)(x+1)} = \frac{1.x-1}{x^2+3} + \frac{0}{x+1}$$

$$\frac{x^2-1}{(x^2+3x+1)} = \frac{x-1}{x^2+3}$$

$$= \frac{x}{x^2+3} - \frac{1}{x^2+3}$$

1.3 APPLICATION OF PARTIAL FRACTION IN CHEMICAL KINETICS AND PHARMACOKINETICS

1. In a second-order kinetics, the differential rate expression is given by the equation

$$r = \frac{dx}{dt} = K_2(a-x)(b-x) \qquad \frac{dx}{(a-x)(b-x)} = Kdt$$

To solve this equation. We have to obtain the partial fraction of

$$\frac{1}{(a-x)(b-x)}$$

As per Partial fraction rule

$$\frac{1}{(a-x)(b-x)} = \frac{A}{a-x} + \frac{B}{b-x} \qquad \text{.....(1)}$$

Take LCM

$$\frac{1}{(a-x)(b-x)} = \frac{A(b-x)+B(a-x)}{(a-x)(b-x)}$$

$$1 = A(b-x) + B(a-x) \qquad \text{.....(2)}$$

Put $b - x = 0 \quad x = b$

$$1 = 0 + B\,(a-b)$$

$$\frac{1}{a-b} = B$$

Put $a - x = 0, x = a$

Take equation (2)

$$1 = A\,(b - x) + B\,(a - x)$$

$$1 = A\,(b - a\,) + .0$$

$$A = \frac{1}{b - a}$$

But

$$\frac{1}{(a - x)(b - x)} = \frac{A}{a - x} + \frac{B}{b - x}$$

Substitute A and B in equation (1)

$$\frac{1}{(a - x)(b - x)} = \frac{\frac{1}{b - a}}{a - x} + \frac{\frac{1}{a - b}}{b - x}$$

$$= \frac{1}{(b - a)(a - x)} + \frac{1}{(a - b)(b - x)}$$

$$= \frac{1}{-(a - b)(a - x)} + \frac{1}{(a - b)(b - x)}$$

$$= \frac{1}{(a - b)(b - x)} - \frac{1}{(a - b)(a - x)}$$

$$= \frac{1}{a - b}\left[\frac{1}{b - x} - \frac{1}{a - x}\right]$$

2. First order Absorption (Infusion Method)

For a drug that enters the body by an apparent first-order absorption process, is eliminated by a first - order process and distributes in the body according to a one - compartment model, is given by equation.

$$\frac{dx}{dt} = K_a X_a - KX$$

It can be reduced into the form $\overline{X} = \dfrac{K_a F X_0}{(S + K)(S + K_a)}$ by applying Laplace transform

To find the value of X, we have to find the partial fraction of the equation

$$\frac{1}{(S + K)(S + K_a)}$$

$$\frac{1}{(S+K)(S+K_a)} = \frac{A}{S+K} + \frac{B}{S+K_a}$$

Take LCM in RHS

$$\frac{1}{(S+K)(S+K_a)} = \frac{A(S+K_a)+B(S+K)}{(S+K)(S+K_a)}$$

$$1 = A(S + K_a) + B(S + K) \qquad \text{.....(1)}$$

Put $S + K = 0 \rightarrow S = -K$

Substitute $S = -K$ in (1)

$$\frac{1}{K_a - K} = A$$

Put $S + K_a = 0 \rightarrow S = -K_a$

Substitute $S = -K_a$ in (1)

$$1 = A\,(S + K_a) + B\,(S + K)$$

$$1 = A - 0 + B\,(-K_a + K)$$

$$B = \frac{1}{K - K_a}$$

$$B = \frac{1}{(K - K_a)}$$

Take

$$\frac{1}{(S+K)(S+K_a)} = \frac{A}{S+K} + \frac{B}{S+K_a}$$

Substitute the values A and B

$$\frac{1}{(S+K)(S+K_a)} = \frac{\frac{1}{K_a - K}}{S+K} + \frac{\frac{1}{K - K_a}}{S+K_a}$$

$$= \frac{1}{(K_a - K)(S+K)} + \frac{1}{(K - K_a)(S+K_a)}$$

$$= \frac{1}{(K_a - K)(S+K)} - \frac{1}{(K_a - K)(S+K_a)}$$

$$\frac{1}{(S+K)(S+K_a)} = \frac{1}{K_a - K}\left[\frac{1}{S+K} - \frac{1}{S+K_a}\right]$$

3. The rapid intravenous injection of a drug that distribute in the body according to two compartment model system with elimination occurring from the central compartment is as shown in model and the amount of drug in the central compartment a_{sc} is given by equation (function)

$$a_{sc} = X_0 \frac{(S+E_2)}{(S+\lambda_1)(S+\lambda_2)}$$

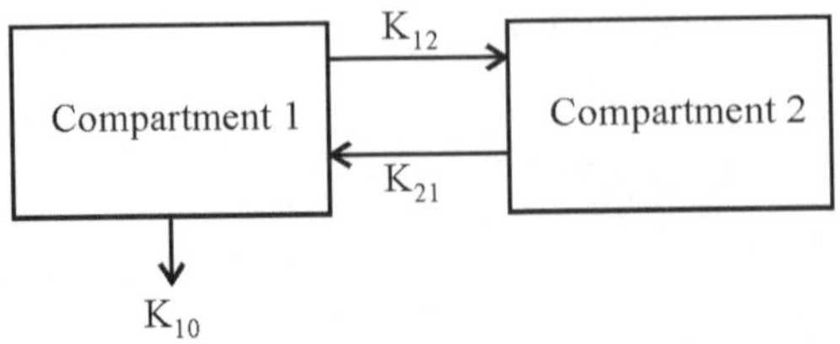

To calculate concentration of drug in the central compartment, the above mentioned equation $\frac{(S+E_2)}{(S+\lambda_1)(S+\lambda_2)}$ has to be resolved into partial fraction.

After resolution into partial fraction, we will arrive into the equation

$$\frac{(S+E_2)}{(S+\lambda_1)(S+\lambda_2)} = \frac{A}{S+\lambda_1} + \frac{B}{S+\lambda_2}$$

$$= \frac{E_2-\lambda_1}{(\lambda_2-\lambda_1)(S+\lambda_1)} - \frac{E_2-\lambda_2}{(\lambda_2-\lambda_1)(S+\lambda_2)}$$

4. The disposition function for the central compartment in three compartmental model is given by the equation.

$$d_{sc} = \frac{(S+E_2)(S+E_3)}{(S+\lambda_1)(S+\lambda_2)(S+\lambda_3)}$$

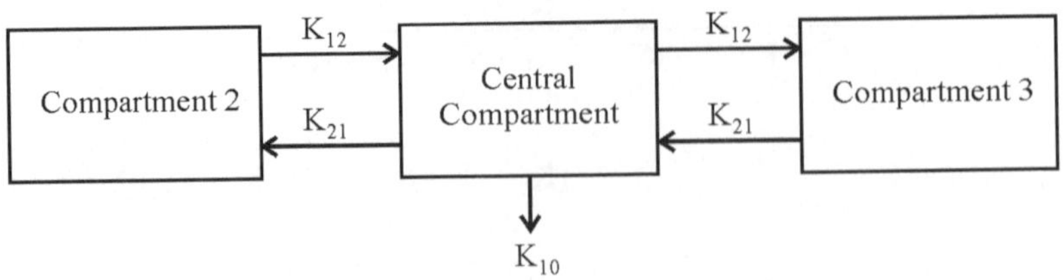

Amount of drug in central compartment a_{sc}, which is product of input and disposition is given by the fraction.

$$a_{sc} = \frac{X_0(S+E_2)(S+E_3)}{(S+\lambda_1)(S+\lambda_2)(S+\lambda_3)}$$

After resolving into partial fraction, the equation will be reduced into the form

$$a_{sc} = \frac{X_0(E_2-\lambda_1)(E_3-\lambda_1)}{(\lambda_2-\lambda_1)(\lambda_3-\lambda_1)}\frac{1}{(S+\lambda_1)} + \frac{X_0(E_2-\lambda_2)(E_3-\lambda_2)}{(\lambda_1-\lambda_2)(\lambda_3-\lambda_2)}\frac{}{(S+\lambda_2)}$$

$$+\frac{X_0(E_2-\lambda_3)(E_3-\lambda_3)}{(\lambda_1-\lambda_3)(\lambda_2-\lambda_3)(S+\lambda_3)}$$

5. When the drug is administered intravenously at a constant rate, rate of change of drug in the body with respect time can be obtained by the Linear differential equation.

$$\frac{dx}{dt} = K_0 - Kx$$

K_0 – is rate of drug infusion

After simplification by applying Laplace Transform

$$\overline{X} = \frac{K_0}{S(S+K)}$$

To calculate total amount of drug in the body, the equation $\frac{K_0}{S(S+K)}$ has to be resolved into partial fraction form

$$\frac{K_0}{S(S+K)} = \frac{A}{S} + \frac{B}{S+K}$$

Take LCM

$$\frac{1}{S(S+K)} = \frac{A(S+K)+B(S)}{S(S+K)}$$

$$1 = A(S+K) + B.S \qquad \text{..... (1)}$$

Put $S = 0$ in (1)

$$1 = A(0+K) + B.0$$

$$1 = A.K$$

$$A = \frac{1}{k}$$

Put $S + K = 0 \rightarrow S = -K$

Substitute $S = -K$ in equation (1)

$$1 = A(S + K) + B.S$$

$$1 = A.0 + B(-K)$$

$$B = -\frac{1}{K}$$

$$\frac{K_0}{S(S+K)} = \frac{A}{S} + \frac{B}{S+K}$$

$$\frac{1}{S(S+K)} = \frac{\frac{1}{K}}{S} + \frac{\frac{-1}{K}}{S+K}$$

$$= \frac{1}{K}.\frac{1}{S} - \frac{1}{K}\frac{1}{S+K}$$

Exercise 1.1

Resolve into Partial Fraction

1. $\frac{3x+5}{(x-1)(x+2)}$
2. $\frac{1}{(x-2)(x-1)^2}$
3. $\frac{2x-3}{(x+5)(x-2)}$
4. $\frac{x+1}{(x)(x+2)(x+4)}$
5. $\frac{3x^2+2x-2}{(x-1)^2(2x-1)}$
6. $\frac{5x^2+1}{x^3-1}$

Answers

1. $\frac{8}{3(x-1)} + \frac{1}{3(x+2)}$
2. $\frac{1}{(x-2)} - \frac{1}{(x-1)} - \frac{1}{(x-1)^2}$
3. $\frac{13}{7(x+5)} + \frac{1}{7(x-2)}$
4. $\frac{-1}{2x} - \frac{2}{3(x-1)} - \frac{1}{6(x+2)}$
5. $\frac{2}{x-1} + \frac{3}{(x-1)^2} - \frac{1}{2x-1}$
6. $\frac{2}{(x-1)} + \frac{3x+1}{(x^2+x+1)}$

CHAPTER 2

LOGARITHMS

2.1 INTRODUCTION

In the absence of calculators and computers, logarithms play an important role in calculations. The operations of multiplication and division are replaced by addition and subtraction and those of raising to a power and extracting a root by multiplication John Napier (1550-1617) introduced the concept of logarithms and Henry Briggs (1556-1631) modified them to suit calculations.

2.1.1 Definition of Logarithm

If a is a positive real number other than 1 such that $a^x = m$, then x is called the logarithm of m to the base a. We write $x = \log_a m$ ($a > 0$, $a \neq 1$)

Thus, if $a^x = m$, then $x = \log_a m$ and

If $x = \log_a(m)$, then $a^x = m$

For example

$2^4 = 16$	$\therefore$	$4 = \log_2 16$; $3^3 = 27 \therefore 3 = \log_3 27$
$10^4 = 10{,}000$	$\therefore$	$4 = \log_{10} (10{,}000)$
$\log_5 25 = 2$	$\because$	$5^2 = 25$
$\log_{\sqrt{2}} 32 = 10$	$\because$	$\log(\sqrt{2})^{10} = 32$

The above examples indicate that indices lead to logarithms and vice-versa.

We define the logarithm as follows:

The logarithm of a number to a given base is the index or the power to which the base should be raised in order to get the number

$\log_a 1 = 0$ $\quad (\because\ a^0 = 1)$ Here $a > 0$, $a \neq 1$

$\log_a a = 1 \qquad (\because\ a^1 = a)$

$\log_a 0 = -\infty \qquad (\because\ a^{-\infty} = \frac{1}{a^{\infty}} = 0)$

for example, $\log_{10}1 = 0$, $\log_e 1 = 0$, $\log_e e = 1$, $\log_{10}10 = 1$

The logarithms to base 10 are called common logarithms. The logarithms to the base e are called Napierian Logarithms or Natural.

[e is called the exponential constant. It is an irrational number lying between 2 and 3].

The graph of $y = \log_{10}x$ when x is a positive real number.

when $x = 1$, $y = \log_{10}1 = 0$

when $x = 10$, $y = \log_{10}10 = 1$

when $x = 100$, $y = \log_{10}100 = 2$ and so on

when $x = \frac{1}{10}$, $y = \log_{10}\left(\frac{1}{10}\right) = -1$

when $x = \frac{1}{100}$, $y = \log_{10}\left(\frac{1}{100}\right) = -2$ and so on

Thus, if $0 < x < 1$, y is negative and if $x > 1$, y is positive. The graph is as shown in Fig. 2.1.

Graph of $y = \log_{10} x$

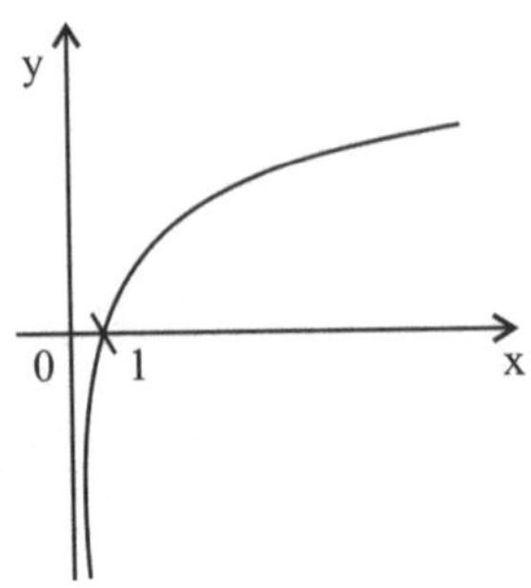

Fig. 2.1

Graph of $y = \log_e x$

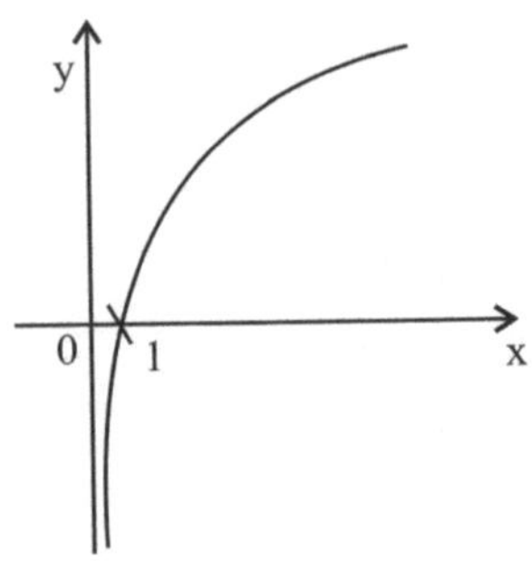

Fig. 2.2

The graph of $y = \log_e x$ when x is a positive real number.

when $x = 1$, $\qquad y = \log_e 1 = 0$

when $x = e$, $\qquad y = \log_e e = 1$

when $x = e^2$, $\qquad y = \log_e e^2 = 2$ and so on

when $x = \frac{1}{e}$, $y = \log_e\left(\frac{1}{e}\right) = -1$

When $0 < x < 1$, y is negative and when $x > 1$, y is positive. The graph is as shown Fig. 2.2

2.2 THEOREMS ON LOGARITHMS

Theorem 1

$$\log_a(mn) = \log_a m + \log_a n$$

Proof: Take $\log_a(mn) = x$, $\log_a m = y$, $\log_a n = z$

Then $a^x = mn$ .....(1)

$a^y = m$ .....(2)

$a^z = n$ .....(3)

Substitute (2), (3) in (1) for m and n, we get,

$$a^x = a^y . a^z \quad \text{i.e., } a^x = a^{y+z} \quad \therefore \quad x = y + z$$

i.e., $\log_a(mn) = \log_a m + \log_a n$

Similarly we have

$$\log_a(mnlp \ldots) = \log_a m + \log_a n + \log_a l + \log_a p + \ldots$$

Note: $\log_a (m + n) \neq \log_a m + \log_a n$ expect in the following cases

Theorem 2

$$\log_a\left(\frac{m}{n}\right) = \log_a m - \log_a n$$

Proof: Take $\log_a\left(\frac{m}{n}\right) = x$, $\log_a m = y$ and $\log_a n = z$

Then $a^x = \frac{m}{n}$ ..... (1)

$a^y = m$ ..... (2)

$a^z = n$ ..... (3)

Substitute for m, n in (1), we get,

$$a^x = \frac{a^y}{a^z} \text{ i.e., } a^x = a^{y-z} \qquad \therefore\ x = y = z$$

$$\therefore \qquad \log_a\left(\frac{m}{n}\right) = \log_a m - \log_a n$$

Theorem 3: $\log_a(m^n) = n \log_a m$

Proof:

Take $\log_a(m^n) = x$ and $\log_a m = y$

Then $m^n = a^x$ ..... (1)

$m = a^y$ ..... (2)

Substitute $m = a^y$ in (1), we get

$(a^y)^n = a^x$ i.e., $a^{ny} = a^x$

$\therefore$ $ny = x$ or $x = ny$

$\therefore$ $\log_a(m^n) = n\log_a m$

Theorem 4: (Theorem on change of base) $\log_a N = \dfrac{\log_e N}{\log_e a}$

Proof: Take $\log_a N = x$, $\log_e N = y$, $\log_e a = z$

Then $a^x = N$ ..... (1)

$e^y = N$ ..... (2)

$e^2 = a$ ..... (3)

From (1) and (2) we get $a^x = e^y$

Put $a = e^z$, we get $(e^z)^x = e^y$

i.e., $e^{zx} = e^y \therefore zx = y$

or $x = \dfrac{y}{z}$ i.e., $\log_a N = \dfrac{\log_e N}{\log_e a}$

Thus we have

(1) $\log_a(mn) = \log_a m + \log_a n$

(2) $\log_a\left(\dfrac{m}{n}\right) = \log_a m - \log_a n$

(3) $\log_a\left(m^n\right) = n\log_a m$

(4) $\log_a N = \dfrac{\log_e N}{\log_e a}$

Note: $\log_a N = \dfrac{\log_N N}{\log_N a}$ [using (4)]

$$= \frac{1}{\log_N a} \quad (\because \quad \log_N N = 1)$$

So, we have $= \log_a N = \dfrac{1}{\log_N a}$

2.3 COMMON LOGARITHMS

Logarithms to the base 10 are called common logarithms. These were first introduced by Henry Briggs in 1615. If '*n*' is the given number and *x* denote the logarithm of '*n*' w.r.t. base 10, then we have $10^x = n$. This equation shows that the common logarithm of a number consists of an integral part and a fractional part and sometimes it can be negative also.

For example, $254 > 10^2$ and $< 10^3$

$\therefore \quad \log_{10} 254 = 2 + \text{a fraction}$

Again, $0.003 > 10^{-3}$ and $< 10^{-2} \therefore \log_{10} 0.003 = -3 + \text{a fraction}$

2.4 CHARACTERISTIC AND MANTISSA

Definition: The integral part of a logarithm is called the **characteristic** and the fractional part is called the **Mantissa.**

To find the characteristic of the logarithm of any number greater than one.

Since $10^0 = 1$, $10^1 = 10$, $10^2 = 100$, $10^3 = 1000$, ... etc, it follows that a number with one digit in its integral part lies between 10^0 and 10^1, a number with two digit in its integral part lies between 10^1 and 10^2; and so on. Hence a number with a digit in its integral part lies between 10^{n-1} and 10^n.

$\therefore$ If *N* is a number whose integral part contains '*n*' digit,

then $N = 10^{(n-1)} + \text{a fraction}$

$\therefore \log_{10} N = (n-1) + \text{a fraction}.$

Hence, the characteristic of a logarithm of a number greater than one is one less than the number of digits in its integral part and is positive.

To find the characteristic of a logarithm of any number less than one (a decimal fraction).

Since $10^0 = 1$, $10^{-1} = 0.1$, $10^{-2} = 0.01$, $10^{-3} = 0.001$, ... etc., it follows that a decimal with no zero immediately after the decimal point lies between 10^{-1} and 10^0; a number two zeros immediately after the decimal point lies between 10^{-2}

and 10^{-1}; and so on. Hence a decimal fraction with n zeros immediately after the decimal point lies between $10^{-(n+1)}$ and 10^{-n}

∴ If D is the decimal fraction with *n* zeros immediately after the decimal point, then

$$D = 10^{-(n+1)} + \text{a fraction}$$

$$\therefore \quad \log_{10} D = -(n+1) + \text{a fraction}$$

Hence, the characteristic of the logarithm of a decimal fraction is one greater than the number of zeros immediately after the decimal point and is negative.

For example,

$\log_{10}58 = 1 + \text{mantissa}$

$\log_{10}7 = 0 + \text{mantissa}$

$\log_{10}123 = 2 + \text{mantissa}$

$\log_{10}0.2 = -1 + \text{mantissa}$

$\log_{10}0.056 = -2 + \text{mantissa}$

$\log_{10}0.00124 = -3 + \text{mantissa}$

2.4.1 Natural Logarithm

Natural logarithm is denoted as *l*n and use e as base, and the value is 2.718282. The natural logarithms is a basic tool in deriving Chemical Kinetics and Pharmacokinetic equations, Natural can be converted to common logarithms, using the equation $2.303 \log(N) = \ln(N)$.

Note: In the case of logarithm of a decimal fraction, the minus is written over the characteristic, and not before it, to indicate that the characteristic alone is negative, and not the whole expression.

For example, $\log_{10}0.0002 = -4 + 0.3010$ which is written as $\log_{10}0.0002 = \bar{4}.3010$ and not as -4.3010 which means that both the integral and the fractional parts are negative.

In working with negative logarithms, sometimes it is necessary to make mantissa positive.

This can be done by adding 1 to mantissa and subtracting 1 from the characteristic.

For example, $-4.7184 = -5 + (1 - 0.7184) = \bar{5}.2816$

To find Mantissa: The mantissa are the same for the logarithms of all numbers which have the same significant digits (drop decimal point and all zeros at the end of the whole number). The mantissa can be obtained by using ready – made four figure logarithmic table. When using four - figure table of logarithms, we use only the first four digits of any whole number. The method of looking at the table is illustrated as follows. Let the first four digits be 2364. Take the first two digit 23, move along the row 23 to column 6 to find 3729. In the same row 23, move further to column 4 of mean difference table to find 11. Add 11 to 3729 to get 3740 which is the required mantissa. If the given number has one digit or two digits, then other digits are taken as zeros and can be proceeded as above.

Anti-logarithmic table: Given logarithm of a number (characteristic + mantissa), we can obtain the number itself by looking at the anti-logarithmic table for the mantissa part in the same way as is explained for finding mantissa of a number. The position of the decimal point is fixed depending upon the characteristic part.

If the characteristic is positive or zero and is '*n*' then put the decimal point after (n + 1) digits. If the characteristic is negative and is '$\bar{n}$', then the decimal point in such way it succeeds by (n – 1) zeros.

For example, Antilog of (1.4581) = 28.72

Here, characteristic is 1 and mantissa is .4581

Similarly, Antilog$(\bar{2}.1342)$ = 0.01362

Worked Examples

1. Find the values of

(i) $\log_{2\sqrt{2}} 64$ (ii) $\log_9 243$ (iii) $\log_{0.1} 100$

Solution: (i) Take $\log_{2\sqrt{2}} 64 = x$, then $(2\sqrt{2})^x = 64$ $\therefore$ $(2^{3/2})^x = 64$

i.e., $2^{3x/2} = 2^6$ $(\because\ 64 = 2^6)$

$\therefore$ $\dfrac{3x}{2} = 6$ or $x = 4$ $\therefore$ $\log_{2\sqrt{2}}(64) = 4$

(ii) Take $\log_9 243 = x$, then $9^x = 243$

i.e., $(3^2)^x = 3^5$ or $3^{2x} = 3^5$ $\therefore$ $x = \dfrac{5}{2}$

i.e., $\log_9 243 = \dfrac{5}{2}$

(iii) Take $\log_{0.1} 100 = x$ $\therefore$ $(0.1)^x$

$$= 100 \text{ i.e., } \left(\frac{1}{10}\right)^x = 10^2$$

$\therefore$ $10^{-x} = 10^2$ or $x = 2$

i.e., $\log_{0.1} 100 = -2$

2. Find x such that (i) $\log_{32} 256 = x$ (ii) $\log_{0.4} x = -3$

Solution: (i) $\log_{32} 256 = x$ means $32^x = 256 \Rightarrow 2^{5x} = 2^8$

$\therefore$ $5x = 8;\ x = \frac{8}{5}$

(ii) $\log_{0.4} x = -3$ means $(0.4)^{-3} = x$

$\therefore$ $x = \left(\frac{4}{10}\right)^{-3} = \left(\frac{2}{5}\right)^{-3} = \left(\frac{5}{2}\right)^3 = \frac{125}{8}$

3. The buffer (Henderson-Hasselbalch) equation for weak base is given by the equation

$$K_b = \frac{(B^+)(OH^-)}{BOH}$$

where B^+ = Salt and BOH = Base Prove that

$$pH = pKw - pKb + \log\frac{base}{salt}$$

Solution:

$$K_b = \frac{(B^+)(OH^-)}{BOH}$$

Take Log both sides of the buffer Equation

$$\log(K_b) = \log((B^+)(OH^-)) - \log(BOH)$$

$$= \log(B^+) + \log(OH^-) - \log(BOH)$$

$$= \log((B^+)(OH^-)) - \log(BOH)$$

$$\log(K_b) = \log\frac{((B^+)(OH^-))}{BOH}$$

Take exp both side

$$K_b = \frac{(B^+)(OH^-)}{BOH}$$

Exercise 2.1

1. Find the value of $\log_4 64$
2. Find the value of $\log \sqrt{\dfrac{24}{35}}$
3. Prove that $\log(x/y) + \log(y/z) + \log(z/x) = 0$
4. Show that $\log_a x \cdot \log_b y = \log_b x \cdot \log_a y$
5. If $x = \log_{2a} a$, $y = \log_{3a} 2a$ and $z = \log_{4a} 3a$. Prove that $xyz + 1 = 2yz$
6. If $\log\left(\dfrac{a+b}{2}\right) = \dfrac{1}{2}(\log^a + \log^b)$. Show that $a = b$
7. If $a^2 + b^2 = 7ab$, show that $\log\left(\dfrac{a+b}{3}\right) = \dfrac{1}{2}(\log a + \log b)$
8. Simplify using table $\sqrt{\dfrac{(0.395)^2(2.45)}{8.034}}$
9. Simplify using table $\left(\dfrac{1}{\sqrt[3]{0.341}}\right)$
10. Show that $1/\log_6 24 + 1/\log_{12} 24 + 1/\log_8 24 = 2$
11. If $a^2 + b^2 = c^2$, Show that $(1/\log_{c+b} a + 1/\log_{c-b} a) = 2$
12. Find the characteristic and mantissa of 0.1362
13. Find the number of digits in $(15)^{16}$
14. Simplify with the use of logarithm table

$$\frac{(3.195)^2 \times (2.27)^3}{\sqrt{(164.3) \times (4.013)^2}}$$

Answers

1.	3	2.	$\bar{1}.9180$	8.	0.2180	9.	1.431
12.	$\bar{1}.1342$	13.	16	14.	1.159		

2.5 APPLICATIONS OF LOGARITHM TO SOLVE PHARMACEUTICAL PROBLEMS

1. If the amount of drug dissolved in body is given by the equation $D_B = D_B^0 e^{-kt}$.

   Prove that $\ln D_B = -kt + \ln D_B^0$ and also prove that $\log D_B = \frac{-kt}{2.303} + \log D_B^0$

   where D_B is concentration of drug in the body at time t and D_B^0 is drug in the body at time $t = 0$

2. If the first Plasma sample is taken at time t_1 and corresponding concentration is c_1 and c_2 is concentration in time t_2 and t is taken as $(t_2 - t_1)$. Then concentration c_2 is given by the equation $c_2 = c_1 e^{-k(t_2 - t_1)}$. Prove that the value of

$$k = \frac{\log c_1 - \log c_2}{(t_2 - t_1)}$$

3. If the rate of the amount of drug excreted in the urine is given by the equation $\frac{du}{dt} = k_e D_B^0 e^{-kt}$. k_e is renal excretion rate constant, D_B is drug in the body at zero hours. Prove that

$$\log \frac{dDu}{dt} = \frac{-kt}{2.303} + \log(k_e D_B^0)$$

4. If drug concentration in multi compartment is $C = A_n e^{-\lambda_n t}$

   Prove that $\log C = \log A_n - \frac{\lambda_n}{2.303}$

5. The function $c = \frac{k_a F X_0}{v(k_a - k)} e^{-kt}$ represents Post absorptive phase of a plasma concentration. Prove that $\log(c) = \log\left(\frac{k_a F X_0}{v(k_a - k)}\right) - \frac{kt}{2.303}$

6. Rate method is used to calculate pharmacokinetics parameter and it is given by the differential equation $\frac{dx_u}{dt} = K_e X_0 e^{-Kt}$. Prove that $\log \frac{dX_u}{dt} = \frac{-kt}{2.3} + \log(k_e X_0)$.

CHAPTER 3

MATRICES AND DETERMINANTS

Expected Learning Outcome

1. Learning the properties of determinants and developing the skills of using them to evaluate a determinant without expansion.
2. Learning different methods of finding inverse of a square matrix.
3. Appreciating the matrix method applied for the solving systems of linear equations.
4. Appreciating the method of solving systems of linear equations by Cramer's rule.
5. Appreciating the application of matrices in solving Pharmacokinetic equation.

3.1 INTRODUCTION

Matrices and determinants are very elegant and powerful mathematical tools used for solving problems that arise not only in mathematics but also in different fields of engineering, Physics, Economics, Pharmaceutical science and statistics etc. In this chapter, we study elementary properties of matrices and determinants and the methods of solving a system of simultaneous linear equations using matrices and determinants and their application in solving two and three compartmental pharmacokinetics equations.

3.2 RECAPITULATION OF TYPES OF MATRICES

A matrix is an arrangement of numbers (real or complex) in rows (horizontal lines) and columns (vertical lines)

$\begin{pmatrix} 2 & 3 & -4 \\ 1 & -2 & 6 \end{pmatrix}$ is a matrix. It has 2 rows and 3 columns

$$\begin{pmatrix} 2 & 3 & -4 \\ 1 & -2 & 6 \end{pmatrix} \begin{matrix} \rightarrow 1^{st} \text{ Row} \\ \rightarrow 2^{nd} \text{ Row} \end{matrix}$$

$$\begin{matrix} \downarrow & \downarrow & \downarrow \\ 1^{st} & 2^{nd} & 3^{rd} \\ \text{col} & \text{col} & \text{col} \end{matrix}$$

The arrangement is enclosed by ordinary brackets or square brackets or pair of double bars. Thus, the above matrix can also be written as

$$\begin{vmatrix} 2 & 3 & -4 \\ 1 & -2 & 6 \end{vmatrix} \text{ or } \begin{vmatrix} 2 & 3 & -4 \\ 1 & -2 & 6 \end{vmatrix}$$

A matrix of order m × n is an arrangement of *mn* numbers (elements) in m rows and n columns

$$\begin{pmatrix} a_{11} & a_{12} & a_{13} & \ldots\ldots\ldots\; a_{1n} \\ a_{21} & a_{22} & a_{23} & \ldots\ldots\ldots\; a_{2n} \\ \ldots & \ldots & \ldots & \ldots\ldots\ldots \\ \ldots & \ldots & \ldots & \ldots\ldots\ldots \\ a_{m1} & a_{m2} & a_{m3} & \ldots\ldots\ldots\; a_{mn} \end{pmatrix} \text{ is a matrix of order } m \times n$$

$$\begin{pmatrix} a_{11} & a_{12} & a_{13} \\ a_{21} & a_{22} & a_{23} \\ a_{31} & a_{32} & a_{33} \end{pmatrix} \text{ is a } 3 \times 3 \text{ matrix}$$

$$\begin{pmatrix} a_{11}\, a_{12}\, a_{13} \\ a_{21}\, a_{22}\, a_{23} \end{pmatrix} \text{ is a } 2 \times 3 \text{ matrix}$$

3.2.1 Types of Matrices

1. **Row matrix or Row vector**: A matrix having only one row is called a row matrix or a row vector.

   Example: $(a_{11} \;\; a_{12} \;\; a_{13})$ is a row matrix of order 1 × 3

   (3 4 –5) is a row matrix of order 1 × 3

2. **Column matrix or Column vector**: A matrix having only one column is called a column matrix or a column vector.

Example: $\begin{pmatrix} a_{11} \\ a_{21} \\ a_{31} \end{pmatrix}$ is a column matrix of order 3 × 1

$\begin{pmatrix} 2 \\ 5 \end{pmatrix}$ is a column matrix of order 2 × 1

3. **Null matrix or Zero matrix**: A matrix in which all the elements are zeros is called a null matrix or zero matrix (void matrix)

Example: $\begin{pmatrix} 000 \\ 000 \end{pmatrix}$ is a zero matrix of order 2 × 3

A zero matrix is usually denoted by O.

4. **Square matrix**: A matrix in which the number of rows is equal to the number of columns is called a square matrix. Otherwise, it is called a rectangular matrix or simply a matrix.

Example: $\begin{pmatrix} 1 & 2 \\ 3 & 6 \end{pmatrix}$ is a square matrix of order 2 × 2 or order 2

$\begin{pmatrix} 1 & 3 & -1 \\ 2 & 4 & 6 \\ 0 & 5 & -5 \end{pmatrix}$ is a square matrix of order 3 × 3 or order 3

In a square matrix the diagonal from left top corner to right bottom corner is called the Principal diagonal or leading diagonal.

5. **Diagonal matrix:** A diagonal matrix is a square matrix in which all elements expect the elements in the principal diagonal are zeros.

Example: $\begin{pmatrix} 3 & 0 \\ 0 & 5 \end{pmatrix}$ and $\begin{pmatrix} 3 & 0 & 0 \\ 0 & 2 & 0 \\ 0 & 0 & 6 \end{pmatrix}$ are diagonal matrices of order 2 and 3 respectively.

Note that $\begin{pmatrix} 0 & 0 & 1 \\ 0 & 5 & 0 \\ 2 & 0 & 0 \end{pmatrix}$ is not a diagonal matrix

6. **Scalar matrix**: It is a diagonal matrix in which all the elements in the principal diagonal are same.

Example: $\begin{pmatrix} 2 & 0 & 0 \\ 0 & 2 & 0 \\ 0 & 0 & 2 \end{pmatrix}$ and $\begin{pmatrix} 8 & 0 \\ 0 & 8 \end{pmatrix}$ are scalar matrices of order 3 and 2 respectively.

7. **Unit matrix or Identity matrix**: A unit matrix is a square matrix in which every element in the principal diagonal is 1 and all other elements are zeros.

Example: $\begin{pmatrix} 1 & 0 \\ 0 & 1 \end{pmatrix}$ and $\begin{pmatrix} 1 & 0 & 0 \\ 0 & 1 & 0 \\ 0 & 0 & 1 \end{pmatrix}$ are unit matrices of order 2 and 3 respectively.

A unit matrix is denoted by I

Note: (i) Every scalar matrix is a diagonal matrix

(ii) Every unit matrix is a scalar matrix as well as a diagonal matrix. But the converse is not true.

(iii) $\begin{pmatrix} 1 & 1 \\ 1 & 1 \end{pmatrix}, \begin{pmatrix} 0 & 1 \\ 1 & 0 \end{pmatrix}, \begin{pmatrix} 1 & 1 \\ 0 & 0 \end{pmatrix}, \begin{pmatrix} 1 & 0 \\ 0 & 0 \end{pmatrix}$ are not unit matrices.

8. **Equal in size matrices**: Two matrices are said to be equal in size if and only if they are of same order.

Example: $A = \begin{pmatrix} 2 & 3 & 4 \\ 1 & 3 & 5 \end{pmatrix}$ and $B = \begin{pmatrix} 3 & -1 & 0 \\ 0 & 2 & 5 \end{pmatrix}$ are equal in size as both A and B are of same order viz 2×3.

Example: $A = \begin{pmatrix} 1 & 2 \\ 5 & 6 \end{pmatrix}$ and $B = \begin{pmatrix} 2 \\ 3 \\ 4 \end{pmatrix}$ are not equal in size as A and B are of different orders.

9. **Equal matrices**: Two matrices are said to be equal if and only if their orders are same and their corresponding elements are equal.

Examples: 1. $A = \begin{pmatrix} 2 & 3 \\ 5 & 7 \end{pmatrix}$ and $B = \begin{pmatrix} 2 & 3 \\ 5 & 7 \end{pmatrix}$

A and B are equal matrices or A = B

2. $\begin{pmatrix} x & 3 & y \\ 4 & 0 & 2 \end{pmatrix}$ and $B = \begin{pmatrix} 1 & 3 & 4 \\ 4 & 0 & 2 \end{pmatrix}$

A = B implies $x = 1, y = 4$

3. $A = \begin{pmatrix} 1 & 2 & 3 \\ 3 & 4 & 5 \end{pmatrix}$ and $B = \begin{pmatrix} 1 & 3 \\ 2 & 4 \\ 3 & 5 \end{pmatrix}$

A and B are not equal as they are of different orders.

3.3 OPERATION ON MATRICES

1. **Scalar multiplication**: A matrix can be multiplied by a scalar (a constant). If A is any matrix and K is any scalar, then KA is a matrix obtained by multiplying every element of A by K.

i.e., if $A = \begin{pmatrix} a_{11} & a_{12} & a_{13} \\ a_{21} & a_{22} & a_{23} \end{pmatrix}$, then

$$KA = \begin{pmatrix} a_{11} & a_{12} & a_{13} \\ a_{21} & a_{22} & a_{23} \end{pmatrix} = \begin{pmatrix} Ka_{11} & Ka_{12} & Ka_{13} \\ Ka_{21} & Ka_{22} & Ka_{23} \end{pmatrix}$$

For example, if $A = \begin{pmatrix} 3 & 4 & 2 \\ 2 & -5 & 6 \end{pmatrix}$, then

(i) $2A = 2\begin{pmatrix} 3 & 4 & 2 \\ 2 & -5 & 6 \end{pmatrix} = \begin{pmatrix} 6 & 8 & 4 \\ 4 & -10 & 12 \end{pmatrix}$

(ii) $-3A = -3\begin{pmatrix} 3 & 4 & 2 \\ 2 & -5 & 6 \end{pmatrix} = \begin{pmatrix} -9 & -12 & -6 \\ -6 & 15 & -18 \end{pmatrix}$

(iii) $\frac{1}{2}A = \frac{1}{2}\begin{pmatrix} 3 & 4 & 2 \\ 2 & -5 & 6 \end{pmatrix} = \begin{pmatrix} \frac{3}{2} & 2 & 1 \\ 1 & -\frac{5}{2} & 3 \end{pmatrix}$

2. **Addition of matrices**: Two matrices can be added or subtracted only if their orders are same. If A and B are matrices of order m × n, then A + B is of same order and it is defined as the matrix obtained by adding the corresponding elements of A and B.

that is if $A = \begin{pmatrix} a_{11} & a_{12} & a_{13} \\ a_{21} & a_{22} & a_{23} \end{pmatrix}$ and $B = \begin{pmatrix} b_{11} & b_{12} & b_{13} \\ b_{21} & b_{22} & b_{23} \end{pmatrix}$,

then
$$A + B = \begin{pmatrix} a_{11} & a_{12} & a_{13} \\ a_{21} & a_{22} & a_{23} \end{pmatrix} + \begin{pmatrix} b_{11} & b_{12} & b_{13} \\ b_{21} & b_{22} & b_{23} \end{pmatrix}$$
$$= \begin{pmatrix} a_{11} + b_{11} & a_{12} + b_{12} & a_{13} + b_{13} \\ a_{21} + b_{21} & a_{22} + b_{22} & a_{23} + b_{23} \end{pmatrix}$$

and
$$A - B = \begin{pmatrix} a_{11} - b_{11} & a_{12} - b_{12} & a_{13} - b_{13} \\ a_{21} - b_{21} & a_{22} - b_{22} & a_{23} - b_{23} \end{pmatrix}$$

For Example if
$$A = \begin{pmatrix} 3 & 4 & 2 \\ 5 & -2 & 6 \end{pmatrix} \text{ and } B = \begin{pmatrix} 2 & -1 & 0 \\ -3 & 2 & 4 \end{pmatrix}, \text{ then}$$
$$A + B = \begin{pmatrix} 3 & 4 & 2 \\ -2 & 5 & 6 \end{pmatrix} + \begin{pmatrix} 2 & -1 & 0 \\ -3 & 2 & 4 \end{pmatrix}$$
$$= \begin{pmatrix} 3+2 & 4-1 & 2+0 \\ 5-3 & -2+2 & 6+4 \end{pmatrix} = \begin{pmatrix} 5 & 3 & 2 \\ 2 & 0 & 10 \end{pmatrix}$$
$$A - B = \begin{pmatrix} 3-2 & 4+1 & 2-0 \\ 5+3 & -2-2 & 6-4 \end{pmatrix} = \begin{pmatrix} 1 & 5 & 2 \\ 8 & -4 & 2 \end{pmatrix}$$

The addition of matrices satisfies certain basic laws. If A, B, C and O are matrices of same order, where O is the null matrix, then

(i) $A + B = B + A$ (Commutative law under matrix addition)

(ii) $A + (B + C) = (A + B) + C$ (Associative law under matrix addition)

(iii) $A + O = O + A = A$ (O is called the identity element under matrix addition)

(iv) $A + B = O$ implies $A = -B$ or $B = -A$

(v) The solution of $A + X = O$ is $X = -A$, where X is of the same order as that of A.

Worked Examples

1. If $A=\begin{pmatrix}0&2&3\\2&1&4\end{pmatrix}$ and $B=\begin{pmatrix}7&6&0\\0&4&1\end{pmatrix}$,

   Find (i) $3A+2B$ (ii) $3B-2A$ (iii) $A+\frac{1}{2}B$

   (i) $3A+2B=3\begin{pmatrix}0&2&3\\2&1&4\end{pmatrix}+2\begin{pmatrix}7&6&0\\0&4&1\end{pmatrix}$

   $$=\begin{pmatrix}0&6&9\\6&3&12\end{pmatrix}+\begin{pmatrix}14&12&0\\0&8&2\end{pmatrix}=\begin{pmatrix}14&18&9\\6&11&14\end{pmatrix}$$

   (ii) $3B-2A=3\begin{pmatrix}7&6&0\\0&4&1\end{pmatrix}+(-2)\begin{pmatrix}0&2&3\\2&1&4\end{pmatrix}$

   $$=\begin{pmatrix}21&18&0\\0&12&3\end{pmatrix}+\begin{pmatrix}0&-4&-6\\-4&-2&-8\end{pmatrix}=\begin{pmatrix}21&14&-6\\-4&10&-5\end{pmatrix}$$

   (iii) $A+\frac{1}{2}B=\begin{pmatrix}0&2&3\\2&1&4\end{pmatrix}+\frac{1}{2}\begin{pmatrix}7&6&0\\0&4&1\end{pmatrix}$

   $$=\begin{pmatrix}0&2&3\\2&1&4\end{pmatrix}+\begin{pmatrix}\frac{7}{2}&3&0\\0&2&\frac{1}{2}\end{pmatrix}=\begin{pmatrix}\frac{7}{2}&5&3\\2&3&\frac{9}{2}\end{pmatrix}$$

2. If $A=\begin{pmatrix}3&5&2\\4&7&6\end{pmatrix}$, $B=\begin{pmatrix}-1&2&5\\4&0&3\end{pmatrix}$ and $C=\begin{pmatrix}0&3&4\\9&8&-7\end{pmatrix}$,

   Find $5A-4B+3C$

   $5A-4B+3C=5\begin{pmatrix}3&5&2\\4&7&6\end{pmatrix}+(-4)\begin{pmatrix}-1&2&5\\4&0&3\end{pmatrix}+3\begin{pmatrix}0&3&4\\9&8&-7\end{pmatrix}$

   $$=\begin{pmatrix}15&25&10\\20&35&30\end{pmatrix}+\begin{pmatrix}4&-8&-20\\-16&0&-12\end{pmatrix}+\begin{pmatrix}0&9&12\\27&24&-21\end{pmatrix}$$

   $$=\begin{pmatrix}15+4+0&25-8+9&10-20+12\\20-16+27&35+0+24&30-12-21\end{pmatrix}$$

   $$=\begin{pmatrix}19&26&2\\31&59&-3\end{pmatrix}$$

3. If $A=\begin{bmatrix}1 & 2\\ -2 & 0\end{bmatrix}$, $B=\begin{bmatrix}3 & 4\\ 0 & -2\end{bmatrix}$, Find 2A + 3B.

$$2A=\begin{bmatrix}2 & 4\\ -4 & 0\end{bmatrix},\ 3B=\begin{bmatrix}9 & 12\\ 0 & -6\end{bmatrix},\ 2A+3B=\begin{bmatrix}11 & 16\\ -4 & -6\end{bmatrix}$$

4. If $A=\begin{bmatrix}3 & 0\\ -3 & 1\\ 4 & 1\end{bmatrix}$, $B=\begin{bmatrix}1 & 2\\ -2 & 1\\ 7 & 2\end{bmatrix}$, $C=\begin{bmatrix}5 & 7\\ 1 & 0\\ 2 & 3\end{bmatrix}$ Find the matrix X such that

2A + 3B – X = C.

2A + 3B – X = C ⇒ X = 2A + 3B – C

$$\Rightarrow \qquad X = 2\begin{bmatrix}3 & 0\\ -3 & 1\\ 4 & 1\end{bmatrix}+3\begin{bmatrix}1 & 2\\ -2 & 1\\ 7 & 2\end{bmatrix}-\begin{bmatrix}5 & 7\\ 1 & 0\\ 2 & 3\end{bmatrix}$$

$$\Rightarrow \qquad X = \begin{bmatrix}6 & 0\\ -6 & 2\\ 8 & 2\end{bmatrix}+\begin{bmatrix}3 & 6\\ -6 & 3\\ 21 & 6\end{bmatrix}-\begin{bmatrix}5 & 7\\ 1 & 0\\ 2 & 3\end{bmatrix}$$

$$\Rightarrow \qquad X = \begin{bmatrix}4 & -1\\ -13 & 5\\ 27 & 5\end{bmatrix}$$

5. Find a, b, c given that

$$4\begin{bmatrix}a & 2 & 3\\ 4 & 5 & -6\\ 7 & -8 & 9\end{bmatrix}-5\begin{bmatrix}3 & 2 & 1\\ 2 & b & -4\\ 9 & -8 & 7\end{bmatrix}=\begin{bmatrix}13 & -2 & 7\\ 6 & -5 & -4\\ -17 & 2c & 1\end{bmatrix}$$

The given matrix equation can be written as

$$\begin{bmatrix}4a & 8 & 12\\ 16 & 20 & -24\\ 28 & -32 & 36\end{bmatrix}+\begin{bmatrix}-15 & -10 & -5\\ -10 & -5b & 20\\ -45 & 40 & -35\end{bmatrix}=\begin{bmatrix}13 & -2 & 7\\ 6 & -5 & -4\\ -17 & 2c & 1\end{bmatrix}$$

i.e.,
$$\begin{bmatrix}4a-15 & -2 & 7\\ 6 & 20-5b & -4\\ -17 & 8 & 1\end{bmatrix}=\begin{bmatrix}13 & -2 & 7\\ 6 & -5 & -4\\ -17 & 2c & 1\end{bmatrix}$$

By equality of matrices, 4a – 15 = 13, 20 – 5b = –5, 8 = 2c

i.e., a = 7, b = 5, c = 4.

6. If $2A+B=\begin{pmatrix} 2 & 3 & 1 \\ 1 & 4 & 0 \end{pmatrix}$ and $3A+2B=\begin{pmatrix} 4 & 6 & 1 \\ 2 & 3 & 5 \end{pmatrix}$ find A and B

$$2A+B=\begin{pmatrix} 2 & 3 & 1 \\ 1 & 4 & 0 \end{pmatrix} \quad .....(1)$$

$$3A+2B=\begin{pmatrix} 4 & 6 & 1 \\ 2 & 3 & 5 \end{pmatrix} \quad .....(2)$$

$$\text{Eq.1. } \times 2 \rightarrow 4A+2B=\begin{pmatrix} 4 & 6 & 2 \\ 2 & 8 & 0 \end{pmatrix}$$

$$\text{Eq.2. } \rightarrow 3A+2B=\begin{pmatrix} 4 & 6 & 1 \\ 2 & 3 & 5 \end{pmatrix}$$

Subtracting eq. (1) and (2),

$$A=\begin{pmatrix} 4 & 6 & 2 \\ 2 & 8 & 0 \end{pmatrix}-\begin{pmatrix} 4 & 6 & 1 \\ 2 & 3 & 5 \end{pmatrix}, \; A=\begin{pmatrix} 0 & 0 & 1 \\ 0 & 5 & -5 \end{pmatrix}$$

Substitute for A in equation (1),

$$B=\begin{pmatrix} 2 & 3 & 1 \\ 1 & 4 & 0 \end{pmatrix}-2\begin{pmatrix} 0 & 0 & 1 \\ 0 & 5 & -5 \end{pmatrix}=\begin{pmatrix} 2 & 3 & -1 \\ 1 & -6 & 10 \end{pmatrix}$$

$$\therefore \quad A=\begin{pmatrix} 0 & 0 & 1 \\ 0 & 5 & -5 \end{pmatrix}, \; B=\begin{pmatrix} 2 & 3 & -1 \\ 1 & -6 & 10 \end{pmatrix}$$

7. Solve for $x : \begin{pmatrix} x^2 & 1 \\ 2 & 3 \end{pmatrix}+\begin{pmatrix} 2x & 3 \\ 1 & 4 \end{pmatrix}=\begin{pmatrix} 3 & 4 \\ 3 & 7 \end{pmatrix}$

The given equation is $\begin{pmatrix} x^2+2x & 4 \\ 3 & 7 \end{pmatrix}=\begin{pmatrix} 3 & 4 \\ 3 & 7 \end{pmatrix}$

$\therefore \quad x^2+2x=3 \qquad \therefore \quad x=-3, x=1$

8. If $\begin{bmatrix} 1 & 0 & 0 \\ 0 & y & 0 \\ 0 & 0 & 1 \end{bmatrix}\begin{bmatrix} x \\ 1 \\ z \end{bmatrix}=\begin{bmatrix} 1 \\ 0 \\ 1 \end{bmatrix}$, then find the values of x, y, z.

$$\begin{bmatrix} 1 & 0 & 0 \\ 0 & y & 0 \\ 0 & 0 & 1 \end{bmatrix}\begin{bmatrix} x \\ 1 \\ z \end{bmatrix}=\begin{bmatrix} 1 \\ 0 \\ 1 \end{bmatrix}; \; \begin{bmatrix} x \\ y \\ z \end{bmatrix}=\begin{bmatrix} 1 \\ 0 \\ 1 \end{bmatrix}$$

$\Rightarrow x=1, y=0$ and $z=1$

9. If $\begin{bmatrix} 2 & 3 \\ 7 & 5 \end{bmatrix} + \begin{bmatrix} 2 & x-2 \\ y-1 & 5 \end{bmatrix} = \begin{bmatrix} 4 & 1 \\ 7 & 10 \end{bmatrix}$, find x and y

$$\begin{bmatrix} 4 & x+1 \\ y+6 & 10 \end{bmatrix} = \begin{bmatrix} 4 & 1 \\ 7 & 10 \end{bmatrix}$$

$\therefore$ $x+1=1$ and $y+6=7$ i.e., $x=0$ and $y=1$

10. If $2A+B=\begin{pmatrix} 1 & -1 \\ 0 & 1 \end{pmatrix}$ and $A-3B=\begin{pmatrix} 0 & 1 \\ 1 & 0 \end{pmatrix}$, find A and B.

Multiply first equation by 3 and add it to the second, we get

$$A = \frac{1}{7}\begin{bmatrix} 3 & -2 \\ 1 & 3 \end{bmatrix}$$

Now, $$B = \begin{bmatrix} 1 & -1 \\ 0 & 1 \end{bmatrix} - \frac{2}{7}\begin{bmatrix} 3 & -2 \\ 1 & 3 \end{bmatrix}$$

$$= \begin{bmatrix} 1-\frac{6}{7} & -1+\frac{4}{7} \\ -\frac{2}{7} & 1-\frac{6}{7} \end{bmatrix} = \begin{bmatrix} \frac{1}{7} & -\frac{3}{7} \\ -\frac{2}{7} & \frac{1}{7} \end{bmatrix}$$

3. **Transpose of a Matrix**: If A is any matrix, then the matrix obtained by interchanging the rows and columns of A is called the transpose of A and it is written as A^1 or A^T.

For example, if $A=\begin{pmatrix} 2 & -3 & 4 \\ 6 & 7 & -8 \end{pmatrix}$, then $A'=\begin{pmatrix} 2 & 6 \\ -3 & 7 \\ 4 & -8 \end{pmatrix}$

Note: A is a matrix of order 2 × 3 and its transpose A' is a matrix of order 3 × 2.

In general, if A is a matrix of order m × n, then its transpose A' is a matrix of order n × m.

Symmetric and Skew-Symmetric Matrices

A square matrix A is called a symmetric matrix if $A' = A$. A square matrix A is called a skew-symmetric matrix if $A' = -A$

Example: $\begin{bmatrix} 2 & 1 \\ 1 & 4 \end{bmatrix}, \begin{bmatrix} -2 & 3 & 1 \\ 3 & 4 & 5 \\ 1 & 5 & 0 \end{bmatrix}$ are symmetric matrices

$\begin{bmatrix} 0 & 2 \\ -2 & 0 \end{bmatrix}, \begin{bmatrix} 0 & -3 & 4 \\ 3 & 0 & -1 \\ -4 & 1 & 0 \end{bmatrix}$ are skew-symmetric matrices

Note:

1. If A is symmetric then $a_{ij} = a_{ji}$ and A is skew-symmetric $a_{ij} = -a_{ji}$ and diagonal elements are zeros.
2. Given a square matrix A, we can express A as the sum of a symmetric matrix and a skew-symmetric matrix in the form $A = \left(\frac{A+A'}{2}\right) + \left(\frac{A-A'}{2}\right)$ where $\frac{A+A'}{2}$ is a symmetric and $\frac{A-A'}{2}$ is a skew-symmetric.

Example: Let $A = \begin{bmatrix} 1 & 2 \\ 3 & 4 \end{bmatrix}$

$$A' = \begin{bmatrix} 1 & 3 \\ 2 & 4 \end{bmatrix}, \frac{A+A'}{2} = \frac{1}{2}\begin{bmatrix} 2 & 5 \\ 5 & 8 \end{bmatrix} = \begin{bmatrix} 1 & \frac{5}{2} \\ \frac{5}{2} & 4 \end{bmatrix}$$

$$\frac{A-A'}{2} = \frac{1}{2}\begin{bmatrix} 0 & -1 \\ 1 & 0 \end{bmatrix} = \begin{bmatrix} 0 & -\frac{1}{2} \\ \frac{1}{2} & 0 \end{bmatrix}$$

we observed that $\begin{bmatrix} 1 & 2 \\ 3 & 4 \end{bmatrix} = \begin{bmatrix} 1 & \frac{5}{2} \\ \frac{5}{2} & 4 \end{bmatrix} + \begin{bmatrix} 0 & -\frac{1}{2} \\ \frac{1}{2} & 0 \end{bmatrix}$

↓ ↓

Symmetric Skew - symmetric

Worked Examples

1. Write the transpose of each of the following matrices

(i) $A=\begin{pmatrix}1 & 4 & 5\\ 2 & 6 & 7\end{pmatrix}$ (ii) $B=\begin{pmatrix}4 & 6 & 3\\ 1 & 0 & 4\\ 0 & 2 & 3\end{pmatrix}$

(i) $A'=\begin{pmatrix}1 & 2\\ 4 & 6\\ 5 & 7\end{pmatrix}$ (ii) $B'=\begin{pmatrix}4 & 1 & 0\\ 6 & 0 & 2\\ 3 & 4 & 3\end{pmatrix}$

2. If $A=\begin{pmatrix}1 & 3 & 4\\ 2 & 1 & 6\end{pmatrix}$, show that $(A')'=A$

$$A=\begin{pmatrix}1 & 3 & 4\\ 2 & 1 & 6\end{pmatrix}\quad A'=\begin{pmatrix}1 & 2\\ 3 & 1\\ 4 & 6\end{pmatrix}\quad (A')'=\begin{pmatrix}1 & 3 & 4\\ 2 & 1 & 6\end{pmatrix}=A$$

That is, the transposed matrix is the matrix itself.

3. If, $A=\begin{bmatrix}2 & 4 & 6\\ 3 & 5 & 7\end{bmatrix}$ show that $(A')'=A$

$$A=\begin{bmatrix}2 & 4 & 6\\ 3 & 5 & 7\end{bmatrix}\quad \therefore A'=\begin{bmatrix}2 & 3\\ 4 & 5\\ 6 & 7\end{bmatrix}\quad \therefore (A')=\begin{bmatrix}2 & 4 & 6\\ 3 & 5 & 7\end{bmatrix}=A\quad \therefore (A')=A$$

4. If $A=\begin{pmatrix}1 & 3 & 4\\ 2 & 1 & 6\end{pmatrix}$ and $B=\begin{pmatrix}2 & -2 & 1\\ 1 & 3 & -2\end{pmatrix}$,

Verify that (a) $(A+B)'=A'+B'$ (b) $(A-B)'=A'-B'$

(a) $$A+B=\begin{pmatrix}1 & 3 & 4\\ 2 & 1 & 6\end{pmatrix}+\begin{pmatrix}2 & -2 & 1\\ 1 & 3 & -2\end{pmatrix}=\begin{pmatrix}3 & 1 & 5\\ 3 & 4 & 4\end{pmatrix}$$

$$\therefore\quad (A+B)'=\begin{pmatrix}3 & 3\\ 1 & 4\\ 5 & 4\end{pmatrix}\qquad \text{.....(1)}$$

$$A' + B' = \begin{pmatrix} 1 & 2 \\ 3 & 1 \\ 4 & 6 \end{pmatrix} + \begin{pmatrix} 2 & 1 \\ -2 & 3 \\ 1 & -2 \end{pmatrix} = \begin{pmatrix} 3 & 3 \\ 1 & 4 \\ 5 & 4 \end{pmatrix} \qquad \text{.....(2)}$$

From (1) and (2), $(A+B)' = A' + B'$

(b) $$A - B = \begin{pmatrix} 1 & 3 & 4 \\ 2 & 1 & 6 \end{pmatrix} - \begin{pmatrix} 2 & -2 & 1 \\ 1 & 3 & -2 \end{pmatrix} = \begin{pmatrix} -1 & 5 & 3 \\ 1 & -2 & 8 \end{pmatrix}$$

$$(A-B)' = \begin{bmatrix} -1 & 1 \\ 5 & -2 \\ 3 & 8 \end{bmatrix}$$

$$(A' - B') = \begin{bmatrix} 1 & 2 \\ 3 & 1 \\ 4 & 6 \end{bmatrix} - \begin{bmatrix} 2 & 1 \\ -2 & 3 \\ 1 & -2 \end{bmatrix} = \begin{bmatrix} -1 & 1 \\ 5 & -2 \\ 3 & 8 \end{bmatrix}$$

$\therefore \quad (A - B)' = A' - B'$

5. If $A = \begin{pmatrix} 2 & 3 \\ 5 & 7 \end{pmatrix}$, find $A + A'$.

$$A = \begin{bmatrix} 2 & 3 \\ 5 & 7 \end{bmatrix} \quad \therefore A' = \begin{bmatrix} 2 & 5 \\ 3 & 7 \end{bmatrix} \quad \therefore A + A' = \begin{bmatrix} 4 & 8 \\ 8 & 14 \end{bmatrix}$$

6. If $A = \begin{pmatrix} 5 & 7 & 9 \\ -3 & 2 & -5 \end{pmatrix}$ and k is a scalar, show that $(KA)' = KA'$.

$$KA = K\begin{pmatrix} 5 & 7 & 9 \\ -3 & 2 & -5 \end{pmatrix} = \begin{pmatrix} 5K & 7K & 9K \\ -3K & 2k & -5K \end{pmatrix}$$

$$(KA)' = \begin{pmatrix} 5k & -3k \\ 7k & 2k \\ 9k & -5k \end{pmatrix} \qquad \text{......(1)}$$

$$KA' = K\begin{bmatrix} 5 & -3 \\ 7 & 2 \\ 9 & -5 \end{bmatrix} = \begin{bmatrix} 5K & -3K \\ 7K & 2K \\ 9K & -5K \end{bmatrix} \qquad \text{.....(2)}$$

From (1) and (2), $(KA)' = KA'$

7. If $A=\begin{pmatrix}1 & 2 & 3 & 0\\ 4 & 1 & 0 & 5\end{pmatrix}$ and $B=\begin{pmatrix}3 & 1\\ -4 & 2\\ 1 & 3\\ 0 & -1\end{pmatrix}$

Find (i) $2A+3B'$ (ii) $3A'-2B$

$$A'=\begin{pmatrix}1 & 4\\ 2 & 1\\ 3 & 0\\ 0 & 5\end{pmatrix},\ B'=\begin{pmatrix}3 & -4 & 1 & 0\\ 1 & 2 & 3 & -1\end{pmatrix}$$

(i) $$2A+3B'=2\begin{pmatrix}1 & 2 & 3 & 0\\ 4 & 1 & 0 & 5\end{pmatrix}+3\begin{pmatrix}3 & -4 & 1 & 0\\ 1 & 2 & 3 & -1\end{pmatrix}=\begin{pmatrix}11 & -8 & 9 & 0\\ 11 & 8 & 9 & 7\end{pmatrix}$$

(ii) $$3A'-2B=3\begin{bmatrix}1 & 4\\ 2 & 1\\ 3 & 0\\ 0 & 5\end{bmatrix}+(-2)\begin{bmatrix}3 & 1\\ -4 & 2\\ 1 & 3\\ 0 & -1\end{bmatrix}=\begin{bmatrix}-3 & 10\\ 14 & -1\\ 7 & -6\\ 0 & 17\end{bmatrix}$$

8. If $A+B=\begin{pmatrix}5 & 3 & 1\\ 2 & 4 & 6\\ 1 & 0 & 2\end{pmatrix}$ and $A-B=\begin{pmatrix}1 & 7 & 5\\ 0 & 2 & 4\\ 5 & 4 & 2\end{pmatrix}$, find A' and B'

$$(A+B)+(A-B)=\begin{bmatrix}5 & 3 & 1\\ 2 & 4 & 6\\ 1 & 0 & 2\end{bmatrix}+\begin{bmatrix}1 & 7 & 5\\ 0 & 2 & 4\\ 5 & 4 & 2\end{bmatrix}$$

$$\therefore\quad 2A=\begin{bmatrix}6 & 10 & 6\\ 2 & 6 & 10\\ 6 & 4 & 4\end{bmatrix}\quad \therefore A=\begin{bmatrix}3 & 5 & 3\\ 1 & 3 & 5\\ 3 & 2 & 2\end{bmatrix}$$

$$B=(A+B)-A=\begin{bmatrix}5 & 3 & 1\\ 2 & 4 & 6\\ 1 & 0 & 2\end{bmatrix}-\begin{bmatrix}3 & 5 & 3\\ 1 & 3 & 5\\ 3 & 2 & 2\end{bmatrix}$$

$$\therefore\ B=\begin{bmatrix}2 & -2 & -2\\ 1 & 1 & 1\\ -2 & -2 & 0\end{bmatrix}\qquad \therefore\ A'=\begin{bmatrix}3 & 1 & 3\\ 5 & 3 & 2\\ 3 & 5 & 2\end{bmatrix},\ B'=\begin{bmatrix}2 & 1 & -2\\ -2 & 1 & -2\\ -2 & 1 & 0\end{bmatrix}$$

4. **Matrix Multiplication:** If A is a matrix of order m × p and B is a matrix of order p × n, then and only then the product AB is defined and its order is m × n. The product AB exists only when the number of columns of A (pre factor) is equal to the number of rows of B (Post factor).

A – m × p (m rows, p columns)

B – p × n (p rows, n columns)

AB – m × n (m rows, n columns)

Examples

(i) If A is a 3 × 2 matrix and B is a 4 × 3 matrix, then AB is not defined but BA is defined, and its order is 4 × 2. AB is not defined because the number of columns of A is not equal to the number of rows of B, BA is defined because the number of columns of B is equal to the number of rows of A

(ii) If A is a m × n matrix and B is a n × p matrix, do AB and BA exist? If so what are their orders?

AB exists and its order is m × p

B – n × p

B – n × p
A – m × n } BA does not exist

Consider $A = \begin{bmatrix} a_{11} & a_{12} & a_{13} \end{bmatrix}$ and $B = \begin{bmatrix} b_{11} \\ b_{12} \\ b_{13} \end{bmatrix}$

Then $AB = \overrightarrow{\begin{pmatrix} a_{11} & a_{12} & a_{13} \end{pmatrix}}_{1\times 3} \begin{bmatrix} b_{11} \\ b_{12} \\ b_{13} \end{bmatrix}_{3\times 1}\downarrow$

$$= \left(a_{11}b_{11} + a_{12}b_{12} + a_{13}b_{13}\right)$$

The elements of the first row of A are multiplied by the corresponding elements of the first column of B and the products are added. The sum is the element in the first row, first column of AB.

Next, consider $A = \begin{pmatrix} a_{11} & a_{12} & a_{13} \\ a_{21} & a_{22} & a_{23} \end{pmatrix}_{2\times3}$ $B = \begin{bmatrix} b_{11} & b_{12} \\ b_{21} & b_{22} \\ b_{31} & b_{32} \end{bmatrix}_{3\times2}$

$$AB = \begin{pmatrix} a_{11} & a_{12} & a_{13} \\ a_{21} & a_{22} & a_{23} \end{pmatrix} \begin{bmatrix} b_{11} & b_{12} \\ b_{21} & b_{22} \\ b_{31} & b_{32} \end{bmatrix}$$

$$= \begin{pmatrix} 1^{st}\ \text{row} \times 1^{st}\ \text{column} & 1^{st}\ \text{row} \times 2^{nd}\ \text{column} \\ 2^{nd}\ \text{row} \times 1^{st}\ \text{column} & 2^{nd}\ \text{row} \times 2^{nd}\ \text{column} \end{pmatrix}$$

$$= \begin{pmatrix} a_{11}b_{11} + a_{12}b_{21} + a_{13}b_{31} & a_{11}b_{12} + a_{12}b_{22} + a_{13}b_{32} \\ a_{21}b_{11} + a_{22}b_{21} + a_{23}b_{31} & a_{21}b_{12} + a_{22}b_{22} + a_{23}b_{32} \end{pmatrix}$$

$$BA = \begin{bmatrix} b_{11} & b_{12} \\ b_{21} & b_{22} \\ b_{31} & b_{32} \end{bmatrix} \begin{pmatrix} a_{11} & a_{12} & a_{13} \\ a_{21} & a_{22} & a_{23} \end{pmatrix}$$

$$= \begin{bmatrix} b_{11}a_{11} + b_{12}a_{21} & b_{11}a_{12} + b_{12}a_{22} & b_{11}a_{13} + b_{12}a_{23} \\ b_{21}a_{11} + b_{22}a_{21} & b_{21}a_{12} + b_{22}a_{22} & b_{21}a_{13} + b_{22}a_{23} \\ b_{31}a_{11} + b_{32}a_{21} & b_{31}a_{12} + b_{32}a_{22} & b_{31}a_{13} + b_{32}a_{23} \end{bmatrix}$$

which is a 3 × 3 matrix

***Note*:**

1. The element in the 8th row and j^{th} column of the new matrix is obtained by multiplying the elements of ith row of the first matrix by the corresponding elements of the jth column of the second matrix and adding these products
2. In general, $AB \neq BA$ i.e., commutative law does not hold good.

Worked Examples

1. If $A = [1\ 3]$ and $B = \begin{bmatrix} 3 & -2 & 1 & -3 \\ -1 & 4 & -3 & 2 \end{bmatrix}$, Find AB

A is a 1 × 2 matrix, B is a 2 × 4 matrix

∴ AB is defined and it is a 1 × 4 matrix

$$AB = \overrightarrow{[1 \quad 3]} \begin{bmatrix} 3 & -2 & 1 & -3 \\ -1 & 4 & -3 & 2 \end{bmatrix}\downarrow$$

$$= [1 \times 3 + 3 \times -1 \quad 1 \times -2 + 34 \quad 1 \times 1 + 3 \times -3 \quad 1 \times -3 + 3 \times 2]$$

$$= [3 - 3 \quad -2 + 12 \quad 1 - 9 - 3 + 6\,] = [\,0 \quad 10 \quad -8 \quad 3]$$

2. If $A = \begin{pmatrix} 1 \\ 3 \end{pmatrix}$ and $B = (1 \quad 6 \quad 7)$, find AB

$A \to 2 \times 1$; B $\therefore$ 1×3 $\therefore$ AB is defined and its order is 2×3

$$AB = \begin{pmatrix} 1 & 6 & 7 \\ 3 & 18 & 21 \end{pmatrix}$$

3. If $AB = \begin{pmatrix} 4 & 3 \\ 1 & 2 \end{pmatrix}$ and $B = \begin{pmatrix} -4 \\ 3 \end{pmatrix}$, find AB.

$$AB = \begin{pmatrix} 4 & 3 \\ 1 & 2 \end{pmatrix}_{2\times2} \begin{pmatrix} -4 \\ 3 \end{pmatrix}_{2\times1}$$

$$= \begin{pmatrix} (4 \times -4) + 3 \times 3 \\ (1 \times -4) + 2 \times 3 \end{pmatrix} = \begin{pmatrix} -16 + 9 \\ -4 + 6 \end{pmatrix} = \begin{pmatrix} -7 \\ 2 \end{pmatrix}_{2\times1}$$

4. If $A = \begin{pmatrix} -1 & 2 \\ 4 & -3 \\ 5 & 6 \end{pmatrix}$ and $B = \begin{pmatrix} 0 & 3 & 5 \\ 4 & 2 & 6 \end{pmatrix}$, find AB and BA.

$A \to 3 \times 2$; $B \to 2 \times 3$ $\therefore AB \to 3 \times 3$; $BA \to 2 \times 2$

$$AB = \begin{bmatrix} -1 & 2 \\ 4 & -3 \\ 5 & 6 \end{bmatrix}\!\rightarrow \begin{pmatrix} 0 & 3 & 5 \\ 4 & 2 & 6 \end{pmatrix}\downarrow$$

$$= \begin{bmatrix} -1\times0+2\times4 & -1\times3+2\times2 & -1\times5+2\times6 \\ 4\times0+(-3)\times4 & 4\times3+(-3)\times2 & 4\times5+(-3)\times6 \\ 5\times0+6\times4 & 5\times3+6\times2 & 5\times5+6\times6 \end{bmatrix}$$

$$= \begin{bmatrix} 8 & 1 & 7 \\ -12 & 6 & 2 \\ 24 & 27 & 61 \end{bmatrix}$$

$$BA = \begin{pmatrix} 0 & 3 & 5 \\ 4 & 2 & 6 \end{pmatrix} \begin{bmatrix} -1 & 2 \\ 4 & -3 \\ 5 & 6 \end{bmatrix}$$

$$= \begin{pmatrix} -0+12+25 & 0-9+30 \\ -4+8+30 & 8-6+36 \end{pmatrix} = \begin{pmatrix} 37 & 21 \\ 34 & 38 \end{pmatrix}$$

Note AB $\neq$ BA

5. If $A = \begin{bmatrix} 3 & -1 & 2 \\ 1 & 2 & 2 \\ 2 & 0 & 5 \end{bmatrix}$, find A^2

A^2 is defined as A × A

$$A^2 = A \times A = \begin{bmatrix} 3 & -1 & 2 \\ 1 & 2 & 2 \\ 2 & 0 & 5 \end{bmatrix} \begin{bmatrix} 3 & -1 & 2 \\ 1 & 2 & 2 \\ 2 & 0 & 5 \end{bmatrix}$$

$$= \begin{bmatrix} 9-1+4 & -3-2+0 & 6-2+10 \\ 3+2+4 & -1+4+0 & 2+4+10 \\ 6+0+10 & -2+0+0 & 4+0+25 \end{bmatrix} = \begin{bmatrix} 12 & -5 & 14 \\ 9 & 3 & 16 \\ 16 & -2 & 29 \end{bmatrix}$$

6. If $A = \begin{pmatrix} -1 & 2 \\ 2 & 4 \end{pmatrix}$ and $B = \begin{pmatrix} 3 & 5 \\ 6 & -7 \end{pmatrix}$, show that $(AB)' = B'A'$

$$AB = \begin{pmatrix} -1 & 2 \\ 2 & 4 \end{pmatrix} \begin{pmatrix} 3 & 5 \\ 6 & -7 \end{pmatrix}$$

$$= \begin{pmatrix} -3+12 & -5-14 \\ 6+24 & 10-28 \end{pmatrix} = \begin{pmatrix} 9 & -19 \\ 30 & -18 \end{pmatrix}$$

$$\therefore \quad (AB)' = \begin{pmatrix} 9 & 30 \\ -19 & -18 \end{pmatrix} \qquad .....(1)$$

$$A' = \begin{pmatrix} -1 & 2 \\ 2 & 4 \end{pmatrix}, \quad B' = \begin{pmatrix} 3 & 6 \\ 5 & -7 \end{pmatrix}$$

$$B'A' = \begin{pmatrix} 3 & 6 \\ 5 & -7 \end{pmatrix} \begin{pmatrix} -1 & 2 \\ 2 & 4 \end{pmatrix}$$

$$=\begin{pmatrix}-3+12 & 6+24\\ -5-14 & 10-28\end{pmatrix}=\begin{pmatrix}9 & 30\\ -19 & -18\end{pmatrix} \quad .....(2)$$

From (1) and (2), it follows $(AB)' = B'\ A'$

Note: $(AB)' = B'\ A'$ is known as reversal law of transposes. In general, if A, B, C..... are square matrices of same order, then

$(ABC...)' = (\ ......\ C'\ B'\ A')$.

7. If $A=\begin{bmatrix}9 & -8 & 7\\ -6 & 5 & -4\\ 3 & -2 & 1\end{bmatrix}$ and $B=\begin{bmatrix}1 & 0 & 0\\ 0 & 1 & 0\\ 0 & 0 & 1\end{bmatrix}$, then find AB and BA.

$$AB=\begin{bmatrix}9 & -8 & 7\\ -6 & 5 & -4\\ 3 & -2 & 1\end{bmatrix}\begin{bmatrix}1 & 0 & 0\\ 0 & 1 & 0\\ 0 & 0 & 1\end{bmatrix}$$

$$=\begin{bmatrix}9+0+0 & 0-8+0 & 0+0+7\\ -6+0+0 & 0+5+0 & 0+0+(-4)\\ 3+0+0 & 0-2+0 & 0+0+1\end{bmatrix}=\begin{bmatrix}9 & -8 & 7\\ -6 & 5 & -4\\ 3 & -2 & 1\end{bmatrix}=A$$

$$BA=\begin{bmatrix}1 & 0 & 0\\ 0 & 1 & 0\\ 0 & 0 & 1\end{bmatrix}\begin{bmatrix}9 & -8 & 7\\ -6 & 5 & -4\\ 3 & -2 & 1\end{bmatrix}$$

$$=\begin{bmatrix}9 & -8 & 7\\ -6 & 5 & -4\\ 3 & -2 & 1\end{bmatrix}=A$$

Note: Here B is a unit matrix and order of A is the same as that of B; AB = BA = A. In general, if A is any matrix and I is a unit matrix such that AI or IA is defined, then AI = A or IA = A.

8. If $A=\begin{pmatrix}3 & 1\\ -1 & 2\end{pmatrix}$, find $A^2-5A+7I$

$$A^2=\begin{pmatrix}3 & 1\\ -1 & 2\end{pmatrix}\begin{pmatrix}3 & 1\\ -1 & 2\end{pmatrix}=\begin{pmatrix}9-1 & 3+2\\ -3-2 & -1+4\end{pmatrix}=\begin{pmatrix}8 & 5\\ -5 & 3\end{pmatrix}$$

$$A^2 - 5A + 7I = \begin{pmatrix} 8 & 5 \\ -5 & 3 \end{pmatrix} - 5\begin{pmatrix} 3 & 1 \\ -1 & 2 \end{pmatrix} + 7\begin{pmatrix} 1 & 0 \\ 0 & 1 \end{pmatrix}$$

$$= \begin{pmatrix} 8-15+7 & 5-5+0 \\ -5+5+0 & 3-10+7 \end{pmatrix} = \begin{pmatrix} 0 & 0 \\ 0 & 0 \end{pmatrix} = 0$$

Thus $A^2 - 5A + 7I$ is a null matrix

9. If $A = \begin{bmatrix} 1 & 2 & -3 \\ 5 & 0 & 2 \\ 1 & -1 & 1 \end{bmatrix}$, $B = \begin{bmatrix} 3 & -1 & 2 \\ 4 & 2 & 5 \\ 2 & 0 & 3 \end{bmatrix}$, and $C = \begin{bmatrix} 4 & 1 & 2 \\ 0 & 3 & 2 \\ 0 & -2 & 3 \end{bmatrix}$

Verify that A(B + C) = AB + AC

$$B + C = \begin{bmatrix} 7 & 0 & 4 \\ 4 & 5 & 7 \\ 2 & -2 & 6 \end{bmatrix}$$

$$A(B + C) = \begin{bmatrix} 1 & 2 & -3 \\ 5 & 0 & 2 \\ 1 & -1 & 1 \end{bmatrix} \begin{bmatrix} 7 & 0 & 4 \\ 4 & 5 & 7 \\ 2 & -2 & 6 \end{bmatrix}$$

$$= \begin{bmatrix} 7+8-6 & 0+10+6 & 4+14-18 \\ 35+0+4 & 0+0-4 & 20+0+12 \\ 7-4+2 & 0-5-2 & 4-7+6 \end{bmatrix} = \begin{bmatrix} 9 & 16 & 0 \\ 39 & -4 & 32 \\ 5 & -7 & 3 \end{bmatrix} \quad .....(1)$$

$$AB = \begin{bmatrix} 1 & 2 & -3 \\ 5 & 0 & 2 \\ 1 & -1 & 1 \end{bmatrix} \begin{bmatrix} 3 & -1 & 2 \\ 4 & 2 & 5 \\ 2 & 0 & 3 \end{bmatrix}$$

$$= \begin{bmatrix} 3+8-6 & -1+4+0 & 2+10-9 \\ 15+0+4 & -5+0+0 & 10+0+6 \\ 3-4+2 & -1-2+0 & 2-5+3 \end{bmatrix} = \begin{bmatrix} 5 & 3 & 3 \\ 19 & -5 & 16 \\ 1 & -3 & 0 \end{bmatrix} \quad .....(2)$$

$$AC = \begin{bmatrix} 1 & 2 & -3 \\ 5 & 0 & 2 \\ 1 & -1 & 1 \end{bmatrix} \begin{bmatrix} 4 & 1 & 2 \\ 0 & 3 & 2 \\ 0 & -2 & 3 \end{bmatrix}$$

$$= \begin{bmatrix} 4+0+0 & 1+6+6 & 2+4-9 \\ 20+0+0 & 5+0-4 & 10+0+6 \\ 4+0+0 & 1-3-2 & 2-2+3 \end{bmatrix} = \begin{bmatrix} 4 & 13 & -3 \\ 20 & 1 & 16 \\ 4 & -4 & 3 \end{bmatrix} \quad \text{.....(3)}$$

Adding (2) and (3)

$$AB + AC = \begin{bmatrix} 5 & 3 & 3 \\ 19 & -5 & 16 \\ 1 & -3 & 0 \end{bmatrix} + \begin{bmatrix} 4 & 13 & -3 \\ 20 & 1 & 16 \\ 4 & -4 & 3 \end{bmatrix} = \begin{bmatrix} 9 & 16 & 0 \\ 39 & -4 & 32 \\ 5 & -7 & 3 \end{bmatrix} \quad \text{.....(4)}$$

From (1) and (4), it follows that A(B + C) = AB + AC. This is known as Left distributive law. Similarly, you can verify that (B + C)A = BA + CA (right distributive law).

10. If $A = \begin{pmatrix} -2 & 1 \\ 1 & -2 \end{pmatrix}$, $B = \begin{pmatrix} 4 \\ 5 \end{pmatrix}$ and $AX = B$, find X

Since A is a 2 × 2 matrix and AX is a 2 × 1 matrix. Let $X = \begin{pmatrix} x \\ y \end{pmatrix}$

Now $AX = B$ implies $\begin{bmatrix} -2 & 1 \\ 1 & -2 \end{bmatrix} \begin{bmatrix} x \\ y \end{bmatrix} = \begin{pmatrix} 4 \\ 5 \end{pmatrix}$

i.e., $\begin{bmatrix} -2x + y \\ x - 2y \end{bmatrix} = \begin{pmatrix} 4 \\ 5 \end{pmatrix}$

By equality of matrices, $-2x + y = 4$ .....(1)

$x - 2y = 5$ .....(2)

Solving (1) and (2), $x = -\frac{13}{3}$, $y = -\frac{14}{3}$

$$X = \begin{pmatrix} x \\ y \end{pmatrix} = \begin{pmatrix} -\frac{13}{3} \\ -\frac{14}{3} \end{pmatrix} = -\frac{1}{3}\begin{pmatrix} 13 \\ 14 \end{pmatrix}$$

11. Find x, y, z given that $\begin{bmatrix} x \\ y \\ z \end{bmatrix} = \begin{bmatrix} 3 & 1 & 3 \\ 2 & 0 & 2 \\ -5 & 1 & -1 \end{bmatrix} \begin{bmatrix} 2 \\ 4 \\ 3 \end{bmatrix}$

$$\begin{bmatrix} x \\ y \\ z \end{bmatrix} = \begin{bmatrix} 3 & 1 & 3 \\ 2 & 0 & 2 \\ -5 & 1 & -1 \end{bmatrix} \begin{bmatrix} 2 \\ 4 \\ 3 \end{bmatrix} = \begin{bmatrix} 6+4+9 \\ 4+0+6 \\ -10+4-3 \end{bmatrix} = \begin{bmatrix} 19 \\ 10 \\ -9 \end{bmatrix} \frac{1}{2}$$

$\therefore \; x = 19, \; y = 10, \; z = -9$

12. If $\begin{pmatrix} \cos\theta & \sin\theta \\ -\sin\theta & \cos\theta \end{pmatrix}$, show that $A^2 = \begin{pmatrix} \cos 2\theta & \sin 2\theta \\ -\sin 2\theta & \cos 2\theta \end{pmatrix}$ and find AA' and $A'A$

$$A^2 = \begin{pmatrix} \cos\theta & \sin\theta \\ -\sin\theta & \cos\theta \end{pmatrix} \begin{pmatrix} \cos\theta & \sin\theta \\ -\sin\theta & \cos\theta \end{pmatrix}$$

$$= \begin{pmatrix} \cos^2\theta - \sin^2\theta & \cos\theta\sin\theta + \sin\theta\cos\theta \\ -\sin\theta\cos\theta - \cos\theta\sin\theta & -\sin^2\theta + \cos^2\theta \end{pmatrix}$$

$$= \begin{pmatrix} \cos 2\theta & \sin 2\theta \\ -\sin 2\theta & \cos 2\theta \end{pmatrix} \quad \because \cos 2\theta - \sin 2\theta = \cos 2\theta, \quad 2\sin\theta\cos\theta = \sin 2\theta$$

$$AA' = \begin{pmatrix} \cos\theta & \sin\theta \\ -\sin\theta & \cos\theta \end{pmatrix} \begin{pmatrix} \cos\theta & -\sin\theta \\ \sin\theta & \cos\theta \end{pmatrix}$$

$$= \begin{pmatrix} \cos^2\theta + \sin^2\theta & -\cos\theta\sin\theta + \sin\theta\cos\theta \\ -\sin\theta\cos\theta + \cos\theta\sin\theta & \sin^2\theta + \cos^2\theta \end{pmatrix}$$

$$= \begin{pmatrix} 1 & 0 \\ 0 & 1 \end{pmatrix} = I$$

$$A'A = \begin{pmatrix} \cos\theta & -\sin\theta \\ \sin\theta & \cos\theta \end{pmatrix} \begin{pmatrix} \cos\theta & \sin\theta \\ -\sin\theta & \cos\theta \end{pmatrix}$$

$$= \begin{pmatrix} \cos^2\theta + \sin^2\theta & \cos\theta\sin\theta - \sin\theta\cos\theta \\ \sin\theta\cos\theta - \cos\theta\sin\theta & \sin^2\theta + \cos^2\theta \end{pmatrix}$$

$$= \begin{pmatrix} 1 & 0 \\ 0 & 1 \end{pmatrix} = I$$

13. Solve for x and y: $\begin{bmatrix} 3 & -4 \\ 9 & 2 \end{bmatrix}\begin{bmatrix} x \\ y \end{bmatrix} = \begin{bmatrix} 10 \\ 2 \end{bmatrix}$

$$3x - 4y = 10$$

$$(9x + 2y = 2) \times 2$$

Adding,

$$\begin{array}{r} 18x + 4y = 4 \\ \hline 21x = 4 \end{array}$$

$$x = \frac{2}{3}$$

∴ $$y = \frac{3x - 10}{4} = \frac{2 - 10}{4} = -2$$

∴ $$x = \frac{2}{3},\ y = -2$$

3.4 DETERMINANTS

If the elements of a matrix are real numbers and order of the matrix is n × n then we denote the set of matrices by the symbol M(n, R). Thus, M(2, R), M(3, R) are the set of all 2 × 2 and 3 × 3 matrices whose elements are real numbers.

Every square matrix is associated with a real number called its determinant. For example, the matrix $\begin{pmatrix} 2 & 3 \\ 1 & 5 \end{pmatrix}$ is associated with the determinant denoted by $|\ |$ whose value is $2 \times 5 - 3 \times 1 = 7$.

A determinant is defined as a (mapping) function from the set of square matrices to set of real numbers. Denoting a determinant as function (mapping) from the set M (2, R) of all 2 × 2 matrices to the set of real numbers. For example,

$\Delta\begin{pmatrix} a_{11} & a_{12} \\ a_{21} & a_{22} \end{pmatrix} = a_{11}a_{22} - a_{21}a_{12}$ which is written as $\begin{vmatrix} a_{11} & a_{12} \\ a_{21} & a_{22} \end{vmatrix}$. The meaning of this statement is that the determinant of the square matrix $\begin{vmatrix} a_{11} & a_{12} \\ a_{21} & a_{22} \end{vmatrix}$ is $(a_{11}a_{22} - a_{21}a_{12})$ which is written as the determinant $\begin{bmatrix} a_{11} & a_{12} \\ a_{21} & a_{22} \end{bmatrix}$.

Similarly, $\Delta : M(3, R) \rightarrow R$. This mapping represents third order determinants is a function from the set M (3, R) of all 3 × 3 determinants to the set of real numbers, for example.

$$(\Delta)=\begin{pmatrix} a_{11} & a_{12} & a_{13} \\ a_{21} & a_{22} & a_{23} \\ a_{31} & a_{32} & a_{33} \end{pmatrix}$$

$$=a_{11}(a_{22}a_{33}-a_{32}a_{23})-a_{12}(a_{21}a_{33}-a_{31}a_{23})+a_{13}(a_{21}a_{32}-a_{31}a_{22})$$

is written as

$$\Delta=\begin{vmatrix} a_{11} & a_{12} & a_{13} \\ a_{21} & a_{22} & a_{23} \\ a_{31} & a_{32} & a_{33} \end{vmatrix}$$

***Note*:** In this notation for the elements (entries), the first suffix represents the row number and second suffix represents the column number. For instance, a_{23} is the element in the 2nd row and 3rd column. In general a_{ij} represents the element in the ith row and j^{th} column.

Examples

(i) $\begin{vmatrix} 1 & 3 \\ 5 & -8 \end{vmatrix}=(1)(-8)-(5)(3)=-23$

(ii) $\begin{vmatrix} 0 & 3 \\ -2 & -5 \end{vmatrix}=(0)(-5)-(-2)(3)=6$

(iii) $\begin{vmatrix} 2 & 4 \\ 3 & 6 \end{vmatrix}=12-12=0$

(iv) $\begin{vmatrix} x & x^2 \\ y & y^2 \end{vmatrix}=xy^2-yx^2=xy(y-x)$

(v) $$\begin{matrix} + & - & + \end{matrix}$$
$$\begin{vmatrix} a_{11} & a_{12} & a_{13} \\ a_{21} & a_{22} & a_{23} \\ a_{31} & a_{32} & a_{33} \end{vmatrix}=a_{11}\begin{vmatrix} a_{22} & a_{23} \\ a_{32} & a_{33} \end{vmatrix}-a_{12}\begin{vmatrix} a_{21} & a_{23} \\ a_{31} & a_{33} \end{vmatrix}+a_{13}\begin{vmatrix} a_{21} & a_{22} \\ a_{31} & a_{32} \end{vmatrix}$$

$$=a_{11}(a_{22}a_{33}-a_{32}a_{23})-a_{12}(a_{21}a_{33}-a_{31}a_{23})+a_{13}(a_{21}a_{32}-a_{31}a_{22})$$

To write expansion, multiply the element a_{11} by the second order determinant which is got by deleting the first row and first column. Next, multiply $-a_{12}$ by determinant obtained by deleting the 1st row and 2nd column.

Then multiply a_{13} by the determinant obtained by deleting 1st row and 3rd column. Sum of these products is the value of the determinant.

$$\Delta = \begin{vmatrix} 6 & 2 & -3 \\ 2 & 3 & 1 \\ 0 & 1 & 5 \end{vmatrix} = 6\begin{vmatrix} 3 & 1 \\ 1 & 5 \end{vmatrix} - 2\begin{vmatrix} 2 & 1 \\ 0 & 5 \end{vmatrix} + (-3)\begin{vmatrix} 2 & 3 \\ 0 & 1 \end{vmatrix}$$

$$= 6(15-1) - 2(10-0) - 3(2-0) = 58$$

Worked Examples

1. Find the value of $\begin{vmatrix} 1 & 6 & 7 \\ 2 & 3 & 0 \\ 0 & 1 & 4 \end{vmatrix}$

$$\begin{matrix} + & - & + \end{matrix}$$

$$\begin{vmatrix} 1 & 6 & 7 \\ 2 & 3 & 0 \\ 0 & 1 & 4 \end{vmatrix} = 1\begin{vmatrix} 3 & 0 \\ 1 & 4 \end{vmatrix} - 6\begin{vmatrix} 2 & 0 \\ 0 & 4 \end{vmatrix} + 7\begin{vmatrix} 2 & 3 \\ 0 & 1 \end{vmatrix}$$

$$= 1(12-0) - 6(8-0) + 7(2-0) = -22$$

2. Evaluate: $\begin{vmatrix} 2 & 0 & -1 \\ 0 & 1 & 5 \\ 1 & 3 & -4 \end{vmatrix}$

$$\begin{matrix} + & - & + \end{matrix}$$

$$\begin{vmatrix} 2 & 0 & -1 \\ 0 & 1 & 5 \\ 1 & 3 & -4 \end{vmatrix} = 2\begin{vmatrix} 1 & 5 \\ 3 & -4 \end{vmatrix} - 0\begin{vmatrix} 0 & 5 \\ 1 & -4 \end{vmatrix} - 1\begin{vmatrix} 0 & 1 \\ 1 & 3 \end{vmatrix}$$

$$= 2(-4-15) - 0 - 1(0-1) = -37$$

3. Solve for x: $\begin{vmatrix} x & 3 \\ 3 & x \end{vmatrix} = 0$

$$\begin{vmatrix} x & 3 \\ 3 & x \end{vmatrix} = 0 \qquad \therefore\ x^2 - 9 = 0 \qquad \therefore\ x = \pm 3$$

4. Solve for x: $\begin{vmatrix} 2 & 3 & 4 \\ -4 & x & -8 \\ 5 & 6 & 7 \end{vmatrix} = 0$

Given equation is $2\begin{vmatrix} x & -8 \\ 6 & 7 \end{vmatrix} - 3\begin{vmatrix} -4 & -8 \\ 5 & 7 \end{vmatrix} + 4\begin{vmatrix} -4 & x \\ 5 & 6 \end{vmatrix} = 0$

i.e., $2(7x + 48) - 3(-28 + 40) + 4(-24 - 5x) = 0$

i.e., $-6x - 36 = 0$

$\therefore \quad x = -6$

5. Solve for x: $\begin{vmatrix} x & 2 & -1 \\ 2 & 5 & x \\ -1 & 2 & x \end{vmatrix} = 0$

$x(5x - 2x) - 2(2x + x) - 1(4 + 5) = 0$

$3x^2 - 6x - 9 = 0$

Solving $x = 3$, $x = -1$

6. If $A = \begin{bmatrix} 1 & 2 \\ 3 & -1 \end{bmatrix}$, $B = \begin{bmatrix} 1 & -4 \\ 3 & -2 \end{bmatrix}$, find $|AB|$.

$$|AB| = \begin{vmatrix} 7 & -8 \\ 0 & -10 \end{vmatrix} = -70$$

7. For what value of x, $\begin{vmatrix} 1 & 6 & 7 \\ 2 & x & 14 \\ 0 & 1 & 4 \end{vmatrix} = 0$

$1(4x - 14) - 6(8 - 0) + 7(2 - 0) = 0$

$4x - 14 - 48 + 14 = 0$

$4x = 48$

$x = 12$

8. Find $|AB|$ if $A = \begin{bmatrix} 1 & 2 \\ 3 & -1 \end{bmatrix}$ and $B = \begin{bmatrix} 1 & 0 \\ -1 & 0 \end{bmatrix}$

$$|AB| = \begin{vmatrix} -1 & 0 \\ 4 & 0 \end{vmatrix} = 0$$

9. For what value of x, $\begin{vmatrix} 2 & 3 & 1 \\ x & 2 & 5 \\ 1 & 3 & 4 \end{vmatrix} = 0$

$$2(8-15)-3(4x-5)+1(3x-2)=0$$
$$-14-12x+15+3x-2=0$$
$$-9x-1=0$$
$$x=-\frac{1}{9}$$

10. If ω is an imaginary cube root of unity, evaluate

$$\begin{vmatrix} 1 & \omega & \omega^2 \\ \omega & \omega^2 & 1 \\ \omega^2 & 1 & \omega \end{vmatrix} = 1(\omega^3-1)-\omega(\omega^2-\omega^2)+\omega^2(\omega-\omega^4)$$

$$=(1-1)-\omega(0)+\omega^2(\omega-\omega)=0 \left[\because \omega^3=1\right]$$

Exercise 3.1

1. Evaluate

(i) $\begin{vmatrix} 4 & 0 \\ 0 & 6 \end{vmatrix}$ (ii) $\begin{vmatrix} 4 & 5 \\ 6 & 7 \end{vmatrix}$ (iii) $\begin{vmatrix} \cos\theta & -\sin\theta \\ \sin\theta & \cos\theta \end{vmatrix}$

(iv) $\begin{bmatrix} x & y \\ y & x \end{bmatrix}$ (v) $\begin{bmatrix} \tan x & \sec x \\ \sec x & \tan x \end{bmatrix}$

2. Solve for x

(i) $\begin{vmatrix} x & 5 \\ 5 & x \end{vmatrix} = 0$ (ii) $\begin{vmatrix} 4 & -x \\ x & -4 \end{vmatrix} = 0$ (iii) $\begin{vmatrix} (2x+1) & 3 \\ -1 & 4 \end{vmatrix} = 0$

(iv) $\begin{vmatrix} 4 & x \\ 6 & 7 \end{vmatrix} = -2$ (v) $\begin{vmatrix} 1 & x \\ x & 1 \end{vmatrix} = 0$

3. Evaluate

(i) $\begin{vmatrix} 2 & 3 & -1 \\ 3 & 4 & -2 \\ -3 & 0 & 2 \end{vmatrix}$ (ii) $\begin{vmatrix} 3 & -5 & 6 \\ 1 & 2 & -1 \\ 2 & 4 & -2 \end{vmatrix}$ (iii) $\begin{vmatrix} 5 & 0 & 0 \\ 0 & 2 & 0 \\ 0 & 0 & 3 \end{vmatrix}$

(iv) $\begin{bmatrix} 2 & 1 & -1 \\ 3 & -2 & -2 \\ 1 & -3 & -3 \end{bmatrix}$ (v) $\begin{bmatrix} \sec x & \sin x & \tan x \\ 0 & 1 & 0 \\ \tan x & \cos x & \sec x \end{bmatrix}$

4. Show that $\begin{vmatrix} a & b & c \\ b & c & a \\ c & a & b \end{vmatrix} = -(a^3 + b^3 + c^3 - 3abc)$

5. Solve for x

(i) $\begin{bmatrix} 1 & 2 & 3 \\ 2 & x & 3 \\ 3 & 4 & 3 \end{bmatrix} = 0$ (ii) $\begin{bmatrix} 1 & 2 & 5 \\ 2 & x & 10 \\ 3 & 0 & -2 \end{bmatrix} = 0$ (iii) $\begin{bmatrix} x & 0 & 1 \\ 0 & x & 0 \\ 1 & 0 & x \end{bmatrix} = 0$

(iv) $\begin{bmatrix} 7 & 4 & 11 \\ -3 & 5 & x \\ -x & 3 & 1 \end{bmatrix} = 0$ (v) $\begin{bmatrix} x & 0 & 2 \\ 2 & 0 & x \\ 0 & x & 0 \end{bmatrix} = 0$ (vi) $\begin{bmatrix} x & 4 & -4 \\ -x & 4 & 4 \\ 4 & -3 & 2 \end{bmatrix} = 0$

6. Show that $\begin{vmatrix} a & h & g \\ h & b & f \\ g & f & c \end{vmatrix} = abc + 2fgh - af^2 - bg^2 - ch^2$

Answers

---

1. (i) 24 (ii) -2 (iii) 1

   (iv) $x^2 - y^2$ (v) -1

2. (i) $x = \pm 5$ (ii) $x = \pm 4$ (iii) $x = -7/8$

3. (i) 4 (ii) 0 (iii) 30

   (iv) 14 (v) 1

5. (i) $x = 3$ (ii) $x = 4$ (iii) $x = 0$

   (iv) $x = 2,\ 13/2$ (v) $x = 0,\ +/-\ 2$ (vi) $x = -8$

3.4.1 Properties of Determinants

Theorem 1: The value of a determinant is not altered when its rows and columns are interchanged. The property is evident in the case of a second order determinant, for

$$\begin{vmatrix} a_{11} & a_{12} \\ a_{21} & a_{22} \end{vmatrix} = a_{11}a_{22} - a_{21}a_{12} = \begin{vmatrix} a_{11} & a_{21} \\ a_{12} & a_{22} \end{vmatrix}$$

We shall prove the property for a third order determinant

$$\text{Take } \Delta = \begin{vmatrix} a_{11} & a_{12} & a_{13} \\ a_{21} & a_{22} & a_{23} \\ a_{31} & a_{32} & a_{33} \end{vmatrix}$$

Interchange the rows and columns and call it as Δ_1

$$\Delta_1 = \begin{vmatrix} a_{11} & a_{21} & a_{31} \\ a_{12} & a_{22} & a_{32} \\ a_{13} & a_{23} & a_{33} \end{vmatrix}$$

To prove that $\Delta = \Delta_1$

Proof: Expand Δ and Δ_1

$$\Delta = a_{11}(a_{22}a_{33} - a_{32}a_{23}) - a_{12}(a_{21}a_{33} - a_{31}a_{23}) + a_{13}(a_{21}a_{32} - a_{31}a_{22})$$

$$= a_{11}a_{22}a_{33} - a_{11}a_{23}a_{32} - a_{12}a_{21}a_{33} + a_{12}a_{23}a_{31} + a_{13}a_{21}a_{32} - a_{13}a_{22}a_{31} \quad .....(1)$$

$$\Delta_1 = a_{11}(a_{22}a_{33} - a_{23}a_{32}) - a_{21}(a_{12}a_{33} - a_{13}a_{32}) + a_{31}(a_{12}a_{23} - a_{13}a_{22})$$

$$= a_{11}a_{22}a_{33} - a_{11}a_{23}a_{32} - a_{12}a_{21}a_{33} + a_{13}a_{21}a_{32} + a_{12}a_{23}a_{31} - a_{13}a_{22}a_{31} \quad .....(2)$$

Note: Write the products so that first suffixes are 1, 2, 3 in order. Comparing the terms in (1) and (2), $\Delta = \Delta_1$.

Note: Since a determinant is not altered in value when its rows and columns are interchanged, all the properties which are true for rows will also be true for columns.

Theorem 2: A determinant changes its sign when any two of its rows (or columns) are interchanged.

$$\text{Take } \Delta = \begin{vmatrix} a_{11} & a_{12} & a_{13} \\ a_{21} & a_{22} & a_{23} \\ a_{31} & a_{32} & a_{33} \end{vmatrix}$$

Let Δ_1 be the determinant obtained by interchanging first and third rows.

$$\text{i.e., } \Delta_1 = \begin{vmatrix} a_{31} & a_{32} & a_{33} \\ a_{21} & a_{22} & a_{23} \\ a_{11} & a_{12} & a_{13} \end{vmatrix}$$

To prove that $\Delta_1 = -\Delta$

$$\Delta = a_{11}(a_{22}a_{33} - a_{32}a_{23}) - a_{12}(a_{21}a_{33} - a_{31}a_{23}) + a_{13}(a_{21}a_{32} - a_{31}a_{22})$$

$$= a_{11}a_{22}a_{33} - a_{11}a_{23}a_{32} - a_{12}a_{21}a_{33} + a_{12}a_{23}a_{31}$$

$$- a_{13}a_{21}a_{32} - a_{13}a_{22}a_{33} \quad .....(1)$$

$$\Delta_1 = a_{31}(a_{22}a_{13} - a_{12}a_{23}) - a_{32}(a_{21}a_{13} - a_{11}a_{23}) + a_{33}(a_{21}a_{12} - a_{11}a_{22})$$

$$= a_{13}a_{22}a_{31} - a_{12}a_{23}a_{31} - a_{13}a_{21}a_{32} + a_{11}a_{23}a_{32}$$

$$+ a_{12}a_{21}a_{33} - a_{11}a_{22}a_{33} \quad .....(2)$$

$$= -[-a_{13}a_{22}a_{31} + a_{12}a_{23}a_{31} + a_{13}a_{21}a_{32} - a_{12}a_{21}a_{33} + a_{11}a_{22}a_{33}$$

Comparing (1) and (2), $\Delta_1 = -\Delta$

Theorem 3: The value of a determinant is zero if any two of its rows (or columns) are identical.

$$\text{i.e., } \Delta = \begin{vmatrix} a_{11} & a_{12} & a_{13} \\ a_{21} & a_{22} & a_{23} \\ a_{11} & a_{12} & a_{13} \end{vmatrix}$$

To prove that $\Delta = 0$

Proof : Let $\Delta = \begin{vmatrix} a_{11} & a_{12} & a_{13} \\ a_{21} & a_{22} & a_{23} \\ a_{11} & a_{12} & a_{13} \end{vmatrix}$ in which two rows are identical,

$$\Delta = a_{11}(a_{22}a_{13} - a_{12}a_{23}) - a_{12}(a_{21}a_{13} - a_{11}a_{23}) + a_{13}(a_{21}a_{12} - a_{11}a_{22})$$

$$= a_{11}a_{22}a_{13} - a_{11}a_{12}a_{23} - a_{12}a_{21}a_{13} + a_{12}a_{11}a_{23} + a_{13}a_{21}a_{12}$$

$$- a_{13}a_{11}a_{22} = 0$$

$\therefore \quad \Delta = 0$

Theorem 4: If every element of any row (or column) of a determinant is multiplied by a constant k, then the whole determinant is multiplied by k.

$$\text{Take } \Delta = \begin{vmatrix} a_{11} & a_{12} & a_{13} \\ a_{21} & a_{22} & a_{23} \\ a_{31} & a_{32} & a_{33} \end{vmatrix}$$

Let Δ_1 be the determinant obtained by multiplying every element of second row by k.

i.e., $\Delta_1 = \begin{vmatrix} a_{11} & a_{12} & a_{13} \\ ka_{21} & ka_{22} & ka_{23} \\ a_{31} & a_{32} & a_{33} \end{vmatrix}$

we have to prove that $\Delta_1 = k\Delta$

Proof: $\Delta = a_{11}(a_{22}a_{33} - a_{32}a_{23}) - a_{12}(a_{21}a_{33} - a_{31}a_{23})$
$+ a_{13}(a_{21}a_{32} - a_{31}a_{22})$ ....(1)

$\Delta_1 = a_{11}(ka_{22}a_{33} - a_{32}ka_{23}) - a_{12}(ka_{21}a_{33} - a_{31}ka_{23})$
$+ a_{13}(ka_{21}a_{32} - a_{31}ka_{22})$
$= a_{11}k(a_{22}a_{33} - a_{32}a_{23}) - a_{12}k(a_{21}a_{33} - a_{31}a_{23})$
$+ a_{13}k(a_{21}a_{32} - a_{31}a_{22})$
$= k[a_{11}(a_{22}a_{33} - a_{32}a_{23}) - a_{12}(a_{21}a_{33} - a_{31}a_{23})$
$+ a_{13}(a_{21}a_{32} - a_{31}a_{22})]$ ....(2)

from (1) and (2), $\Delta_1 = k\Delta$

Hence, $\begin{vmatrix} a_{11} & a_{12} & a_{13} \\ ka_{21} & ka_{22} & ka_{23} \\ a_{31} & a_{32} & a_{33} \end{vmatrix} = k\begin{vmatrix} a_{11} & a_{12} & a_{13} \\ a_{21} & a_{22} & a_{23} \\ a_{31} & a_{32} & a_{33} \end{vmatrix}$

This means if their is a common factor k in any row (or column) of determinant, then k can be taken outside the determinant.

For example, $\begin{vmatrix} 2 & 3 & -1 \\ 4 & 6 & -2 \\ 3 & 0 & 11 \end{vmatrix} = 2\begin{vmatrix} 2 & 3 & -1 \\ 2 & 3 & -1 \\ 3 & 0 & 11 \end{vmatrix}$ by taking out 2 from second row

$= 2 \times 0$ (it is because two rows are same)

$= 0$

Theorem 5: If each element of any row (or column) of a determinant is the sum of two terms, then the determinant can be expressed as the sum of two determinants.

To prove that

$$\begin{vmatrix} a_{11}+x_{11} & a_{12}+x_{12} & a_{13}+x_{13} \\ a_{21} & a_{22} & a_{23} \\ a_{31} & a_{32} & a_{33} \end{vmatrix} = \begin{vmatrix} a_{11} & a_{12} & a_{13} \\ a_{21} & a_{22} & a_{23} \\ a_{31} & a_{32} & a_{33} \end{vmatrix} + \begin{vmatrix} x_{11} & x_{12} & x_{13} \\ a_{21} & a_{22} & a_{23} \\ a_{31} & a_{32} & a_{33} \end{vmatrix}$$

$$\text{LHS} = \begin{vmatrix} a_{11}+x_{11} & a_{12}+x_{12} & a_{13}+x_{13} \\ a_{21} & a_{22} & a_{23} \\ a_{31} & a_{32} & a_{33} \end{vmatrix}$$

$$= (a_{11}+x_{11})(a_{22}a_{33} - a_{32}a_{33}) - (a_{12}+x_{12})(a_{21}a_{33} - a_{31}a_{23}) + (a_{13}+x_{13})(a_{21}a_{32} - a_{31}a_{22})$$

$$= [a_{11}(a_{22}a_{33} - a_{32}a_{33}) - a_{12}(a_{21}a_{33} - a_{31}a_{23}) + a_{13}(a_{21}a_{32} - a_{31}a_{22})]$$

$$+ [x_{11}(a_{22}a_{33} - a_{31}a_{23}) - x_{12}(a_{21}a_{33} - a_{31}a_{23}) + x_{13}(a_{21}a_{32} - a_{31}a_{22})]$$

$$= \begin{vmatrix} a_{11} & a_{12} & a_{13} \\ a_{21} & a_{22} & a_{23} \\ a_{31} & a_{32} & a_{33} \end{vmatrix} + \begin{vmatrix} x_{11} & x_{12} & x_{13} \\ a_{21} & a_{22} & a_{23} \\ a_{31} & a_{32} & a_{33} \end{vmatrix} = \text{RHS}$$

Note: Similarly,

$$\begin{vmatrix} a_{11}+x_{11} & a_{12}+x_{12} & a_{13}+x_{13} \\ a_{21}+x_{21} & a_{22}+x_{22} & a_{23}+x_{23} \\ a_{31} & a_{32} & a_{33} \end{vmatrix}$$

$$= \begin{vmatrix} a_{11} & a_{12} & a_{13} \\ a_{21}+x_{21} & a_{22}+x_{22} & a_{23}+x_{23} \\ a_{31} & a_{32} & a_{33} \end{vmatrix} + \begin{vmatrix} a_{11} & a_{12} & a_{13} \\ a_{21}+x_{21} & a_{22}+x_{22} & a_{23}+x_{23} \\ a_{31} & a_{32} & a_{33} \end{vmatrix}$$

$$= \begin{vmatrix} a_{11} & a_{12} & a_{13} \\ a_{21} & a_{22} & a_{23} \\ a_{31} & a_{32} & a_{33} \end{vmatrix} + \begin{vmatrix} a_{11} & a_{12} & a_{13} \\ x_{21} & x_{22} & x_{23} \\ a_{31} & a_{32} & a_{33} \end{vmatrix} + \begin{vmatrix} x_{11} & x_{12} & x_{13} \\ a_{21} & a_{22} & a_{23} \\ a_{31} & a_{32} & a_{33} \end{vmatrix} + \begin{vmatrix} x_{11} & x_{12} & x_{13} \\ x_{21} & x_{22} & x_{23} \\ a_{31} & a_{32} & a_{33} \end{vmatrix}$$

Theorem 6: The value of a determinant is not altered, if to the elements of any row (or column) the same multiplies of the corresponding elements of any row (or column) are added.

$$\text{Let } \Delta = \begin{vmatrix} a_{11} & a_{12} & a_{13} \\ a_{21} & a_{22} & a_{23} \\ a_{31} & a_{32} & a_{33} \end{vmatrix}$$

Let Δ_1 be the determinant obtained when *k* times the elements of second row are added to the elements of first row.

i.e., $$\Delta = \begin{vmatrix} a_{11}+ka_{21} & a_{12}+ka_{22} & a_{13}+ka_{23} \\ a_{21} & a_{22} & a_{23} \\ a_{31} & a_{32} & a_{33} \end{vmatrix}$$

To prove that $\Delta_1 = \Delta$

Proof:

$$\Delta_1 = \begin{vmatrix} a_{11}+ka_{21} & a_{12}+ka_{22} & a_{13}+ka_{23} \\ a_{21} & a_{22} & a_{23} \\ a_{31} & a_{32} & a_{33} \end{vmatrix}$$

$$= \begin{vmatrix} a_{11} & a_{12} & a_{13} \\ a_{21} & a_{22} & a_{23} \\ a_{31} & a_{32} & a_{33} \end{vmatrix} + \begin{vmatrix} ka_{21} & ka_{22} & ka_{23} \\ a_{21} & a_{22} & a_{23} \\ a_{31} & a_{32} & a_{33} \end{vmatrix} \text{ by theorem 5}$$

$$= \Delta + k \begin{vmatrix} a_{21} & a_{22} & a_{23} \\ a_{21} & a_{22} & a_{23} \\ a_{31} & a_{32} & a_{33} \end{vmatrix} \text{ by theorem 4}$$

$$= \Delta + k(0) = \Delta \qquad \therefore\ \Delta_1 = \Delta$$

Note: (i) Similarly, $\begin{vmatrix} a_{11} & a_{12} & a_{13} \\ a_{21} & a_{22} & a_{23} \\ a_{31} & a_{32} & a_{33} \end{vmatrix} = \begin{vmatrix} a_{11}+ka_{12} & a_{12} & a_{13} \\ a_{21}+ka_{22} & a_{22} & a_{23} \\ a_{31}+ka_{32} & a_{32} & a_{33} \end{vmatrix}$

(ii) The above property is very important as we use it while evaluating determinants. A determinant is not changed if we add (k = 1) any row to any other or if we subtract (k = – 1) any row from any other row.

Theorem 7: If all the elements in a row (or column) of a determinant are zeros, then the determinant is zero.

Take $\Delta = \begin{vmatrix} a_{11} & a_{12} & a_{13} \\ a_{21} & a_{22} & a_{23} \\ 0 & 0 & 0 \end{vmatrix}$ in which all elements in the third row are zeros. By expanding Δ, we get $\Delta = 0$.

Theorem 8: In a determinant, if all the elements on one side of the principal diagonal are zeros, then the value of the determinant is equal to the product of the elements in the principal diagonal.

To prove that $\begin{vmatrix} a_{11} & a_{12} & a_{13} \\ 0 & a_{22} & a_{23} \\ 0 & 0 & a_{33} \end{vmatrix} = a_{11}a_{22}a_{33}$

Proof: $\text{LHS} = a_{11}(a_{22}a_{33} - 0) - a_{12}(0 - 0) + a_{13}(0 - 0)$

$= a_{11}\, a_{22}\, a_{33} = \text{RHS}$

Examples

1. $\begin{vmatrix} 2 & 3 & -4 \\ 0 & 5 & 6 \\ 0 & 0 & 3 \end{vmatrix} = 2 \times 5 \times 3 = 30$

2. $\begin{vmatrix} 3 & 0 & 0 \\ 4 & 1 & 0 \\ 3 & 7 & -6 \end{vmatrix} = -18$

Worked Examples

1. Show that $\begin{vmatrix} a-b-c & 2a & 2a \\ 2b & b-c-a & 2b \\ 2c & 2c & c-a-b \end{vmatrix} = (a+b+c)^3$

$$\text{LHS} = \begin{vmatrix} a-b-c & 2a & 2a \\ 2b & b-c-a & 2b \\ 2c & 2c & c-a-b \end{vmatrix} \quad \text{Take } R_1' = R_1 + R_2 + R_3$$

$$= \begin{vmatrix} a+b+c & a+b+c & a+b+c \\ 2b & b-c-a & 2b \\ 2c & 2c & c-a-b \end{vmatrix}$$

$$= (a+b+c)\begin{vmatrix} 1 & 1 & 1 \\ 2b & b-c-a & 2b \\ 2c & 2c & c-a-b \end{vmatrix}$$

Take $C_2' = C_2 - C_1,\ C_3' = C_3 - C_1$

$$= (a+b+c)\begin{vmatrix} 1 & 0 & 0 \\ 2b & b-c-a-2b & 0 \\ 2c & 0 & c-a-b-2c \end{vmatrix}$$

$$= (a+b+c)\begin{vmatrix} 1 & 0 & 0 \\ 2b & -c-a-b & 0 \\ 2c & 0 & -a-b-c \end{vmatrix}$$

$= (a + b + c)\,(-c - a - b)\,(-a - b - c)$

$= (a + b + c)\,(-1)\,(c + a + b)\,(-1)\,(a + b + c)$

$= (a + b + c)^3 = \text{RHS}$

2. Show that $\begin{vmatrix} 1 & a & a^2 \\ 1 & b & b^2 \\ 1 & c & c^2 \end{vmatrix} = (a-b)\,(b-c)\,(c-a)$

$$\text{LHS} = \begin{vmatrix} 1 & a & a^2 \\ 1 & b & b^2 \\ 1 & c & c^2 \end{vmatrix} \text{ Take } R_2' = R_2 - R_1,\ R_3' = R_3 - R_1$$

$$= \begin{vmatrix} 1 & a & a^2 \\ 0 & b-a & b^2-a^2 \\ 0 & c-a & c^2 \end{vmatrix} = \begin{vmatrix} 1 & a & a^2 \\ 0 & b-a & (b+a)(b-a) \\ 0 & c-a & (c+a)(c-a) \end{vmatrix}$$

$$= (b-a)(c-a)\begin{vmatrix} 1 & a & a^2 \\ 0 & 1 & b+a \\ 0 & 1 & c+a \end{vmatrix} \qquad \text{Take } R_3' = R_3 - R_2$$

$$= (b-a)(c-a)\begin{vmatrix} 1 & a & a^2 \\ 0 & 1 & b+a \\ 0 & 0 & c-b \end{vmatrix}$$

$= (b - a)\,(c - a)\,(c - b) = (-1)\,(a - b)(c - a)$

$= (a - b)(c - a)\,(c - b) = (-)\,(a - b)(c - a)\,(-1)\,(b - c)$

$= (a - b)\,(b - c)\,(c - a) = \text{RHS}$

3. Show that $\begin{vmatrix} 1 & a & a^2 \\ 1 & b & b^2 \\ 1 & c & c^2 \end{vmatrix} = (a - b)(b - c)(c - a)(a + b + c)$

$$\text{LHS} = \begin{vmatrix} 1 & a & a^2 \\ 1 & b & b^2 \\ 1 & c & c^2 \end{vmatrix} \text{ Take } R_2' = R_2 - R_1, \quad R_3' = R_3 - R_1$$

$$= \begin{vmatrix} 1 & a & a^3 \\ 0 & b-a & b^3 - a^3 \\ 0 & c-a & c^3 - a^3 \end{vmatrix} = \begin{vmatrix} 1 & a & a^3 \\ 0 & b-c & (b-c)(b^2+ba+a^2) \\ 0 & c-a & (c-a)(c^2+ca+a^2) \end{vmatrix}$$

$$\because x^3 - y^3 = (x-y)(x^2+xy+y^2)$$

$$= (b-c)(c-a)\begin{vmatrix} 1 & a & a^3 \\ 0 & 1 & b^2+ba+a^2 \\ 0 & 1 & c^2+ca+a^2 \end{vmatrix} \qquad \text{Take } R_3' = R_3 - R_2$$

$$= (b-a)(c-a)\begin{vmatrix} 1 & a & a^3 \\ 0 & 1 & b^2+ba+a^2 \\ 0 & 0 & (c^2-b^2)+(ca-ba) \end{vmatrix}$$

$$= (b - a)(c - a)[(c^2 - b^2) + (ca - ba)]$$

$$= (b - a\ (c - a)[(c + b)(c - b) + a(c - b)]$$

$$= (a - b)(b - c)(c - a)(a + b + c) = \text{RHS}$$

4. Show that $\begin{vmatrix} a+b+2c & a & b \\ c & b+c+2a & b \\ c & a & c+a+2b \end{vmatrix} = 2(a+b+c)^3$

Taking $C_1' = C_1 + C_2 + C_3$

$$\text{LHS} = \begin{vmatrix} 2a+2b+2c & a & b \\ 2a+2b+2c & b+c+2a & b \\ 2a+2b+2c & a & c+a+2b \end{vmatrix}$$

$$= 2(a+b+c)\begin{vmatrix} 1 & a & b \\ 1 & b+c+2a & b \\ 1 & a & c+a+2b \end{vmatrix}$$

taking $R_1' = R_2 - R_1,\ R_3' = R_3 - R_1$

$$= 2(a+b+c)\begin{vmatrix} 1 & a & b \\ 0 & b+c+a & 0 \\ 0 & 0 & c+a+b \end{vmatrix}$$

$$= 2\,(a+b+c)\,(b+c+a)\,(c+a+b) = 2(a+b+c)^3 = \text{RHS}$$

5. Show that $\begin{vmatrix} -a^2 & ab & ac \\ ab & -b^2 & bc \\ ac & bc & -c^2 \end{vmatrix} = 4a^2b^2c^2$

$$\text{LHS} = \begin{vmatrix} -a^2 & ab & ac \\ ab & -b^2 & bc \\ ac & bc & -c^2 \end{vmatrix}$$

takeout a, b, c from R_1, R_2, R_3 respectively

$$= abc\begin{vmatrix} -a & b & c \\ a & -b & c \\ a & b & -c \end{vmatrix}$$

take out, a, b, c from C_1, C_2, C_3 respectively

$$= (abc)(abc)\begin{vmatrix} -1 & 1 & 1 \\ 1 & -1 & 1 \\ 1 & 1 & -1 \end{vmatrix}$$

$$= a^2b^2c^2\,[-1\,(1-1) - 1\,(-1-1) + 1\,(1+1)]$$

$$= a^2b^2c^2\,[4] = 4a^2b^2c^2 = \text{RHS}$$

6. Show that $\begin{vmatrix} x & y & y \\ y & x & y \\ y & y & x \end{vmatrix} = 9x + 2y)(x - y)^2$

$$\text{LHS} = \begin{vmatrix} x & y & y \\ y & x & y \\ y & y & x \end{vmatrix} \quad \text{adding } C_1 + C_2 + C_3 = C_1'$$

$$= \begin{vmatrix} x+2y & y & y \\ x+2y & x & y \\ x+2y & y & x \end{vmatrix} \quad \text{taking} \quad R_2' = R_2 - R_1, \quad R_3' = R_3 - R_1$$

$$= \begin{vmatrix} x+2y & y & y \\ 0 & x-y & 0 \\ 0 & 0 & x-y \end{vmatrix} = (x+2y)(x-y)(x-y)$$

$$= (x + 2y)\,(x - y)^2 = \text{RHS}$$

7. Show that $\begin{vmatrix} 1+a & 1 & 1 \\ 1 & 1+b & 1 \\ 1 & 1 & 1+c \end{vmatrix} = abc\left(1+\frac{1}{a}+\frac{1}{b}+\frac{1}{c}\right)$

$$\text{LHS} = (1 + a)\,[(1 + b)\,(1 + c) - 1] -1\,[(1+c) - 1\,] + 1\,[1 - (1 + b)]$$

$$= (1 + a)\,[\,b + c + bc] - c - b$$

$$= b + c + bc + ab + ac + abc - c - b = abc + bc + ac + ab$$

$$= abc\left(1+\frac{1}{a}+\frac{1}{b}+\frac{1}{c}\right) = \text{RHS}$$

8. Prove that $\begin{vmatrix} 1 & b+c & b^2+c^2 \\ 1 & c+a & c^2+a^2 \\ 1 & a+b & a^2+b^2 \end{vmatrix} = (a-b)(b-c)(c-a)$

$$\text{LHS} = \begin{vmatrix} 1 & b+c & b^2+c^2 \\ 1 & c+a & c^2+a^2 \\ 1 & a+b & a^2+b^2 \end{vmatrix} \qquad \text{Taking } R_2' = R_2 - R_1\; R_3' = R_3 - R_1$$

$$=\begin{vmatrix}1 & b+c & b^2+c^2\\0 & a-b & a^2-b^2\\0 & a-c & a^2-c^2\end{vmatrix}$$

$$=(a-b)(a-c)\begin{vmatrix}1 & b+c & b^2+c^2\\0 & 1 & a+b\\0 & 1 & a+c\end{vmatrix} \quad \text{taking } R_3' = R_3 - R_2$$

$$=(a-b)(a-c)\begin{vmatrix}1 & b+c & b^2+c^2\\0 & 1 & a+b\\0 & 0 & c-b\end{vmatrix} = (a-b)(a-c)(c-b)$$

$$=(a-b)(a-c)(c-b) = \text{RHS}$$

9. If $abc = -1$ Prove that $\begin{vmatrix}a^3+1 & a^2 & a\\b^3+1 & b^2 & b\\c^3+1 & c^2 & c\end{vmatrix} = 0$

given that a, b, c are all different.

$$\text{LHS} = \begin{vmatrix}a^3+1 & a^2 & a\\b^3+1 & b^2 & b\\c^3+1 & c^2 & c\end{vmatrix} = \begin{vmatrix}a^3 & a^2 & a\\b^3 & b^2 & b\\c^3 & c^2 & c\end{vmatrix} + \begin{vmatrix}1 & a^2 & a\\1 & b^2 & b\\1 & c^2 & c\end{vmatrix}$$

$$= abc\begin{vmatrix}a^2 & a & 1\\b^2 & b & 1\\c^2 & c & 1\end{vmatrix} + \begin{vmatrix}1 & a^2 & a\\1 & b^2 & b\\1 & c^2 & c\end{vmatrix}$$

$$= abc\begin{vmatrix}a^2 & a & 1\\b^2 & b & 1\\c^2 & c & 1\end{vmatrix} \times \begin{vmatrix}1 & a^2 & a\\1 & b^2 & b\\1 & c^2 & c\end{vmatrix} \quad \text{by interchanging } C_1 \text{ and } C_2$$

$$= abc\begin{vmatrix}a^2 & a & 1\\b^2 & b & 1\\c^2 & c & 1\end{vmatrix} + \begin{vmatrix}a^2 & a & 1\\b^2 & b & 1\\c^2 & c & 1\end{vmatrix} \quad \text{by interchanging } C_2 \text{ and } C_3$$

$$= 0 = \text{RHS} \quad (\because abc = -1)$$

10. Show that $\begin{vmatrix} a & a+1 & a+2 \\ a+3 & a+4 & a+5 \\ a+6 & a+7 & a+8 \end{vmatrix} = 0$

$$\text{Det} = \begin{vmatrix} a & a+1 & a+2 \\ a+3 & a+4 & a+5 \\ a+6 & a+7 & a+8 \end{vmatrix} \quad \text{Taking } R_2' = R_2 - R_1 \quad R_3' = R_3 - R_1$$

$$= \begin{vmatrix} a & a+1 & a+2 \\ 3 & 3 & 3 \\ 6 & 6 & 6 \end{vmatrix} = 2\begin{vmatrix} a & a+1 & a+2 \\ 3 & 3 & 3 \\ 3 & 3 & 3 \end{vmatrix} = 0$$

11. Solve for $x = \begin{vmatrix} x+3 & 5 & 7 \\ 3 & x+5 & 7 \\ 3 & 5 & x+7 \end{vmatrix} = 0$

Taking $C_1' = C_1 + C_2 + C_3$

$$\begin{vmatrix} x+15 & 5 & 7 \\ x+15 & x+5 & 7 \\ x+15 & 5 & x+7 \end{vmatrix} = 0$$

i.e., $(x+15)\begin{vmatrix} 1 & 5 & 7 \\ 1 & x+5 & 7 \\ 1 & 5 & x+7 \end{vmatrix} = 0$

Taking $R_2' = R_2 - R_1; \quad R_3' = R_3 - R_1$

i.e., $(x+15)\begin{vmatrix} 1 & 5 & 7 \\ 0 & x & 0 \\ 0 & 0 & x \end{vmatrix} = 0$

i.e., $(x + 15)\, x^2 = 0$

$\therefore\ x + 15 = 0, \quad x^2 = 0 \qquad$ i.e., $x = -15, \quad x = 0$

12. Solve for x: $\begin{vmatrix} x & -6 & -1 \\ 2 & -3x & x-3 \\ -3 & 2x & x+2 \end{vmatrix} = 0$

Take $C_1' = C_1 + C_3$

$$\begin{vmatrix} x-1 & -6 & -1 \\ x-1 & -3x & x-3 \\ x-1 & 2x & x+2 \end{vmatrix} = 0$$

i.e., $$(x-1)\begin{vmatrix} 1 & -6 & -1 \\ 1 & -3x & x-3 \\ 1 & 2x & x+2 \end{vmatrix} = 0$$

Taking $R_2\,(-3\,-2) = R_2' - R_1;\quad R_3' = R_3 - R_1$

$$(x-1)\begin{vmatrix} 1 & -6 & -1 \\ 0 & -3x+6 & x-2 \\ 0 & 2x+6 & x+3 \end{vmatrix} = 0$$

$$(x-1)\begin{vmatrix} 1 & -6 & -1 \\ 0 & -3(x-2) & (x-2) \\ 0 & 2(x+3) & (x+3) \end{vmatrix} = 0$$

$$(x-1)(x-2)(x+3)\begin{vmatrix} 1 & -6 & -1 \\ 0 & -3 & 1 \\ 0 & 2 & 1 \end{vmatrix} = 0 \quad (x-1)(x-2)(x+3)[-5] = 0$$

$\therefore$ $x-1=0,\ x-2=0,\ x+3=0$, i.e., $x=1,\ x=2,\ x=-3$

3.4.2 Product of Determinants

Theorem 9: If A and B are two square matrices of same order, then $\Delta(AB) = \Delta(A)\,\Delta(B)$.

Proof: Take $A = \begin{pmatrix} a_{11} & a_{12} \\ a_{21} & a_{22} \end{pmatrix}$, $B = \begin{pmatrix} b_{11} & b_{12} \\ b_{21} & b_{22} \end{pmatrix}$

$\Delta(A) = a_{11}a_{22} - a_{12}a_{21},\quad \Delta(B) = b_{11}b_{22} - b_{12}b_{21}$

$$AB = \begin{pmatrix} a_{11}b_{11} + a_{12}b_{21} & a_{11}b_{12} + a_{12}b_{22} \\ a_{21}b_{11} + a_{22}b_{21} & a_{21}b_{12} + a_{22}b_{22} \end{pmatrix}$$

$$\begin{aligned} \Delta(AB) &= (a_{11}b_{11} + a_{12}b_{21})\,(a_{21}b_{12} + a_{22}b_{22}) \\ &\quad - (a_{11}b_{12} + a_{12}b_{22})\,(a_{21}b_{11} + a_{22}b_{21}) \\ &= \cancel{a_{11}b_{11}a_{21}b_{12}} + a_{11}b_{11}\,a_{22}b_{22} + a_{12}b_{21}\,a_{21}b_{12} \\ &\quad + \cancel{a_{12}b_{21}a_{22}b_{22}} - \cancel{a_{11}b_{12}a_{21}b_{11}} \end{aligned}$$

$$- a_{11}b_{12}a_{22}b_{21} - a_{12}b_{22}a_{21}b_{11} - \cancel{a_{12}b_{22}a_{22}b_{21}}$$

$$= (a_{11}a_{22} - a_{12}a_{21})\,(b_{11}b_{22} - b_{12}b_{21}) = \Delta(A)\,\Delta(B).$$

$$\therefore \qquad \Delta(AB) = \Delta(A)\,\Delta(B).$$

Note: (i) $\Delta(A) = |A|$

(ii) The value of a determinant is not altered when its rows and columns are interchanged (Theorem 1) Hence to find the product of two determinants, we can use row by column or row by row or column by column multiplication method

---

Worked Examples

---

1. If $A = \begin{pmatrix} 1 & 2 \\ 3 & 4 \end{pmatrix}$, $B = \begin{pmatrix} 5 & 6 \\ 7 & 8 \end{pmatrix}$, Prove that $\Delta(A).\ \Delta(B) = \Delta(AB)$

$$\Delta(A) = \begin{bmatrix} 1 & 2 \\ 3 & 4 \end{bmatrix} = 4 - 6 = -2$$

$$\Delta(B) = \begin{bmatrix} 5 & 6 \\ 7 & 8 \end{bmatrix} = 40 - 42 = -2$$

$$\Delta(A).\Delta(B) = 4 \qquad \text{.....(1)}$$

$$AB = \begin{pmatrix} 1 & 2 \\ 3 & 4 \end{pmatrix}\begin{pmatrix} 5 & 6 \\ 7 & 8 \end{pmatrix} = \begin{pmatrix} 19 & 22 \\ 43 & 50 \end{pmatrix}$$

$$\Delta AB = \begin{vmatrix} 19 & 22 \\ 43 & 50 \end{vmatrix} = 950 - 946 = 4 \qquad \text{.....(2)}$$

From (1) and (2) we get $\Delta(A).\ \Delta(B) = \Delta(AB)$

2. If $A = \begin{bmatrix} 1 & 2 \\ 3 & -1 \end{bmatrix}$, $B = \begin{bmatrix} 1 & -4 \\ 3 & -2 \end{bmatrix}$, Find $|AB|$

$$|AB| = |A||B| = \begin{vmatrix} 1 & 2 \\ 3 & -1 \end{vmatrix}\begin{vmatrix} 1 & -4 \\ 3 & -2 \end{vmatrix} = (-1-6)(-2+12) = -70$$

3. If $A = \begin{bmatrix} 3 & 8 \\ 1 & 4 \end{bmatrix}$, $B = \begin{bmatrix} 1 & 2 \\ 3 & -1 \end{bmatrix}$, Verify |AB| = |BA|

$$AB = \begin{bmatrix} 3 & 8 \\ 1 & 4 \end{bmatrix}\begin{bmatrix} 1 & 2 \\ 3 & -1 \end{bmatrix} = \begin{bmatrix} 27 & -2 \\ 13 & -2 \end{bmatrix}$$

$$|AB| = \begin{vmatrix} 27 & -2 \\ 13 & -2 \end{vmatrix} = -54 + 26 = -28 \qquad .....(1)$$

$$\therefore \quad |BA| = \begin{bmatrix} 1 & 2 \\ 3 & -1 \end{bmatrix}\begin{bmatrix} 3 & 8 \\ 1 & 4 \end{bmatrix} = \begin{bmatrix} 5 & 16 \\ 8 & 20 \end{bmatrix} \qquad .....(2)$$

From (1) and (2) |AB| = |BA|

Note: This result holds good also when A and B are square matrices of order n.

4. Find |AB| if $A = \begin{bmatrix} 1 & 2 \\ 3 & -1 \end{bmatrix}$, $B = \begin{bmatrix} 1 & 0 \\ -1 & 0 \end{bmatrix}$

$$|AB| = |A|\,|B| = \begin{vmatrix} 1 & 2 \\ 3 & -1 \end{vmatrix}\begin{vmatrix} 1 & 0 \\ -1 & 0 \end{vmatrix} = (-7)(0) = 0$$

5. Prove that $\begin{vmatrix} x & y \\ z & t \end{vmatrix}^2 = \begin{vmatrix} x^2+z^2 & xy+zt \\ xy+zt & y^2+t^2 \end{vmatrix}$

$$LHS = \begin{vmatrix} x & y \\ z & t \end{vmatrix}\begin{vmatrix} x & y \\ z & t \end{vmatrix}$$

Multiply by column method

$$= \begin{vmatrix} x^2+z^2 & xy+zt \\ xy+zt & y^2+t^2 \end{vmatrix} = RHS$$

6. Prove that $\begin{vmatrix} -3 & 5 \\ 1 & 0 \end{vmatrix}\begin{vmatrix} 7 & 2 \\ 4 & -1 \end{vmatrix} = \begin{vmatrix} -11 & -17 \\ 7 & 4 \end{vmatrix} = 75$

$$LHS = \begin{vmatrix} -3 & 5 \\ 1 & 0 \end{vmatrix}\begin{vmatrix} 7 & 2 \\ 4 & -1 \end{vmatrix}$$

Multiply by row by row method

$$= \begin{vmatrix} -21+10 & -12-5 \\ 7+0 & 4+0 \end{vmatrix}$$

$$= \begin{vmatrix} -11 & -17 \\ 7 & 4 \end{vmatrix} = -44+119 = 75 = \text{RHS}$$

7. If $A = \begin{pmatrix} a & ib \\ ib & a \end{pmatrix}, B = \begin{pmatrix} c & id \\ id & c \end{pmatrix}$, prove that $(a^2 + b^2)(c^2 + d^2) = \alpha^2 + \beta^2$

where $\alpha = ac - bd$, $\beta = ad + bc$

We know that $|A|\,|B| = |AB|$

$$\therefore \quad \begin{pmatrix} a & ib \\ ib & a \end{pmatrix}\begin{pmatrix} c & id \\ id & c \end{pmatrix} = \begin{vmatrix} ac-bd & i(ad+bc) \\ i(ad+bc) & ac-bd \end{vmatrix}$$

i.e., $(a^2 + b^2)(c^2 + d^2) = (ac - bd)^2 + (ad + bc)^2 = \alpha^2 + \beta^2$

8. Prove that $2\begin{vmatrix} 1 & a & a^2 \\ 1 & b & b^2 \\ 1 & c & c^2 \end{vmatrix} = \begin{vmatrix} 0 & (a-b)^2 & (a-c)^2 \\ (b-a)^2 & 0 & (b-c)^2 \\ (c-a)^2 & (c-b)^2 & 0 \end{vmatrix}$

$$\text{LHS} = 2\begin{vmatrix} 1 & a & a^2 \\ 1 & b & b^2 \\ 1 & c & c^2 \end{vmatrix}\begin{vmatrix} 1 & a & a^2 \\ 1 & b & b^2 \\ 1 & c & c^2 \end{vmatrix}$$

In the first determinant interchange 1st and 3rd columns and multiply the elements of 2nd column by –2

$$= \begin{vmatrix} a^2 & -2a & 1 \\ b^2 & -2b & 1 \\ c^2 & -2c & 1 \end{vmatrix}\begin{vmatrix} 1 & a & a^2 \\ 1 & b & b^2 \\ 1 & c & c^2 \end{vmatrix} \text{ Multiply by row by row method}$$

$$= \begin{vmatrix} a^2-2a^2+a^2 & a^2-2ab+b^2 & a^2-2ac+c^2 \\ b^2-2ab+a^2 & b^2-2b^2+b^2 & b^2-2bc+c^2 \\ c^2-2ac+a^2 & c^2-2bc+b^2 & c^2-2c^2+c^2 \end{vmatrix}$$

$$= \begin{vmatrix} 0 & (a-b)^2 & (a-c)^2 \\ (b-a)^2 & 0 & (b-c)^2 \\ (c-a)^2 & (c-b)^2 & 0 \end{vmatrix} = \text{RHS}$$

9. If $S_n = a^n + b^n + c^n$, prove that $\begin{vmatrix} S_0 & S_1 & S_2 \\ S_1 & S_2 & S_3 \\ S_2 & S_3 & S_4 \end{vmatrix} = [(a-b)(b-c)(c-a)]^2$

Let $$\Delta = \begin{vmatrix} 1 & 1 & 1 \\ a & b & c \\ a^2 & b^2 & c^2 \end{vmatrix}$$

We know that $\Delta = (a-b)\,b-c)(c-a)$

Now, $$\Delta^2 = \begin{vmatrix} 1 & 1 & 1 \\ a & b & c \\ a^2 & b^2 & c^2 \end{vmatrix} \begin{vmatrix} 1 & 1 & 1 \\ a & b & c \\ a^2 & b^2 & c^2 \end{vmatrix}$$

Multiplying by row by row method

$$= \begin{vmatrix} 1+1+1 & a+b+c & a^2+b^2+c^2 \\ a+b+c & a^2+b^2+c^2 & a^3+b^3+c^3 \\ a^2+b^2+c^2 & a^3+b^3+c^3 & a^4+b^4+c^4 \end{vmatrix}$$

$$= \begin{vmatrix} 3 & S_1 & S_2 \\ S_1 & S_2 & S_3 \\ S_2 & S_3 & S_4 \end{vmatrix} = \begin{vmatrix} S_0 & S_1 & S_2 \\ S_1 & S_2 & S_3 \\ S_2 & S_3 & S_4 \end{vmatrix}$$

$$\therefore \qquad \begin{vmatrix} S_0 & S_1 & S_2 \\ S_1 & S_2 & S_3 \\ S_2 & S_3 & S_4 \end{vmatrix} = \Delta^2 = [(a-b)(b-c)(c-a)]^2$$

Exercise 3.2

1. Find the value of $\begin{vmatrix} 3 & -2 \\ 1 & 6 \end{vmatrix}$

2. Evaluate A^2 given that $A = \begin{vmatrix} 1 & -1 \\ -1 & 1 \end{vmatrix}$

3. Find the value of $\begin{vmatrix} 1 & 1 & -1 \\ 1 & 2 & 3 \\ 2 & 4 & 6 \end{vmatrix}$

4. Find the value of $\begin{vmatrix} 41 & 42 & 43 \\ 44 & 45 & 46 \\ 47 & 48 & 49 \end{vmatrix}$

5. If $A = \begin{bmatrix} \sin\theta & -\cos\theta \\ \cos\theta & \sin\theta \end{bmatrix}$, find det A

6. Find x given that

(i) $\begin{vmatrix} 2 & x \\ 4 & 8 \end{vmatrix} = 0$ (ii) $\begin{vmatrix} 2x+1 & 5 \\ -5 & 2 \end{vmatrix} = 0$ (iii) $\begin{vmatrix} 2 & x \\ 3 & -5 \end{vmatrix} = \begin{vmatrix} 2 & -1 \\ 3 & -5 \end{vmatrix}$

7. Evaluate $\begin{vmatrix} 4223 & 4225 \\ 4228 & 4230 \end{vmatrix}$

8. If $\Delta = \begin{vmatrix} a_{11} & a_{12} \\ a_{21} & a_{22} \end{vmatrix}$, then find $\begin{vmatrix} ka_{11} & ka_{12} \\ ka_{21} & ka_{22} \end{vmatrix}$ in terms of Δ

9. Evaluate

(i) $\begin{vmatrix} 441 & 442 & 443 \\ 445 & 446 & 447 \\ 449 & 450 & 451 \end{vmatrix}$ (ii) $\begin{vmatrix} 86 & 87 & 88 \\ 87 & 88 & 89 \\ 88 & 89 & 90 \end{vmatrix}$ (iii) $\begin{vmatrix} 4 & 4^2 & 4^3 \\ 4^2 & 4^3 & 4^4 \\ 4^3 & 4^4 & 4^5 \end{vmatrix}$

10. Show that $\begin{vmatrix} 1+x & 2 & 3 \\ 1 & 2+x & 3 \\ 1 & 2 & 3+x \end{vmatrix} = x^2(x+6)$

11. Prove that $\begin{vmatrix} 1 & 1 & 1 \\ bc & ca & ab \\ b+c & c+a & a+b \end{vmatrix} = (a-b)(b-c)(c-a)$

12. Prove that $\begin{vmatrix} 1 & 1 & 1 \\ a & b & c \\ bc & ca & ab \end{vmatrix} = (a-b)(b-c)(c-a)$

13. Show that $\begin{vmatrix} 0 & ab^2 & ac^2 \\ a^2b & 0 & bc^2 \\ a^2c & b^2c & 0 \end{vmatrix} = 2a^3b^3c^3$

14. Show that $\begin{vmatrix} b+c & a & a \\ b & c+a & b \\ c & c & a+b \end{vmatrix} = 4abc$

15. Show that $\begin{vmatrix} 1 & a & b+c \\ 1 & b & c+a \\ 1 & c & a+b \end{vmatrix} = 0$

16. Given $1 + \omega + \omega^2 = 0$ and $\omega^3 = 1$, show that $\begin{vmatrix} 1 & \omega^3 & \omega^2 \\ \omega^3 & 1 & \omega \\ \omega^2 & \omega & 1 \end{vmatrix} = 3$

17. If a, b, c are all different and $\begin{vmatrix} a & a^2 & a^3-1 \\ b & b^2 & b^3-1 \\ c & c^2 & c^3-1 \end{vmatrix} = 0$ prove that $abc = 1$

18. Prove that $\begin{vmatrix} bc & a & a^2 \\ ca & b & b^2 \\ ab & c & c^2 \end{vmatrix} = \begin{vmatrix} 1 & a^2 & a^3 \\ 1 & b^2 & b^3 \\ 1 & c^2 & c^3 \end{vmatrix} = (a-b)(b-c)(c-a)(ab+bc+ca)$

19. Solve for x

(i) $\begin{vmatrix} x+1 & 2 & 3 \\ a & x+2 & 3 \\ 1 & 2 & x+3 \end{vmatrix} = 0$ (ii) $\begin{vmatrix} a-x & a+x & a+x \\ a+x & a-x & a+x \\ a+x & a+x & a-x \end{vmatrix} = 0$

(iii) $\begin{vmatrix} x+2 & 3 & 4 \\ 2 & x+3 & 4 \\ 2 & 3 & x+4 \end{vmatrix} = 0$ (iv) $\begin{vmatrix} a-x & b & c \\ a & b-x & c \\ a & b & c-x \end{vmatrix} = 0$

Answers

1. 20 2. 0 3. 0
4. 0 5. 1
6. (i) $x = 4$, (ii) $x = -27/4$, (iii) $x = -1$
7. 0
9. (i) 0 (ii) 0 (iii) 0
19. (i) $x = 0, -6$ (ii) $x = 0$ (iii) $x = 0$ (iv) $x = a + b + c$

3.5 MINORS AND CO-FACTORS

Consider a square matrix $A = \begin{bmatrix} a_{11} & a_{12} & a_{13} \\ a_{21} & a_{22} & a_{23} \\ a_{31} & a_{32} & a_{33} \end{bmatrix}$ ..... (1)

The determinant of this matrix is $|A| = \begin{vmatrix} a_{11} & a_{12} & a_{13} \\ a_{21} & a_{22} & a_{23} \\ a_{31} & a_{32} & a_{33} \end{vmatrix}$ ..... (2)

If the row and the column containing the element a_{11} (i.e., 1st row and 1st column) are removed, we get the second order determinant $\begin{vmatrix} a_{22} & a_{23} \\ a_{32} & a_{33} \end{vmatrix}$ which is called the minor of the element a_{11}.

So the minor of an element is a determinant of a matrix obtained by deleting the row and the column containing that element. If the minors are multiplied by proper signs (+ or –), we get the Co-factors.

The signs to be multiplied are given by the rule $\begin{vmatrix} + & - & + \\ - & + & - \\ + & - & + \end{vmatrix}$

That is, we take + sign if the sum of the suffixes is even and – sign if the sum of the suffixes is odd.

(i) The minor of a_{12} is $\begin{vmatrix} a_{21} & a_{23} \\ a_{31} & a_{33} \end{vmatrix}$ and its co-factor is

$$(-1)^{1+2}\begin{vmatrix} a_{21} & a_{23} \\ a_{31} & a_{33} \end{vmatrix} = -\begin{vmatrix} a_{21} & a_{23} \\ a_{31} & a_{33} \end{vmatrix}$$

(ii) The minor of a_{23} is $\begin{vmatrix} a_{22} & a_{23} \\ a_{32} & a_{33} \end{vmatrix}$ and its co-factor is $-\begin{vmatrix} a_{11} & a_{12} \\ a_{31} & a_{32} \end{vmatrix}$

The co-factors of the elements a_{11}, a_{12} etc are denoted by A_{11}, A_{12} etc.,

The co-factors of the elements of A are:

$$A_{11} = \text{co-factor (CF) of } a_{11} = +\begin{vmatrix} a_{22} & a_{23} \\ a_{32} & a_{33} \end{vmatrix}$$

$$A_{12} = \text{co-factor } a_{12} = -\begin{vmatrix} a_{21} & a_{23} \\ a_{31} & a_{33} \end{vmatrix}$$

$$A_{13} = \text{co-factor of } a_{13} = +\begin{vmatrix} a_{21} & a_{22} \\ a_{31} & a_{32} \end{vmatrix}$$

$$A_{21} = \text{co-factor of } a_{21} = -\begin{vmatrix} a_{12} & a_{13} \\ a_{32} & a_{33} \end{vmatrix}$$

$$A_{22} = \text{co-factor of } a_{22} = -\begin{vmatrix} a_{11} & a_{13} \\ a_{31} & a_{33} \end{vmatrix}$$

$$A_{23} = \text{co-factor of } a_{23} = -\begin{vmatrix} a_{11} & a_{12} \\ a_{31} & a_{32} \end{vmatrix}$$

$$A_{31} = \text{co-factor of } a_{31} = +\begin{vmatrix} a_{12} & a_{13} \\ a_{22} & a_{23} \end{vmatrix}$$

$$A_{32} = \text{co-factor of } a_{32} = -\begin{vmatrix} a_{11} & a_{13} \\ a_{21} & a_{23} \end{vmatrix}$$

$$A_{33} = \text{co-factor of } a_{33} = +\begin{vmatrix} a_{11} & a_{12} \\ a_{21} & a_{22} \end{vmatrix}$$

Note:

1. In general, the co-factor of a_{ij} is got by deleting the ith row and j^{th} column and is denoted by A_{ij}.
2. The sign of the co-factor of a_{ij} is given by $(-1)^{i+j}$.

Examples

(i) Write the co-factors of the elements 6, 2 and 8 in $\begin{vmatrix} 3 & -4 & 6 \\ 2 & 5 & 7 \\ 9 & 8 & 0 \end{vmatrix}$

$$\text{Co – factor of 6 is } +\begin{vmatrix} 2 & 5 \\ 9 & 8 \end{vmatrix} = 16 - 45 = -29$$

$$\text{Co – factor of 2 is } -\begin{vmatrix} -4 & 6 \\ 8 & 0 \end{vmatrix} = -(0 - 48) = 48$$

Co – factor of 8 is $-\begin{vmatrix} 3 & 6 \\ 2 & 7 \end{vmatrix} = -(21-12) = -9$

(ii) Write the co-factors of 2 and 3 in $\begin{vmatrix} 2 & -5 \\ 3 & 4 \end{vmatrix} \begin{vmatrix} + & - \\ - & + \end{vmatrix}$

Co – factor of 2 = + |4| = 4

Co – factor of 3 = – |–5| = 5

Adjoint or Adjugate of a Square Matrix

Consider a square matrix $A = \begin{bmatrix} a_{11} & a_{12} & a_{13} \\ a_{21} & a_{22} & a_{23} \\ a_{31} & a_{32} & a_{33} \end{bmatrix}$

The matrix formed by the C.F.'s is $\begin{bmatrix} A_{11} & A_{12} & A_{13} \\ A_{21} & A_{22} & A_{23} \\ A_{31} & A_{32} & A_{33} \end{bmatrix}$

The transpose of this matrix is C.F is $\begin{bmatrix} A_{11} & A_{21} & A_{31} \\ A_{12} & A_{22} & A_{32} \\ A_{13} & A_{23} & A_{33} \end{bmatrix}$

This is called the adjoint of the matrix *A*.

Definition: The adjoint of a square matrix A is the transpose of the matrix formed by the co-factors of the elements of A and it is written as adj. A.

Important Properties

1. The sum of the products of the elements of any row (or column) of |A| with the corresponding co-factors of the same row (or column) is always equal to |A|

   i.e., $a_{11}A_{11} + a_{12}A_{12} + a_{13}A_{13} = |A|$

   $$\text{LHS} = a_{11}\begin{vmatrix} a_{22} & a_{23} \\ a_{32} & a_{33} \end{vmatrix} - a_{12}\begin{vmatrix} a_{21} & a_{23} \\ a_{31} & a_{33} \end{vmatrix} + a_{13}\begin{vmatrix} a_{21} & a_{22} \\ a_{31} & a_{32} \end{vmatrix}$$

   $$= a_{11}(a_{22}a_{33} - a_{32}a_{23}) - a_{12}(a_{21}a_{33} - a_{31}a_{23}) + a_{13}(a_{21}a_{32} - a_{31}a_{22})$$

   $$= |A| = \text{RHS}$$

Similarly, $a_{21}A_{21} + a_{22}A_{22} + a_{23}A_{23} = |A|$;

$A_{31}A_{31} + a_{32}A_{32} + a_{33}A_{33} = |A|$ and so on

2. The sum of the products of the elements of any row (or column) of |A| with the corresponding co-factors of any other row (or column) is always zero.

i.e., $a_{11}A_{11} + a_{12}A_{12} + a_{13}A_{13} = 0$

$$\because \quad -a_{11}\begin{vmatrix} a_{12} & a_{13} \\ a_{32} & a_{33} \end{vmatrix} + a_{12}\begin{vmatrix} a_{11} & a_{13} \\ a_{31} & a_{33} \end{vmatrix} - a_{13}\begin{vmatrix} a_{11} & a_{12} \\ a_{31} & a_{32} \end{vmatrix}$$

$$= -a_{11}(a_{12}a_{33} - a_{32}a_{13}) + a_{12}(a_{11}a_{33} - a_{31}a_{13}) - a_{13}(a_{11}a_{32} - a_{31}a_{12}) = 0$$

Similarly, $a_{11}A_{31} + a_{12}A_{32} + a_{13}A_{33} = 0$ and so on

Worked Examples

1. Find the adjoint of $\begin{bmatrix} 1 & 4 & -2 \\ -2 & -5 & 4 \\ 1 & -2 & 1 \end{bmatrix}$

Let

$$A = \begin{bmatrix} 1 & 4 & -2 \\ -2 & -5 & 4 \\ 1 & -2 & 1 \end{bmatrix} \qquad \text{.....(1)}$$

$$|A| = \begin{vmatrix} 1 & 4 & -2 \\ -2 & -5 & 4 \\ 1 & -2 & 1 \end{vmatrix}$$

Co-factors are

$$A_{11} = +\begin{vmatrix} -5 & 4 \\ -2 & 1 \end{vmatrix} = 3$$

$$A_{12} = -\begin{vmatrix} -2 & 4 \\ 1 & 1 \end{vmatrix} = 6$$

$$A_{13} = +\begin{vmatrix} -2 & -5 \\ 1 & -2 \end{vmatrix} = 9$$

$$A_{21} = +\begin{vmatrix} 4 & -2 \\ -2 & 1 \end{vmatrix} = 0$$

$$A_{22} = +\begin{vmatrix} 1 & -2 \\ 1 & 1 \end{vmatrix} = 3$$

$$A_{23} = +\begin{vmatrix} 1 & 4 \\ 1 & -2 \end{vmatrix} = 6$$

$$A_{31} = +\begin{vmatrix} 4 & -2 \\ -5 & 4 \end{vmatrix} = 6$$

$$A_{32} = +\begin{vmatrix} 1 & -2 \\ -2 & 4 \end{vmatrix} = 0$$

$$A_{33} = +\begin{vmatrix} 1 & 4 \\ -2 & -5 \end{vmatrix} = 3$$

$$\text{adj } A = \begin{bmatrix} A_{11} & A_{21} & A_{31} \\ A_{12} & A_{22} & A_{32} \\ A_{13} & A_{23} & A_{33} \end{bmatrix} = \begin{bmatrix} 3 & 0 & 6 \\ 6 & 3 & 0 \\ 9 & 6 & 3 \end{bmatrix} \qquad \text{..... (2)}$$

Note: According to the important property stated above,

$a_{11}A_{11} + a_{12}A_{12} + a_{13}A_{13} = |A|$

R_1 in (1) × C_1 in (2) = $1 \times 3 + 4 \times 6 + (-2) \times 9 = 9$

R_2 in (1) × C_2 in (2) = $-2 \times 0 + (-5) \times 3 + 4 \times 6 = 9$

R_3 in (1) × C_3 in (2) = $1 \times 6 - 2 \times 0 + 1 \times 3 = 9$

Further, R_1 in (1) × C_2 in (2) = $1 \times 0 + 4 \times 3 + (-2) \times 6 = 12 - 12 = 0$ and so on

2. Find the adjoint of $A = \begin{bmatrix} 1 & -2 & 3 \\ 0 & 2 & 1 \\ -4 & 5 & 2 \end{bmatrix}$ and verify that A. (adj. A) = (adj. A)

(A) = |A| [where I is the unit matrix of order 3]

$$A = \begin{bmatrix} 1 & -2 & 3 \\ 0 & 2 & 1 \\ -4 & 5 & 2 \end{bmatrix} \begin{vmatrix} + & - & + \\ - & + & - \\ + & - & + \end{vmatrix}$$

$$A_{11} = +\begin{vmatrix} 2 & 1 \\ 5 & 2 \end{vmatrix} = -1$$

$$A_{12} = -\begin{vmatrix} 0 & 1 \\ -4 & 2 \end{vmatrix} = -4$$

$$A_{13} = +\begin{vmatrix} 0 & 2 \\ -4 & 5 \end{vmatrix} = 8$$

$$A_{21} = -\begin{vmatrix} -2 & 3 \\ 5 & 2 \end{vmatrix} = 19$$

$$A_{22} = +\begin{vmatrix} 1 & 3 \\ -4 & 2 \end{vmatrix} = 14$$

$$A_{23} = -\begin{vmatrix} 1 & -2 \\ -4 & 5 \end{vmatrix} = 3$$

$$A_{31} = +\begin{vmatrix} -2 & 3 \\ 2 & 1 \end{vmatrix} = -8$$

$$A_{32} = -\begin{vmatrix} 1 & 3 \\ 0 & 1 \end{vmatrix} = -1$$

$$A_{33} = +\begin{vmatrix} 1 & -2 \\ 0 & 2 \end{vmatrix} = 2$$

$$\text{adj } A = \begin{bmatrix} A_{11} & A_{21} & A_{31} \\ A_{12} & A_{22} & A_{32} \\ A_{13} & A_{23} & A_{33} \end{bmatrix} = \begin{bmatrix} -1 & 19 & -8 \\ -4 & 14 & -1 \\ 8 & 3 & 2 \end{bmatrix}$$

$$|A| = a_{11}A_{11} + a_{12}A_{12} + a_{13}A_{13} = 1(-1) + (-2)(-4) + 3(8) = 31$$

$$A.\ \text{adj}.\ A = \begin{bmatrix} 1 & -2 & 3 \\ 0 & 2 & 1 \\ -4 & 5 & 2 \end{bmatrix} \begin{bmatrix} -1 & 19 & -8 \\ -4 & 14 & -1 \\ 8 & 3 & 2 \end{bmatrix}$$

$$= \begin{bmatrix} 31 & 0 & 1 \\ 0 & 31 & 0 \\ 0 & 0 & 31 \end{bmatrix} = 31\begin{bmatrix} 1 & 0 & 0 \\ 0 & 1 & 0 \\ 0 & 0 & 1 \end{bmatrix} = |A|I$$

$$\text{adj. A.A} = \begin{bmatrix} -1 & 19 & -8 \\ -4 & 14 & -1 \\ 8 & 3 & 2 \end{bmatrix} \begin{bmatrix} 1 & -2 & 3 \\ 0 & 2 & 1 \\ -4 & 5 & 2 \end{bmatrix}$$

$$= \begin{bmatrix} 31 & 0 & 0 \\ 0 & 31 & 0 \\ 0 & 0 & 31 \end{bmatrix} = 31 \begin{bmatrix} 1 & 0 & 0 \\ 0 & 1 & 0 \\ 0 & 0 & 1 \end{bmatrix} = |A|I$$

Thus, A. adj. A = adj. A.A = |A| I

3. To find the adjoint of a second order square matrix by inspection.

$$\text{Let} \quad A = \begin{pmatrix} a_{11} & a_{12} \\ a_{21} & a_{22} \end{pmatrix} \begin{vmatrix} + & - \\ - & + \end{vmatrix}$$

A_{11} = co-factor of $a_{11} = a_{22}$; A_{12} = co-factor of $a_{12} = -a_{21}$;

A_{21} = co-factor of $a_{21} = -a_{12}$; A_{22} = co-factor of $a_{22} = a_{11}$

$$\text{Adj. A} = \begin{pmatrix} A_{11} & A_{21} \\ A_{12} & A_{22} \end{pmatrix} = \begin{pmatrix} a_{22} & -a_{12} \\ -a_{21} & a_{11} \end{pmatrix}$$

Thus, if $A = \begin{pmatrix} a_{11} & a_{12} \\ a_{21} & a_{22} \end{pmatrix}$ then adj. $A = \begin{pmatrix} a_{22} & -a_{12} \\ -a_{21} & a_{11} \end{pmatrix}$

Note: To get adj.A, principal diagonal terms are interchanged and the signs of other terms are changed.

For example, $A = \begin{pmatrix} 2 & 3 \\ 5 & -6 \end{pmatrix} \Rightarrow \text{adj } A = \begin{pmatrix} -6 & -3 \\ -5 & 2 \end{pmatrix}$;

$$B = \begin{pmatrix} 3 & -4 \\ 2 & 3 \end{pmatrix} \Rightarrow \text{adj } B = \begin{pmatrix} 3 & 4 \\ -2 & 3 \end{pmatrix}$$

4. If $A = \begin{pmatrix} 5 & 3 \\ -2 & 4 \end{pmatrix}$ and $B = \begin{pmatrix} 2 & -3 \\ 4 & 8 \end{pmatrix}$, verify that (adj.A). (adj.B) = adj. (BA)

$$A = \begin{pmatrix} 5 & 3 \\ -2 & 4 \end{pmatrix}, \quad B = \begin{pmatrix} 2 & -3 \\ 4 & 8 \end{pmatrix}$$

$$\therefore \quad \text{adj. A} = \begin{pmatrix} 4 & -3 \\ 2 & 5 \end{pmatrix}, \text{adj. B} = \begin{pmatrix} -8 & 3 \\ -4 & 2 \end{pmatrix}$$

$$\therefore \qquad (\text{adj. A})(\text{adj.B}) = \begin{pmatrix} 4 & -3 \\ 2 & 5 \end{pmatrix} \begin{pmatrix} -8 & 3 \\ -4 & 2 \end{pmatrix}$$

$$= \begin{pmatrix} -20 & 6 \\ -36 & 16 \end{pmatrix} \qquad \text{.....(1)}$$

$$\text{BA} = \begin{pmatrix} 2 & -3 \\ 4 & -8 \end{pmatrix} \begin{pmatrix} 5 & 3 \\ -2 & 4 \end{pmatrix}$$

$$= \begin{pmatrix} 10+6 & 6-12 \\ 20+16 & 12-32 \end{pmatrix} = \begin{pmatrix} 16 & -6 \\ 36 & -20 \end{pmatrix}$$

$$\therefore \qquad \text{adj.(BA)} = \begin{pmatrix} -20 & 16 \\ -36 & 16 \end{pmatrix} \qquad \text{.....(2)}$$

From (1) and (2), it follows (adj.A) (adj.B) = adj. (BA)

Note: This result holds good also when A and B are square matrices of order n.

5. If $A = \begin{bmatrix} 1 & -3 \\ 2 & 0 \end{bmatrix}$, write adj.(A)

$$\text{adj. (A)} = \begin{bmatrix} 0 & 3 \\ -2 & 1 \end{bmatrix}$$

6. If $A = \begin{pmatrix} a & b \\ c & d \end{pmatrix}$, $B = \begin{pmatrix} 1 & 0 \\ 0 & 1 \end{pmatrix}$, find adj. (AB)

$$\text{AB} = \begin{pmatrix} a & b \\ c & d \end{pmatrix} \begin{pmatrix} 1 & 0 \\ 0 & 1 \end{pmatrix} = \begin{pmatrix} a & b \\ c & d \end{pmatrix}$$

$$\text{adj. (AB)} = \begin{pmatrix} d & -b \\ -c & a \end{pmatrix}$$

7. If $A = \begin{bmatrix} 2 & -1 & 3 \\ -1 & 4 & 2 \\ 0 & -3 & 1 \end{bmatrix}$, $B = [-1 \ \ 2 \ \ -1]$, find B (adj.A)

$$\text{adj. A} = \begin{bmatrix} 10 & -8 & 14 \\ 1 & 2 & -7 \\ 3 & 6 & 7 \end{bmatrix}$$

$$B\,(\text{adj.}A) = [-1 \quad 2 \quad -1]\begin{bmatrix} 10 & -8 & -14 \\ 1 & 2 & -7 \\ 3 & 6 & 7 \end{bmatrix}$$

$$= [-10+2-3 \quad 8+4-6 \quad 14-14-7] = [-11 \quad 6 \quad -7]$$

If A is a Square Matrix of Order 3, then

(adj. A). A = A . (adj. A) = |A| I

$$\text{Take } A = \begin{bmatrix} a_{11} & a_{12} & a_{13} \\ a_{21} & a_{22} & a_{23} \\ a_{31} & a_{32} & a_{33} \end{bmatrix}, \text{ then adj } A = \begin{bmatrix} A_{11} & A_{21} & A_{31} \\ A_{12} & A_{22} & A_{32} \\ A_{13} & A_{23} & A_{33} \end{bmatrix}$$

$$A.\,(\text{adj. }A) = \begin{bmatrix} a_{11} & a_{12} & a_{13} \\ a_{21} & a_{22} & a_{23} \\ a_{31} & a_{32} & a_{33} \end{bmatrix}\begin{bmatrix} A_{11} & A_{21} & A_{31} \\ A_{12} & A_{22} & A_{32} \\ A_{13} & A_{23} & A_{33} \end{bmatrix}$$

$$= \begin{bmatrix} (a_{11}A_{11}+a_{12}A_{12}+a_{13}A_{13}) & (a_{11}A_{21}+a_{12}A_{22}+a_{13}A_{23}) & (a_{11}A_{31}+a_{12}A_{32}+a_{13}A_{33}) \\ (a_{21}A_{11}+a_{22}A_{12}+a_{23}A_{13}) & (a_{21}A_{21}+a_{22}A_{22}+a_{23}A_{23}) & (a_{11}A_{31}+a_{22}A_{32}+a_{23}A_{33}) \\ (a_{31}A_{11}+a_{32}A_{12}+a_{33}A_{13}) & (a_{31}A_{21}+a_{32}A_{22}+a_{33}A_{23}) & (a_{31}A_{31}+a_{32}A_{32}+a_{33}A_{33}) \end{bmatrix}$$

$$= \begin{bmatrix} (a_{11}A_{11}+a_{12}A_{12}+a_{13}A_{13}) & (a_{11}A_{21}+a_{12}A_{22}+a_{13}A_{23}) & (a_{11}A_{31}+a_{12}A_{32}+a_{13}A_{33}) \\ (a_{21}A_{11}+a_{22}A_{12}+a_{23}A_{13}) & (a_{21}A_{21}+a_{22}A_{22}+a_{23}A_{23}) & (a_{11}A_{31}+a_{22}A_{32}+a_{23}A_{33}) \\ (a_{31}A_{11}+a_{32}A_{12}+a_{33}A_{13}) & (a_{31}A_{21}+a_{32}A_{22}+a_{33}A_{23}) & (a_{31}A_{31}+a_{32}A_{32}+a_{33}A_{33}) \end{bmatrix}$$

$$= \begin{bmatrix} |A| & 0 & 0 \\ 0 & |A| & 0 \\ 0 & 0 & |A| \end{bmatrix} = |A|\begin{bmatrix} 1 & 0 & 0 \\ 0 & 1 & 0 \\ 0 & 0 & 1 \end{bmatrix} = |A|\,I$$

Similarly, it can be shown that (adj. A). A = |A| I

∴ (adj. A) .A = A. (adj. A) = |A| I

Singular and Non-Singular Matrices

A square matrix A is said to be singular if |A| = 0.

$$\text{For example, } A = \begin{pmatrix} 2 & 3 \\ 4 & 6 \end{pmatrix}, \; |A| = \begin{vmatrix} 2 & 3 \\ 4 & 6 \end{vmatrix} = 0$$

Therefore A is a singular matrix

A square matrix A is said to be non-singular if $|A| \neq 0$

For example, $A = \begin{pmatrix} 2 & 5 \\ -1 & 6 \end{pmatrix}$, $|A| = \begin{vmatrix} 2 & 5 \\ -1 & 6 \end{vmatrix} = 17 \neq 0$

Therefore A is a non-singular matrix

Worked Examples

1. Find whether each of the following matrices is singular or non-singular.

(i) $\begin{pmatrix} 2 & 1 \\ 1 & 3 \end{pmatrix}$, (ii) $\begin{pmatrix} x & x \\ x & x \end{pmatrix}$, (iii) $\begin{pmatrix} 4 & 10 & 11 \\ 7 & 6 & 2 \\ 1 & 5 & 4 \end{pmatrix}$, (iv) $\begin{pmatrix} 1 & 3 & 0 \\ 2 & 1 & 0 \\ 3 & 3 & 0 \end{pmatrix}$

(i) $|A| = \begin{vmatrix} 2 & 1 \\ 1 & 3 \end{vmatrix} = 6 - 2 = 5 \neq 0$ $\quad\therefore$ A is non – singular.

(ii) $|A| = \begin{vmatrix} x & x \\ x & x \end{vmatrix} = 0$ $\quad\therefore$ A is singular.

(iii) $|A| = \begin{vmatrix} 4 & 10 & 11 \\ 7 & 6 & 2 \\ 1 & 5 & 4 \end{vmatrix} = 115 \neq 0$ $\quad\therefore$ A is non – singular.

(iv) $|A| = \begin{vmatrix} 1 & 3 & 0 \\ 2 & 1 & 0 \\ 3 & 3 & 0 \end{vmatrix} = 0$ $\quad\therefore$ A is singular.

2. If $A = \begin{bmatrix} 3 & 2 & x \\ 4 & 1 & -1 \\ 0 & 3 & 4 \end{bmatrix}$ is a singular matrix, find x ?

Since A is singular, $|A| = 0$ i.e., $\begin{vmatrix} 3 & 2 & x \\ 4 & 1 & -1 \\ 0 & 3 & 4 \end{vmatrix} = 0$

i.e., $3(4 + 3) - 2(16 - 0) + x(12 - 0) = 0 \Rightarrow x = \frac{11}{12}$

3. If the matrix $\begin{bmatrix} 5x & 2 \\ -10 & 1 \end{bmatrix}$ is singular, find the value of x? $\begin{vmatrix} 5x & 2 \\ -10 & 1 \end{vmatrix} = 0$

   i.e., $5x + 20 = 0$

   i.e., $5x = -20$

   i.e., $x = -4$

3.6 INVERSE OF A MATRIX

If A and B are two non-singular matrices of same order and if AB = BA = I, then A and B are called inverses of each other. That is, A is the inverse of B and B is the inverse of A.

Then $B = A^{-1}$ or $A = B^{-1}$

Note that AB = BA = I can be written as

$$AA^{-1} = A^{-1}A = I \text{ and } BB^{-1} = B^{-1}B = I$$

For example, Let $A = \begin{pmatrix} 2 & -3 \\ 3 & -5 \end{pmatrix}$ and $B = \begin{pmatrix} 5 & -3 \\ 3 & -2 \end{pmatrix}$

$$AB = \begin{pmatrix} 2 & -3 \\ 3 & -5 \end{pmatrix}\begin{pmatrix} 5 & -3 \\ 3 & -2 \end{pmatrix} = \begin{pmatrix} 1 & 0 \\ 0 & 1 \end{pmatrix} = I$$

$$BA = \begin{pmatrix} 5 & -3 \\ 3 & -2 \end{pmatrix}\begin{pmatrix} 2 & -3 \\ 3 & -5 \end{pmatrix} = \begin{pmatrix} 1 & 0 \\ 0 & 1 \end{pmatrix} = I$$

i.e., AB = BA = I $\therefore$ A and B are inverses of each other

i.e., $\begin{pmatrix} 5 & -3 \\ 3 & -2 \end{pmatrix} = \begin{pmatrix} 2 & -3 \\ 3 & -5 \end{pmatrix}^{-1}$

Note:

(a) Inverse of a square matrix A exists if and only if A is non-singular i.e., $|A| \neq 0$

(b) Inverse of a square matrix, if it exists, is unique

(c) A singular matrix has no inverse.

To Find the Inverse of a Non-Singular Matrix A

If A is a square matrix, A. adj(A) = adj(A).A = |A| I ..... (1)

Since A is non-singular, $|A| \neq 0$. Divide (1) by |A|,

$$\frac{A.adj.A}{|A|} = \frac{adj.A.A}{|A|} = \frac{|A|I}{|A|}$$

i.e., $$A.\left(\frac{adj.A}{|A|}\right) = \left(\frac{adj.A}{|A|}\right).A = I \quad \text{..... (2)}$$

compare this with $A.\ A^{-1} = A^{-1}\ .\ A = I$ ..... (3)

Hence $$A^{-1} = \frac{adj.A}{|A|}$$

i.e., $$A^{-1} = \frac{1}{|A|}.adj.A$$

If A and B are non-singular matrices of same order, then prove that $(AB)^{-1} = B^{-1}A^{-1}$

Consider $(AB)\ (B^{-1}A^{-1}) = A\ [B(B^{-1}A^{-1})]$ by associative law

$= A[(BB^{-1})A^{-1}]$ by associative law

$= A[I\ A^{-1}]$ $\qquad \because BB^{-1} = I$

$= A\ A^{-1}$ $\qquad \because I\ A^{-1} = A^{-1}$

$= I$ $\qquad \because AA^{-1} = I$

$\therefore \quad (AB)(B^{-1}A^{-1}) = I$ .....(1)

Similarly, it can be proved that $(B^{-1}\ A^{-1})\ (AB) = I$ .....(2)

From (1) and (2), $(AB)\ (A^{-1}B^{-1}) = (B^{-1}\ A^{-1})\ (AB)$

This means that inverse of AB is $B^{-1}A^{-1}$ i.e., $(AB)^{-1} = B^{-1}A^{-1}$

This is known as reversal law of inverses.

Similarly, if A, B, C, are non-singular matrices of same order, then $(ABC\ \ldots)^{-1} = (\ldots\ C^{-1}B^{-1}A^{-1})$

Worked Examples

1. Find the inverse of $\begin{bmatrix} 1 & 2 & -1 \\ -1 & 1 & 2 \\ 2 & -1 & 1 \end{bmatrix}$

Let $A = \begin{bmatrix} 1 & 2 & -1 \\ -1 & 1 & 2 \\ 2 & -1 & 1 \end{bmatrix}$, then $A^{-1} = \frac{1}{|A|}\text{ adj.}A$

$$A_{11} = \begin{vmatrix} 1 & 2 \\ -1 & 1 \end{vmatrix} = 3$$

$$A_{12} = \begin{vmatrix} -1 & 2 \\ 2 & 1 \end{vmatrix} = 5$$

$$A_{13} = \begin{vmatrix} -1 & 1 \\ 2 & -1 \end{vmatrix} = -1$$

$$A_{21} = \begin{vmatrix} 2 & -1 \\ -1 & 1 \end{vmatrix} = -1$$

$$A_{22} = \begin{vmatrix} 1 & -1 \\ 2 & 1 \end{vmatrix} = 3$$

$$A_{23} = \begin{vmatrix} 1 & 2 \\ 2 & -1 \end{vmatrix} = 5$$

$$A_{31} = \begin{vmatrix} 2 & -1 \\ 1 & 2 \end{vmatrix} = 5$$

$$A_{32} = \begin{vmatrix} 1 & -1 \\ -1 & 2 \end{vmatrix} = -1$$

$$A_{33} = \begin{vmatrix} 1 & 2 \\ -1 & 1 \end{vmatrix} = 3$$

$$A = \begin{bmatrix} A_{11} & A_{12} & A_{13} \\ A_{21} & A_{22} & A_{23} \\ A_{31} & A_{32} & A_{33} \end{bmatrix} = \begin{bmatrix} 3 & 5 & -1 \\ -1 & 3 & 5 \\ 5 & -1 & 3 \end{bmatrix}$$

$$|A| = a_{11} A_{11} + a_{12} A_{12} + a_{13} A_{13}$$
$$= 1(3) + 2(5) + (-1)(-1) = 14$$

So, $$A^{-1} = \frac{1}{|A|}\text{ adj.}A = \frac{1}{14}\begin{bmatrix} 3 & 5 & -1 \\ -1 & 3 & 5 \\ 5 & -1 & 3 \end{bmatrix}$$

2. If $A = \begin{bmatrix} 1 & 3 & 4 \\ 1 & 4 & 5 \\ 2 & 5 & 7 \end{bmatrix}$, show A^{-1} does not exist

Here, $|A| = \begin{bmatrix} 1 & 3 & 4 \\ 1 & 4 & 5 \\ 2 & 5 & 7 \end{bmatrix} = \begin{bmatrix} 1 & 3 & 1 \\ 1 & 4 & 1 \\ 2 & 5 & 2 \end{bmatrix}$ taking $C_3' = C_3 - C_2$

$= 0$ (As two columns are identical)

$\therefore \quad |A| = 0$

So, A^{-1} does not exist

3. Find the inverse of $A = \begin{bmatrix} \cos\theta & -\sin\theta & 0 \\ \sin\theta & \cos\theta & 0 \\ 0 & 0 & 1 \end{bmatrix}$

$$A_{11} = \begin{vmatrix} \cos\theta & 0 \\ 0 & 1 \end{vmatrix} = \cos\theta$$

$$A_{12} = \begin{vmatrix} \sin\theta & 0 \\ 0 & 1 \end{vmatrix} = -\sin\theta$$

$$A_{13} = \begin{vmatrix} \sin\theta & \cos\theta \\ 0 & 0 \end{vmatrix} = 0$$

$$A_{21} = \begin{vmatrix} -\sin\theta & 0 \\ 0 & 1 \end{vmatrix} = \sin\theta$$

$$A_{22} = \begin{vmatrix} \cos\theta & 0 \\ 0 & 1 \end{vmatrix} = 0$$

$$A_{23} = \begin{vmatrix} \cos\theta & -\sin\theta \\ 0 & 0 \end{vmatrix} = 0$$

$$A_{31} = \begin{vmatrix} -\sin\theta & 0 \\ \cos\theta & 0 \end{vmatrix} = 0$$

$$A_{32} = \begin{vmatrix} \cos\theta & 0 \\ \sin\theta & 0 \end{vmatrix} = 0$$

$$A_{33} = \begin{vmatrix} \cos\theta & -\sin\theta \\ \sin\theta & \cos\theta \end{vmatrix} = \cos^2\theta + \sin^2\theta = 1$$

$$\therefore \quad \text{adj. } A = \begin{bmatrix} A_{11} & A_{12} & A_{13} \\ A_{21} & A_{22} & A_{23} \\ A_{31} & A_{32} & A_{33} \end{bmatrix} = \begin{bmatrix} \cos\theta & -\sin\theta & 0 \\ \sin\theta & \cos\theta & 0 \\ 0 & 0 & 1 \end{bmatrix}$$

$$|A| = a_{11} A_{11} + a_{12} A_{12} + a_{13} A_{13} = \cos^2\theta + \sin^2\theta = 1$$

$$\therefore \quad A^{-1} = \frac{1}{|A|}\text{adj.}A = \frac{1}{1}\begin{bmatrix} \cos\theta & \sin\theta & 0 \\ -\sin\theta & \cos\theta & 0 \\ 0 & 0 & 1 \end{bmatrix} = \begin{bmatrix} \cos\theta & \sin\theta & 0 \\ -\sin\theta & \cos\theta & 0 \\ 0 & 0 & 1 \end{bmatrix}$$

Note: that A^{-1} is the transpose of A in this case.

Orthogonal matrices

A square matrix A is called orthogonal matrix if $AA^{-1} = I = A^{-1}A$.

That is, A^{-1} is the inverse of A.

In the above example, $A^{-1} \begin{bmatrix} \cos & \sin & 0 \\ -\sin & \cos & 0 \\ 0 & 0 & 1 \end{bmatrix}$

4. Find the inverse of $\begin{bmatrix} a & 0 & 0 \\ 0 & b & 0 \\ 0 & 0 & c \end{bmatrix}$ where a, b, c are non zero real numbers

$$A = \begin{bmatrix} a & 0 & 0 \\ 0 & b & 0 \\ 0 & 0 & c \end{bmatrix}$$

$A_{11} = bc$ $\qquad A_{21} = 0$ $\qquad A_{31} = 0$

$A_{12} = 0$ $\qquad A_{22} = ac$ $\qquad A_{32} = 0$

$A_{13} = 0$ $\qquad A_{23} = 0$ $\qquad A_{33} = ab$

$$\therefore \quad \text{adj.}A = \begin{bmatrix} bc & 0 & 0 \\ 0 & ac & 0 \\ 0 & 0 & ab \end{bmatrix}; \ |A| = abc$$

$$\therefore \quad A^{-1} = \frac{1}{abc}\begin{bmatrix} bc & 0 & 0 \\ 0 & ac & 0 \\ 0 & 0 & ab \end{bmatrix} = \begin{bmatrix} \frac{1}{a} & 0 & 0 \\ 0 & \frac{1}{b} & 0 \\ 0 & 0 & \frac{1}{c} \end{bmatrix}$$

Note: Find the inverse of $\begin{bmatrix} 1 & 0 & 0 \\ 0 & 2 & 0 \\ 0 & 0 & 3 \end{bmatrix}$

$$\text{Inverse} = \begin{bmatrix} \frac{1}{1} & 0 & 0 \\ 0 & \frac{1}{2} & 0 \\ 0 & 0 & \frac{1}{3} \end{bmatrix}$$

5. Find the inverse of $\begin{bmatrix} 2 & 3 \\ 2 & 5 \end{bmatrix}$

Let $\quad A = \begin{pmatrix} 2 & 3 \\ 2 & 5 \end{pmatrix}$, adj $A = \begin{bmatrix} 5 & -3 \\ -2 & 2 \end{bmatrix}$

$$|A| = \begin{vmatrix} 2 & 3 \\ 2 & 5 \end{vmatrix} = 10 - 6 = 4$$

So, $\quad A^{-1} = \frac{1}{|A|}\text{adj}.A = \frac{1}{4}\begin{pmatrix} 5 & -3 \\ -2 & 2 \end{pmatrix} = \begin{pmatrix} \frac{5}{4} & -\frac{3}{4} \\ -\frac{1}{2} & \frac{1}{2} \end{pmatrix}$

6. If $A = \begin{pmatrix} 2 & -1 \\ -1 & 2 \end{pmatrix}$, show that $A^2 - 4A + 3I = 0$ and hence find A^{-1}

$$A^2 = \begin{pmatrix} 2 & -1 \\ -1 & 2 \end{pmatrix}\begin{pmatrix} 2 & -1 \\ -1 & 2 \end{pmatrix} = \begin{pmatrix} 5 & -4 \\ -4 & 5 \end{pmatrix}$$

$$A^2 - 4A + 3I = \begin{pmatrix} 5 & -4 \\ -4 & 5 \end{pmatrix} + (-4)\begin{pmatrix} 2 & -1 \\ -1 & 2 \end{pmatrix} + \begin{pmatrix} 1 & 0 \\ 0 & 1 \end{pmatrix}$$

$$= \begin{pmatrix} 5-8+3 & -4+4+0 \\ -4+4+0 & 5-8+3 \end{pmatrix} = \begin{pmatrix} 0 & 0 \\ 0 & 0 \end{pmatrix} = 0$$

$\therefore \quad A^2 - 4A + 3I = 0$

A^{-1} exists as $|A| \neq 0$. Multiply (1) by A^{-1}

$$A^2 A^{-1} - 4A A^{-1} + 3I A^{-1} = 0$$

$$AI - 4I + 3A^{-1} = 0 \qquad (\because AA^{-1} = I)$$

$$A - 4I + 3A^{-1} = 0 \qquad (\because AI = A)$$

$$3A^{-1} = 4I - A = 4\begin{pmatrix} 1 & 0 \\ 0 & 1 \end{pmatrix} - \begin{pmatrix} 2 & -1 \\ -1 & 2 \end{pmatrix} = \begin{pmatrix} 2 & 1 \\ 1 & 2 \end{pmatrix}$$

$$\therefore \quad A^{-1} = \frac{1}{3}\begin{pmatrix} 2 & 1 \\ 1 & 2 \end{pmatrix}$$

7. If $A = \begin{pmatrix} 1 & -2 & 2 \\ 0 & 2 & -3 \\ 3 & -2 & 4 \end{pmatrix}$ and $\begin{pmatrix} -2 \\ 2 \\ 0 \end{pmatrix}$, find $A^{-1}B$

$$\text{adj. } A = \begin{pmatrix} 2 & 4 & 2 \\ -9 & -2 & 3 \\ -6 & -4 & 2 \end{pmatrix}$$

$$|A| = 1(8-6) + 2(0+9) + 2(0-6)$$

$$= 2 + 12 - 12 = 8$$

$$\therefore \quad A^{-1} = \frac{1}{8}\begin{pmatrix} 2 & 4 & 2 \\ -9 & -2 & 3 \\ -6 & -4 & 2 \end{pmatrix}$$

$$A^{-1}B = \frac{1}{8}\begin{pmatrix} 2 & 4 & 2 \\ -9 & -2 & 3 \\ -6 & -4 & 2 \end{pmatrix}\begin{pmatrix} -2 \\ 2 \\ 0 \end{pmatrix} = \frac{1}{8}\begin{pmatrix} -4+8 \\ 18-4 \\ 12-8 \end{pmatrix} = \frac{1}{8}\begin{pmatrix} 4 \\ 14 \\ 4 \end{pmatrix} = \begin{pmatrix} \frac{1}{2} \\ \frac{7}{4} \\ \frac{1}{2} \end{pmatrix}$$

8. If AX = B, where $A=\begin{pmatrix}3 & -1 & 2\\ 2 & 1 & -1\\ 1 & 3 & -5\end{pmatrix}$, $B=\begin{pmatrix}13\\ 3\\ -8\end{pmatrix}$, $X=\begin{pmatrix}x\\ y\\ z\end{pmatrix}$, find the value of x, y, z by using inverse of A.

$$\text{adj. } A=\begin{pmatrix}-2 & 1 & -1\\ 9 & -17 & 7\\ 5 & -10 & 5\end{pmatrix}$$

$$|A| = 3(-5+3) + 1(-10+1) + 2(6-1)$$

$$= -6 - 9 + 10 = -5$$

$$A^{-1} = \frac{1}{|A|}\text{adj.}A$$

$$= -\frac{1}{5}\begin{pmatrix}-2 & 1 & -1\\ 9 & -17 & 7\\ 5 & -10 & 5\end{pmatrix}$$

Now. AX = B $\quad\therefore\ X = A^{-1}B$

$$X=-\frac{1}{5}\begin{pmatrix}-2 & 1 & -1\\ 9 & -17 & 7\\ 5 & -10 & 5\end{pmatrix}\begin{pmatrix}13\\ 3\\ -8\end{pmatrix}$$

i.e.,
$$X=-\frac{1}{5}\begin{pmatrix}-26+3+8\\ 117-51-56\\ 65-30-40\end{pmatrix}=-\frac{1}{5}\begin{pmatrix}-15\\ 10\\ -5\end{pmatrix}=\begin{pmatrix}3\\ -2\\ 1\end{pmatrix}$$

$\therefore\quad x = 3, y = -2, z = 1$

Exercise 3.3

I 1. If $A=\begin{bmatrix}3 & -2\\ 2 & 2\end{bmatrix}$, find adj. A

2. If $A=\begin{bmatrix}3 & 0\\ 0 & 2\end{bmatrix}$, find adj. A

3. Find A^{-1} given that

(i) $A = \begin{bmatrix} 4 & -1 \\ -7 & 2 \end{bmatrix}$

4. Show that if $A = \begin{bmatrix} -3 & 4 \\ 3 & -4 \end{bmatrix}$, then A^{-1} does not exist

5. If $A = \begin{bmatrix} 1 & 2 & 3 \\ 2 & x & 3 \\ 3 & 4 & 5 \end{bmatrix}$ is singular, find x

6. If $A = \begin{bmatrix} 3 & 4 \\ 4 & 5 \end{bmatrix}$, find A^{-1}

7. If $A = \begin{bmatrix} 1 & 0 \\ 0 & 1 \end{bmatrix}$, find $A.A^{-1}$

II 1. Find the adjoint of:

(i) $\begin{bmatrix} 1 & -2 & 3 \\ 0 & 2 & 1 \\ -4 & 5 & 2 \end{bmatrix}$ (ii) $\begin{bmatrix} 1 & 2 & 2 \\ 1 & 3 & 4 \\ 1 & 4 & 3 \end{bmatrix}$

2. If $A = \begin{pmatrix} 1 & 3 \\ 5 & 7 \end{pmatrix}$ and $B = \begin{pmatrix} -1 & 2 \\ 3 & -4 \end{pmatrix}$, find adj.(AB)

3. If $A = \begin{pmatrix} 4 & 1 \\ -3 & 2 \end{pmatrix}$ and $B = \begin{pmatrix} 0 & 2 \\ 1 & -1 \end{pmatrix}$,

Verify that adj.(AB) = (adj.B)(adj.A)

4. Find whether each of the following matrices is singular or non-singular:

(i) $\begin{pmatrix} 2 & 3 \\ -1 & 5 \end{pmatrix}$ (ii) $\begin{pmatrix} 2 & -1 \\ -2 & 1 \end{pmatrix}$ (iii) $\begin{pmatrix} 3 & 5 \\ -1 & 6 \end{pmatrix}$ (iv) $\begin{bmatrix} 1 & 2 & 3 \\ 2 & 3 & 4 \\ 3 & 4 & 5 \end{bmatrix}$

5. Find the inverse of each of the following

(i) $\begin{bmatrix} 1 & 2 & 3 \\ 1 & 3 & 3 \\ 2 & 4 & 3 \end{bmatrix}$ (ii) $\begin{bmatrix} 1 & 2 & -3 \\ 0 & 1 & 2 \\ 0 & 0 & 1 \end{bmatrix}$ (iii) $\begin{pmatrix} 2 & -1 \\ 3 & 4 \end{pmatrix}$

6. If $A = \begin{bmatrix} 3 & 1 & 2 \\ -2 & -1 & 1 \\ 3 & 0 & 2 \end{bmatrix}$, find $(A')^{-1}$

7. If $A = \begin{bmatrix} 1 & 2 \\ 3 & 4 \end{bmatrix}$ and $B = \begin{bmatrix} 5 & 6 \\ 7 & 8 \end{bmatrix}$, Verify that $(AB)^{-1} = B^{-1}A^{-1}$

8. If $A = \begin{bmatrix} 1 & -2 & 2 \\ 0 & 2 & -3 \\ 3 & -2 & 4 \end{bmatrix}$ and $B = \begin{pmatrix} -2 \\ 2 \\ -5 \end{pmatrix}$, find $A^{-1}B$

Answers

I 1. $\begin{bmatrix} 2 & 2 \\ -2 & 3 \end{bmatrix}$ 2. $\begin{bmatrix} 6 & 0 \\ 0 & 6 \end{bmatrix}$ 3. $\begin{bmatrix} 2 & 7 \\ 1 & 4 \end{bmatrix}$

4. X= 5/2 5. $\begin{bmatrix} -5 & 4 \\ 4 & -3 \end{bmatrix}$ 6. $\begin{bmatrix} 1 & 0 \\ 0 & 1 \end{bmatrix}$

II 1. (i) $\begin{bmatrix} -1 & 19 & -8 \\ -4 & 14 & -1 \\ 8 & 3 & 2 \end{bmatrix}$ (ii) $\begin{bmatrix} -7 & 2 & 2 \\ 1 & 3 & -2 \\ 1 & -2 & 1 \end{bmatrix}$

2. $\begin{bmatrix} -18 & 10 \\ -16 & 8 \end{bmatrix}$

4. (i) Non singular (ii) Singular (iii) Non singular (iv) Singular

5. (i) $\frac{1}{3}\begin{bmatrix} 3 & -6 & 3 \\ -3 & 3 & 0 \\ 2 & 0 & -1 \end{bmatrix}$ (ii) $\begin{bmatrix} 1 & -2 & 7 \\ 0 & 1 & -2 \\ 0 & 0 & 1 \end{bmatrix}$ (iii) $\frac{1}{11}\begin{bmatrix} 4 & 1 \\ -3 & 2 \end{bmatrix}$

6. $\frac{1}{7}\begin{bmatrix} -2 & 7 & 3 \\ -2 & 0 & 3 \\ 3 & -7 & -1 \end{bmatrix}$

8. $\begin{bmatrix} \frac{-3}{8} \\ \frac{-1}{8} \\ \frac{-3}{8} \end{bmatrix}$

3.7 SOLUTION OF SYSTEM OF LINEAR OF EQUATIONS USING MATRIX METHOD

To solve $a_1x + b_1y + c_1z = d_1$

$a_2x + b_2y + c_2z = d_2$ using matrix method.

$a_3x + b_3y + c_3z = d_3$

Let $A = \begin{pmatrix} a_1 & b_1 & c_1 \\ a_2 & b_2 & c_2 \\ a_3 & b_3 & c_3 \end{pmatrix}$, $X = \begin{pmatrix} x \\ y \\ z \end{pmatrix}$, $D = \begin{pmatrix} d_1 \\ d_2 \\ d_3 \end{pmatrix}$

The given set of equations can be written as AX = D ..... (1)

Assume that $|A| = 0$

Then, A^{-1} exists

Multiply on left side of (1) by A^{-1}

$A^{-1}(AX) = A–1D$ or $(A–1A)X = A^{-1}D$ (by associative law)

$IX = A^{-1}D$ (it is because $A^{-1}A = I$) or $X = A^{-1}D$ (it is because $IX = X$)

The solution is given by $\begin{bmatrix} x \\ y \\ z \end{bmatrix} = A^{-1}D$

Worked Examples

1. Solve by matrix method

$x + 2y = -3$

$2x - 3y = 8$

Let $A = \begin{pmatrix} 1 & 2 \\ 2 & -3 \end{pmatrix}, \; B = \begin{pmatrix} -3 \\ 8 \end{pmatrix}, \; X = \begin{pmatrix} x \\ y \end{pmatrix}$

Given equation reduce to the matrix equation

$AX = B$ so that $X = A^{-1}B$

Now, $$A^{-1} = \frac{1}{-7}\begin{pmatrix} -3 & -2 \\ -2 & 1 \end{pmatrix}$$

$\therefore$ $$X = -\frac{1}{7}\begin{pmatrix} -3 & -2 \\ -2 & 1 \end{pmatrix}\begin{pmatrix} -3 \\ 8 \end{pmatrix}$$

$$= -\frac{1}{7}\begin{pmatrix} -7 \\ 14 \end{pmatrix} = \begin{pmatrix} 1 \\ -2 \end{pmatrix}$$

$\therefore$ $$\begin{pmatrix} x \\ y \end{pmatrix} = \begin{pmatrix} 1 \\ -2 \end{pmatrix} \text{ i.e., } x = 1, y = -2$$

2. Solve using matrix method

$$x + y + z = 3; \quad 3x + 4y + 7z = 14; \quad x - y + z = 1$$

$$A = \begin{bmatrix} 1 & 1 & 1 \\ 3 & 4 & 7 \\ 1 & -1 & 1 \end{bmatrix}, \quad X = \begin{bmatrix} x \\ y \\ z \end{bmatrix}, \quad D = \begin{bmatrix} 3 \\ 14 \\ 1 \end{bmatrix}$$

The solution is $X = A^{-1}D$

$$A_{11} = \begin{vmatrix} 4 & 7 \\ -1 & 1 \end{vmatrix} = 11$$

$$A_{12} = -\begin{vmatrix} 3 & 7 \\ 1 & 1 \end{vmatrix} = 4$$

$$A_{13} = \begin{vmatrix} 3 & 4 \\ 1 & -1 \end{vmatrix} = -7$$

$$A_{21} = -\begin{vmatrix} 1 & 1 \\ -1 & 1 \end{vmatrix} = -2$$

$$A_{22} = \begin{vmatrix} 1 & 1 \\ 1 & 1 \end{vmatrix} = 0$$

$$A_{23} = -\begin{vmatrix} 1 & 1 \\ 1 & -1 \end{vmatrix} = 2$$

$$A_{31} = \begin{vmatrix} 1 & 1 \\ 4 & 7 \end{vmatrix} = 3$$

$$A_{32} = -\begin{vmatrix} 1 & 1 \\ 3 & 7 \end{vmatrix} = -4$$

$$A_{33} = \begin{vmatrix} 1 & 1 \\ 3 & 4 \end{vmatrix} = 1$$

$$\therefore \quad \text{adj.}A = \begin{bmatrix} 11 & -2 & 3 \\ 4 & 0 & -4 \\ -7 & 2 & 1 \end{bmatrix}$$

$$|A| = 1\,(11) - 1\,(-4) + 1\,(-7) = 8$$

$$A^{-1} = \frac{1}{8}\begin{bmatrix} 11 & -2 & 3 \\ 4 & 0 & -4 \\ -7 & 2 & 1 \end{bmatrix}$$

$$X = A^{-1}D = \frac{1}{8}\begin{bmatrix} 11 & -2 & 3 \\ 4 & 0 & -4 \\ -7 & 2 & 1 \end{bmatrix}\begin{bmatrix} 3 \\ 14 \\ 1 \end{bmatrix}$$

$$= \frac{1}{8}\begin{bmatrix} 33 - 28 + 3 \\ 12 + 0 - 4 \\ -21 + 28 + 1 \end{bmatrix} = \frac{1}{8}\begin{bmatrix} 8 \\ 8 \\ 8 \end{bmatrix} = \begin{bmatrix} 1 \\ 1 \\ 1 \end{bmatrix}$$

$\therefore\ x = 1, y = 1, z = 1$

3. Solve the equations using matrix method:

$x - y - 2x = 3$

$2x + y + z = 5$

$4x - y - 2z = 1$

Take $A = \begin{bmatrix} 1 & -1 & -2 \\ 2 & 1 & 1 \\ 4 & -1 & -2 \end{bmatrix}, \ X = \begin{bmatrix} x \\ y \\ z \end{bmatrix}, \ D = \begin{bmatrix} 3 \\ 5 \\ 1 \end{bmatrix}$

The solution is $X = A^{-1}D$

$$A_{11} = \begin{vmatrix} 1 & 1 \\ -1 & -2 \end{vmatrix} = -1$$

$$A_{12} = -\begin{vmatrix} 2 & 1 \\ 4 & -2 \end{vmatrix} = 8$$

$$A_{13} = \begin{vmatrix} 2 & 1 \\ 4 & -1 \end{vmatrix} = -6$$

$$A_{21} = -\begin{vmatrix} -1 & -2 \\ -1 & -2 \end{vmatrix} = 0$$

$$A_{22} = \begin{vmatrix} 1 & -2 \\ 4 & -2 \end{vmatrix} = 6$$

$$A_{23} = -\begin{vmatrix} 1 & -1 \\ 4 & -1 \end{vmatrix} = -3$$

$$A_{31} = \begin{vmatrix} -1 & -2 \\ 1 & 1 \end{vmatrix} = 1$$

$$A_{32} = -\begin{vmatrix} 1 & -2 \\ 2 & 1 \end{vmatrix} = -5$$

$$A_{33} = \begin{vmatrix} 1 & -1 \\ 2 & 1 \end{vmatrix} = 3$$

$\therefore$ $\text{adj.}A = \begin{bmatrix} -1 & 0 & 1 \\ 8 & 6 & -5 \\ -6 & -3 & 3 \end{bmatrix}, \ |A| = R_1 \text{ of } A \times C_1 \text{ of adj.}A$

$$= -1 - 8 + 12 = 3$$

$$A^{-1} = \frac{1}{3}\begin{bmatrix} -1 & 0 & 1 \\ 8 & 6 & -5 \\ -6 & -3 & 3 \end{bmatrix}$$

$$X = A^{-1}D = \frac{1}{3}\begin{bmatrix} -1 & 0 & 1 \\ 8 & 6 & -5 \\ -6 & -3 & 3 \end{bmatrix}\begin{bmatrix} 3 \\ 5 \\ 1 \end{bmatrix}$$

$$= \frac{1}{3}\begin{bmatrix} -3+0+1 \\ 24+30-5 \\ -18-15+3 \end{bmatrix} = \frac{1}{3}\begin{bmatrix} -2 \\ 49 \\ -30 \end{bmatrix} = \begin{bmatrix} -\frac{2}{3} \\ \frac{49}{3} \\ -10 \end{bmatrix}$$

$$\therefore \; x = -\frac{2}{3}, \; y = \frac{49}{3}, \; z = -10$$

4. Solve the following using matrix method

   $x - y - 2z = 3;\ 2x + y + z = 5;\ 4x - y - 2z = 11$

$$A = \begin{bmatrix} 1 & -1 & -2 \\ 2 & 1 & 1 \\ 4 & -1 & -2 \end{bmatrix}, \; X = \begin{bmatrix} x \\ y \\ z \end{bmatrix}, \; D = \begin{bmatrix} 3 \\ 5 \\ 11 \end{bmatrix}$$

The solution is $X = A^{-1}D$

$$A_{11} = \begin{vmatrix} 1 & 1 \\ -1 & -2 \end{vmatrix} = -2+1 = -1$$

$$A_{12} = -\begin{vmatrix} 2 & 1 \\ 4 & -2 \end{vmatrix} = -(-4-4) = 8$$

$$A_{13} = \begin{vmatrix} 2 & 1 \\ 4 & -1 \end{vmatrix} = -6$$

$$A_{21} = -\begin{vmatrix} -1 & -2 \\ -1 & -2 \end{vmatrix} = 0$$

$$A_{22} = \begin{vmatrix} 1 & -2 \\ 4 & -2 \end{vmatrix} = 6$$

$$A_{23} = -\begin{vmatrix} 1 & -1 \\ 4 & -1 \end{vmatrix} = -3$$

$$A_{31} = \begin{vmatrix} -1 & -2 \\ 1 & 1 \end{vmatrix} = 1$$

$$A_{32} = -\begin{vmatrix} 1 & -2 \\ 2 & 1 \end{vmatrix} = -5$$

$$A_{33} = \begin{vmatrix} 1 & -1 \\ 2 & 1 \end{vmatrix} = 3$$

$$\therefore \qquad \text{adj.}A = \begin{bmatrix} -1 & 0 & 1 \\ 8 & 6 & -5 \\ -6 & -3 & 3 \end{bmatrix},$$

$$|A| = 1(-1) - (-1)(-8) + (-2)(-6) = 3$$

$$A^{-1} = \frac{1}{3}\begin{bmatrix} -1 & 0 & 1 \\ 8 & 6 & -5 \\ -6 & -3 & 3 \end{bmatrix}$$

$$X = A^{-1}D = \frac{1}{3}\begin{bmatrix} -1 & 0 & 1 \\ 8 & 6 & -5 \\ -6 & -3 & 3 \end{bmatrix}\begin{bmatrix} 3 \\ 5 \\ 11 \end{bmatrix}$$

$$= \frac{1}{3}\begin{bmatrix} -3+0+11 \\ 24+30-55 \\ -18-15+33 \end{bmatrix} = \frac{1}{3}\begin{bmatrix} 8 \\ -1 \\ 0 \end{bmatrix} = \begin{bmatrix} \frac{8}{3} \\ -\frac{1}{3} \\ 0 \end{bmatrix}$$

$$\therefore \qquad x = \frac{8}{3}, \; y = \frac{1}{3}, \; z = 0$$

5. Solve the following equations by matrix method.

$7x + 6x - 5z = 30;\ 3x - 4y + z = 0;\ x + 2y - 3z = 10$

Let $$A = \begin{pmatrix} 7 & 6 & -5 \\ 3 & -4 & 1 \\ 1 & 2 & -3 \end{pmatrix},\ B = \begin{pmatrix} 30 \\ 0 \\ 10 \end{pmatrix},\ X = \begin{pmatrix} x \\ y \\ z \end{pmatrix}$$

The solution $X = A^{-1} B$

$$\text{adj. } A = \begin{pmatrix} 10 & 8 & -14 \\ 10 & -16 & -22 \\ 10 & -8 & -46 \end{pmatrix}$$

$$|A| = 7(12 - 2) - 6(-9 - 1) - 5(6 + 4) = 70 + 60 - 50 = 80$$

$$\therefore \quad A^{-1} = \frac{1}{|A|} \text{adj.} A = \frac{1}{80}\begin{pmatrix} 10 & 8 & -14 \\ 10 & -16 & -22 \\ 10 & -8 & -46 \end{pmatrix}$$

$$X = A^{-1}B = \frac{1}{80}\begin{pmatrix} 10 & 8 & -14 \\ 10 & -16 & -22 \\ 10 & -8 & -46 \end{pmatrix}\begin{pmatrix} 30 \\ 0 \\ 10 \end{pmatrix}$$

$$= \frac{1}{80}\begin{pmatrix} 300-140 \\ 300-220 \\ 300-460 \end{pmatrix} = \frac{1}{80}\begin{pmatrix} 160 \\ 80 \\ -160 \end{pmatrix} = \begin{pmatrix} 2 \\ 1 \\ -2 \end{pmatrix}$$

$\therefore\ x = 2, y = 1, z = -2$

6. Solve by matrix method

$3x + y + 2z = 3$

$2x - 3y - z = -3$

$x + 2y + z = 4$

Let $$A = \begin{pmatrix} 3 & 1 & 2 \\ 2 & -3 & -1 \\ 1 & 2 & 1 \end{pmatrix},\ B = \begin{pmatrix} 3 \\ -3 \\ 4 \end{pmatrix},\ X = \begin{pmatrix} x \\ y \\ z \end{pmatrix}$$

The solution $X = A^{-1} B$

$$\text{adj. } A = \begin{pmatrix} -1 & 3 & 5 \\ -3 & 1 & -7 \\ 7 & -5 & -11 \end{pmatrix}$$

$$|A| = 3(-3+2) - 1(2+1) + 2(4+3) = -3 - 3 + 14 = 8$$

$$\therefore \qquad A^{-1} = \frac{1}{|A|} \text{adj.} A = \frac{1}{8}\begin{pmatrix} -1 & 3 & 5 \\ -3 & 1 & 7 \\ 7 & -5 & -11 \end{pmatrix}$$

Now, $$X = A^{-1}B = \frac{1}{8}\begin{pmatrix} -1 & 3 & 5 \\ -3 & 1 & 7 \\ 7 & -5 & -11 \end{pmatrix}\begin{pmatrix} 3 \\ -3 \\ 4 \end{pmatrix} = \frac{1}{8}\begin{pmatrix} -3-9+20 \\ -9-3+28 \\ 21+15-44 \end{pmatrix}$$

$$= \frac{1}{8}\begin{pmatrix} 8 \\ 16 \\ -8 \end{pmatrix} = \begin{pmatrix} 1 \\ 20 \\ -1 \end{pmatrix} = \begin{pmatrix} 2 \\ 1 \\ -2 \end{pmatrix}$$

$\therefore\ x = 1, y = 2, z = -1$

7. Solve the following by matrix method:

$x + y - 2z = 0$

$2x - y + z = 2$

$x + 2y - z = 2$

Let $$A = \begin{pmatrix} 1 & 1 & -2 \\ 2 & -1 & 1 \\ 1 & 2 & -1 \end{pmatrix},\ B = \begin{pmatrix} 0 \\ 2 \\ 2 \end{pmatrix},\ X = \begin{pmatrix} x \\ y \\ z \end{pmatrix}$$

The solution $X = A^{-1} B$

$$\text{adj. } A = \begin{pmatrix} -1 & 3 & -1 \\ 3 & 1 & -5 \\ 5 & -1 & -3 \end{pmatrix}$$

$$|A| = 1\,(1-2) - 1\,(-2-1) - 2\,(4+1) = -1 + 3 - 10 = -8$$

$$A^{-1} = \frac{1}{|A|} \text{ adj. } A = \frac{1}{-8}\begin{pmatrix} -1 & -3 & -1 \\ 3 & 1 & -5 \\ 5 & -1 & -3 \end{pmatrix}$$

$$\therefore \quad X = A^{-1}B = \frac{-1}{8}\begin{pmatrix} -1 & -3 & -1 \\ 3 & 1 & -5 \\ 5 & -1 & -3 \end{pmatrix}\begin{pmatrix} 0 \\ 2 \\ 2 \end{pmatrix} = -\frac{1}{8}\begin{pmatrix} -6-2 \\ 2-10 \\ -2-6 \end{pmatrix}$$

$$\text{i.e.,} \quad X = \begin{pmatrix} 1 \\ 1 \\ 1 \end{pmatrix}$$

$\therefore$ $x = 1, y = 1, z = 1$

8. Solve by matrix method: $x + y + z = 4$, $2x - y - z = 2$, $x + 2y - z = 9$

$$\text{Let} \quad A = \begin{pmatrix} 1 & 1 & 1 \\ 2 & -1 & -1 \\ 1 & 2 & -1 \end{pmatrix}, \quad B = \begin{pmatrix} 4 \\ 2 \\ 9 \end{pmatrix}, \quad X = \begin{pmatrix} x \\ y \\ z \end{pmatrix}$$

Given equations reduce to the matrix equation $AX = B$ so that $X = A^{-1}B$

To find A^{-1}

$$\text{adj } A = \begin{pmatrix} 3 & 3 & 0 \\ 1 & -2 & 3 \\ 5 & -1 & -3 \end{pmatrix}$$

$$|A| = 1(1+2) - 1(-2+1) + 1(4+1) = 3 + 1 + 5 = 9$$

$$\therefore \quad A^{-1} = \frac{1}{9}\begin{pmatrix} 3 & 3 & 0 \\ 1 & -2 & 3 \\ 5 & -1 & -3 \end{pmatrix}$$

$$\therefore \quad X = A^{-1}B = \frac{1}{9}\begin{pmatrix} 3 & 3 & 0 \\ 1 & -2 & 3 \\ 5 & -1 & -3 \end{pmatrix}\begin{pmatrix} 4 \\ 2 \\ 9 \end{pmatrix} = \frac{1}{9}\begin{pmatrix} 18 \\ 27 \\ -9 \end{pmatrix} = \begin{pmatrix} 2 \\ 3 \\ -1 \end{pmatrix}$$

$\therefore$ $x = 2, y = 3, z = -1$

3.7.1 Cramer's Rule

To solve simultaneous linear equations using determinants

$a_1x + b_1y + c_1z = d_1$

To solve $a_2x + b_2y + c_2z = d_2$ using determinants

$a_3x + b_3y + c_3z = d_3$

$$\text{Consider } \Delta = \begin{vmatrix} a_1 & b_1 & c_1 \\ a_2 & b_2 & c_2 \\ a_3 & b_3 & c_3 \end{vmatrix}$$

Multiply both side by z,

$$x\Delta = x\begin{vmatrix} a_1 & b_1 & c_1 \\ a_2 & b_2 & c_2 \\ a_3 & b_3 & c_3 \end{vmatrix} = \begin{vmatrix} a_1x & b_1 & c_1 \\ a_2x & b_2 & c_2 \\ a_3x & b_3 & c_3 \end{vmatrix}$$

Add y times C_2 and z times C_3 to C_1

$$x\Delta = \begin{vmatrix} a_1x + b_1y + c_1z & b_1 & c_1 \\ a_2x + b_2y + c_2z & b_2 & c_2 \\ a_3x + b_3y + c_3z & b_3 & c_3 \end{vmatrix}$$

i.e., $x\Delta = \begin{vmatrix} d_1 & b_1 & c_1 \\ d_2 & b_2 & c_2 \\ d_3 & b_3 & c_3 \end{vmatrix}$ by using the given equations

i.e., $x\Delta = \Delta_1$ (say) $\quad \therefore \quad x = \dfrac{\Delta_1}{\Delta}$

Similarly, $y = \dfrac{\Delta_2}{\Delta}$ where $\Delta_2 = \begin{vmatrix} a_1 & d_1 & c_1 \\ a_2 & d_2 & c_2 \\ a_3 & d_3 & c_3 \end{vmatrix}$

and $y = \dfrac{\Delta_3}{\Delta}$ where $\Delta_3 = \begin{vmatrix} a_1 & b_1 & d_1 \\ a_2 & b_2 & d_2 \\ a_3 & b_3 & d_3 \end{vmatrix}$

To apply the rule, remember the following points

1. First, write the given equations in order so that the constant terms are all on right side.
2. Take Δ as the determinant formed by the coefficients of x, y, z.

3. In Δ, replace the first column by constant terms of the equation. Call this Δ_1
4. In Δ, replace the second column by constant terms and call it Δ_2
5. In Δ, replace the third column by constant terms and call it Δ_3
6. The solution is $x=\frac{\Delta_1}{\Delta}$, $y=\frac{\Delta_2}{\Delta}$, $z=\frac{\Delta_3}{\Delta}$ $(\Delta \neq 0)$ incase $\Delta = 0$, there is no unique solution.

Worked Examples

1. Solve using Cramer's rule

   $x + y + z = 7;\ 2x + 3y + 2z = 17;\ 4x + 9y + z = 37$

   $$\text{Here, } \Delta = \begin{vmatrix} 1 & 1 & 1 \\ 2 & 3 & 2 \\ 4 & 9 & 1 \end{vmatrix} = 1(3-18) - 1(2-8) + 1(18-12) = -3$$

   $$\Delta_1 = \begin{vmatrix} 7 & 1 & 1 \\ 17 & 3 & 2 \\ 37 & 9 & 1 \end{vmatrix} = 7(3-18) - 1(17-74) + 1(153-111) = -6$$

   $$\Delta_2 = \begin{vmatrix} 1 & 7 & 1 \\ 2 & 17 & 2 \\ 4 & 37 & 1 \end{vmatrix} = 1(17-74) - 7(2-8) + 1(74-68) = -9$$

   $$\Delta_3 = \begin{vmatrix} 1 & 1 & 7 \\ 2 & 3 & 17 \\ 4 & 9 & 37 \end{vmatrix} = 1(111-153) - 1(74-68) + 7(18-12) = -6$$

   $$x = \frac{\Delta_1}{\Delta} = \frac{-6}{-3} = 2,\quad y = \frac{\Delta_2}{\Delta} = \frac{-9}{-3} = 3,\quad z = \frac{\Delta_3}{\Delta} = \frac{-6}{-3} = 2$$

   $\therefore$ (x, y, z) = (2, 3, 2)

   Verification: Substitute for x, y, z in the given equations

   $2 + 3 + 2 = 7,\ 4 + 9 + 4 = 17,\ 8 + 27 + 2 = 37$

2. Solve by Cramer's rule

   $5y + 2x + z = -1;\ x + 7y - 6z = -18;\ 3y + 6z = 6$

$$\text{Here, } \Delta = \begin{vmatrix} 2 & 5 & 1 \\ 1 & 7 & -6 \\ 0 & 3 & 6 \end{vmatrix} = 2(42+18) - 5(6-0) + 13(3-0) = 93$$

$$\Delta_1 = \begin{vmatrix} -1 & 5 & 1 \\ -18 & 7 & -6 \\ 9 & 3 & 6 \end{vmatrix} = -1(42+18) - 5(-108+54) + 1(-54-63) = 93$$

$$\Delta_2 = \begin{vmatrix} 2 & -1 & 1 \\ 1 & -18 & -6 \\ 0 & 9 & 6 \end{vmatrix} = 2(-108+54) + 1(6-0) + 1(9-0) = -93$$

$$\Delta_3 = \begin{vmatrix} 2 & 5 & -1 \\ 1 & 7 & -18 \\ 0 & 3 & 9 \end{vmatrix} = 2(63+54) - 5(9-0) - 1(3-0) = 186$$

$$x = \frac{\Delta_1}{\Delta} = \frac{93}{93} = 1, \quad y = \frac{\Delta_2}{\Delta} = \frac{-93}{93} = -1, \quad z = \frac{\Delta_3}{\Delta} = \frac{186}{93} = 2$$

$\therefore$ (x, y, z) = (1, –1, 2)

3. Solve using determinants

   $4(y - x) = 5z - 22$; $3z + 4x = 6y + 2$; $z - 3y = 14 - 10x$

$$\text{Here, } \Delta = \begin{vmatrix} -4 & 4 & -5 \\ 4 & -6 & 3 \\ 10 & -3 & 1 \end{vmatrix} = -4(-6+9) - 4(4-30) - 5(-12+60) = 148$$

$$\Delta_1 = \begin{vmatrix} 22 & 4 & -5 \\ 2 & -6 & 3 \\ 14 & -3 & 1 \end{vmatrix} = -22(-6+9) - 4(2-42) - 5(-6+84) = -296$$

$$\Delta_2 = \begin{vmatrix} -4 & -22 & -5 \\ 4 & 2 & 3 \\ 10 & 14 & 1 \end{vmatrix} = -4(2-42) + 22(4-30) - 5(56-20) = -592$$

$$\Delta_3 = \begin{vmatrix} -4 & 4 & -22 \\ 4 & -6 & 2 \\ 10 & -3 & 14 \end{vmatrix} = -4(-84+6) - 4(56-20) - 22(-12+60) = -888$$

$$x=\frac{\Delta_1}{\Delta}=\frac{-296}{-148}=2,\quad y=\frac{\Delta_2}{\Delta}=\frac{-592}{-148}=4,\quad z=\frac{\Delta_3}{\Delta}=\frac{-888}{-148}=6$$

$\therefore$ (x, y, z) = (2, 4, 6)

4. Solve by Cramer's rule:

   3x + 4y = 7; 7x – y = 6;

$$\Delta=\begin{vmatrix}3 & 4\\ 7 & -1\end{vmatrix}=-3-28=-31$$

$$\Delta_1=\begin{vmatrix}7 & 4\\ 6 & -1\end{vmatrix}=-7-24=-31$$

$$\Delta_2=\begin{vmatrix}3 & 7\\ 7 & 6\end{vmatrix}=18-49=-31$$

$$x=\frac{\Delta_1}{\Delta}=\frac{-31}{-31}=1,\quad y=\frac{\Delta_2}{\Delta}=\frac{-31}{-31}=1,$$

   $\therefore$ Solution is x = 1, y = 1

5. Solve by Cramer's rule

   2x + y = 1; x – 3y = 4

$$\Delta=\begin{vmatrix}2 & 1\\ 1 & -3\end{vmatrix}=-6-1=-7$$

$$\Delta_1=\begin{vmatrix}1 & 1\\ 4 & -3\end{vmatrix}=-3-4=-7$$

$$\Delta_2=\begin{vmatrix}2 & 1\\ 1 & 4\end{vmatrix}=8-1=7$$

$$x=\frac{\Delta_1}{\Delta}=\frac{-7}{-7}=1,\quad y=\frac{\Delta_2}{\Delta}=\frac{7}{-7}=-1,$$

   $\therefore$ Solution is x = 1, y = –1

6. Solve by Cramer's rule:

   x – 3y = 5; 3x – y – 7 = 0

$$\Delta = \begin{vmatrix} 1 & -3 \\ 3 & -1 \end{vmatrix} = -1+9=8$$

$$\Delta_1 = \begin{vmatrix} 5 & -3 \\ 7 & -1 \end{vmatrix} = -5+21=16$$

$$\Delta_2 = \begin{vmatrix} 1 & 5 \\ 3 & 7 \end{vmatrix} = 7-15=-8$$

$$x = \frac{\Delta_1}{\Delta} = \frac{16}{8} = 2, \quad y = \frac{\Delta_2}{\Delta} = \frac{-8}{8} = -1,$$

$\therefore$ Solution is $x = 2, y = -1$

7. Solve by Cramer's rule

   $2x - 3y = 5; 7x - y = 8$

$$\Delta = \begin{vmatrix} 2 & -3 \\ 7 & -1 \end{vmatrix} = -2+21=19$$

$$\Delta_1 = \begin{vmatrix} 5 & -3 \\ 8 & -1 \end{vmatrix} = -5+24=19$$

$$\Delta_2 = \begin{vmatrix} 2 & 5 \\ 7 & 8 \end{vmatrix} = 16-35=-19$$

$$x = \frac{\Delta_1}{\Delta} = \frac{19}{19} = 1, \quad y = \frac{\Delta_2}{\Delta} = \frac{-19}{19} = -1,$$

$\therefore$ Solution is $x = 1, y = -1$

Exercise 3.4

---

1. Solve the following by matrix method

   (i) $x + y + z = 3$

   $2x - y + z = 2$

   $x - 2y + 3z = 2$

   (ii) $2x - y = 7$

   $x + 3y = 21$

(iii) $2x + 8y + 5z = 5$

$x + y - z = -2$

$x + 2y - z = 2$

2. Solve by Cramer's rule

(i) $5x + 3y= 1$

$2x + 3y = -1$

(ii) $y - 3x = 1$

$6x - 5y + 8 = 0$

(iii) $3x + 2y + 5z = 32$

$2x + 5y + 3z = 31$

$5x + 3y + 2z = 32$

(iv) $7x + 6y - 5z = 30$

$3x - 4y + z =32$

$x + 2y - 3z = 32$

Answers

1. (i) $x = x, y = 1, z = 1$ (ii) $x = 6, y = 5$ (iii) $x = -3, y = 2, z = -1$

2. (i) $x = \frac{2}{3}\ y = \frac{-7}{9}$ (ii) $x = \frac{47}{14}\ y = \frac{41}{14}$ (iii) $x = \frac{5}{13}\ y = \frac{18}{13}\ z = \frac{24}{13}$

3.8 CHARACTERISTIC EQUATION AND ROOTS OF A SQUARE MATRIX

If A is any square matrix and I is the identity matrix of the order same as that of A, then $|A - \lambda I| = 0$ where λ is a constant is called the characteristic equation of A. The root of this equation $|A - \lambda I| = 0$ are called the characteristic roots or Eigen values or latent roots of square matrix A.

Worked Examples

1. If $A=\begin{bmatrix}2 & 5\\4 & 5\end{bmatrix}$, Find the characteristic roots of A.

$$A-\lambda I=\begin{bmatrix}2 & 5\\4 & 5\end{bmatrix}-\lambda\begin{bmatrix}1 & 0\\0 & 1\end{bmatrix}$$

$$=\begin{bmatrix}2-\lambda & 5\\4 & 5-\lambda\end{bmatrix} \text{ is the characteristic matrix}$$

Now, $\begin{bmatrix}2-\lambda & 5\\4 & 5-\lambda\end{bmatrix}=0$ is the characteristic equation of A

Solving this equation i.e., $(2-\lambda)(5-\lambda)-20=0$

i.e., $10-7\lambda+\lambda^2-20=0$

i.e., $\lambda^2-7\lambda-10=0$

$$\lambda=\frac{7\pm\sqrt{49+40}}{2}=\frac{7\pm\sqrt{89}}{2}$$

$\therefore$ $\quad \dfrac{7+\sqrt{89}}{2}$ and $\dfrac{7-\sqrt{89}}{2}$

are the characteristic roots of the square matrix A.

2. If $A=\begin{bmatrix}2 & 2 & 1\\1 & 3 & 1\\1 & 2 & 2\end{bmatrix}$, find the characteristic roots of A.

$$A-\lambda I=\begin{bmatrix}2 & 2 & 1\\1 & 3 & 1\\1 & 2 & 2\end{bmatrix}-\lambda\begin{bmatrix}1 & 0 & 0\\0 & 1 & 0\\0 & 0 & 1\end{bmatrix}$$

is the characteristic matrix

i.e., $\begin{bmatrix}2-\lambda & 2 & 1\\1 & 3-\lambda & 1\\1 & 2 & 2-\lambda\end{bmatrix}$ is the characteristic matrix

$$|A-\lambda I|=0\Rightarrow\begin{bmatrix}2-\lambda & 2 & 1\\1 & 3-\lambda & 1\\1 & 2 & 2-\lambda\end{bmatrix}=0$$

is the characteristic equation of A.

Expanding the above determinants, we get

$$(2-\lambda)[(3-\lambda)(2-\lambda)-2]-2(2-\lambda-1)+1(2-3+\lambda)=0$$

i.e., $(2-\lambda)[6-5\lambda+\lambda^2-2]-2[1-\lambda]+1(-1+\lambda)=0$

i.e., $(2-\lambda)(4-5\lambda+\lambda^2)-2+2\lambda-1+\lambda=0$

i.e, $8-4\lambda-10\lambda+5\lambda^2+2\lambda^2-\lambda^3-3+3\lambda=0$

i.e., $-\lambda^3+7\lambda^2-11\lambda+5=0$

i.e., $\lambda^3-7\lambda^2+11\lambda-5=0$

by inspection, $\lambda = 1$ is a root (it is because $1-7+11-5=0$)

Divided the equation by $\lambda-1$,

$$(\lambda-1)\overline{)\,\lambda^3-7\lambda^2+11\lambda-5\,}((\lambda^2-6\lambda+5)$$
$$\lambda^3-\lambda^2$$
$$-6\lambda^2+11\lambda-5$$
$$-6\lambda^2+6\lambda$$
$$5\lambda-5$$
$$5\lambda-5$$
$$0$$

The reduced equation $\lambda^2-6\lambda+5=0$

i.e., $(\lambda-5)(\lambda-1)$ $\therefore\ \lambda=1, \lambda=5$

$\therefore$ the characteristic roots of the square matrix A are 1, 1, 5

3. If $A=\begin{bmatrix}2 & -1\\ 0 & 1\end{bmatrix}$, fin the characteristic roots of A.

$$A-\lambda I=\begin{bmatrix}2 & -1\\ 0 & 1\end{bmatrix}-\lambda\begin{bmatrix}1 & 0\\ 0 & 1\end{bmatrix}=\begin{bmatrix}2-\lambda & -1\\ 0 & 1-\lambda\end{bmatrix}$$

Now, $|A-\lambda I|=0 \Rightarrow \begin{bmatrix}2-\lambda & -1\\ 0 & 1-\lambda\end{bmatrix}=0$

i.e., $(2-\lambda)(1-\lambda)=0$ $\therefore\ \lambda=2$ or $\lambda=1$

$\therefore$ the characteristic roots are 1 and 2

4. If $A = \begin{bmatrix} 1 & 0 & -1 \\ 1 & 2 & 1 \\ 2 & 2 & 3 \end{bmatrix}$, Find the characteristic roots of A.

$$A - \lambda I = \begin{bmatrix} 1 & 0 & -1 \\ 1 & 2 & 1 \\ 2 & 2 & 3 \end{bmatrix} - \lambda \begin{bmatrix} 1 & 0 & 0 \\ 0 & 1 & 0 \\ 0 & 0 & 1 \end{bmatrix} = \begin{bmatrix} 1-\lambda & 0 & -1 \\ 1 & 2-\lambda & 1 \\ 2 & 2 & 3-\lambda \end{bmatrix}$$

$\therefore$ $$|A - \lambda I| = 0 \Rightarrow \begin{vmatrix} 1-\lambda & 0 & -1 \\ 1 & 2-\lambda & 1 \\ 2 & 2 & 3-\lambda \end{vmatrix} = 0$$

i.e., $(1-\lambda)[(2-\lambda)(3-\lambda)-2] - 0 - 1[(2-4+2\lambda)] = 0$

i.e., $(1-\lambda)[6-5\lambda+\lambda^2-2] + 2 - 2\lambda] = 0$

i.e., $(1-\lambda)(4-5\lambda+\lambda^2) + 2 - 2\lambda = 0$

i.e, $4-4\lambda-5\lambda+5\lambda^2+\lambda^2-\lambda^3+2-2\lambda = 0$

i.e., $-\lambda^3+6\lambda^2-11\lambda+6=0$

i.e., $\lambda^3-6\lambda^2+11\lambda-6=0$

$\lambda = 1$ is a root bu inspection

Divided the equation by $\lambda - 1$, we get

$\lambda^2 - 5\lambda + 6 = 0$

i.e., $(\lambda-2)(\lambda-3) = 0 \quad \therefore \lambda = 2, \lambda = 3$

$\therefore$ The characteristic roots of A are 1, 2, 3

3.9 CAYLEY – HAMILTON THEOREM

Statement: Every square matrix satisfies its characteristic equation

Worked Examples

1. Verify Cayley-Hamilton theorem for the square matrix $\begin{bmatrix} 1 & 2 \\ 2 & 1 \end{bmatrix}$

Take $A = \begin{bmatrix} 1 & 2 \\ 2 & 1 \end{bmatrix}$

The characteristic equation of A is given by

$$|A - \lambda I| = 0$$

i.e., $$\begin{vmatrix} 1-\lambda & 2 \\ 2 & 1-\lambda \end{vmatrix} = 0$$

i.e., $(1-\lambda)^2 - 4 = 0$

i.e., $1 - 2\lambda + \lambda^2 - 4 = 0$

i.e., $\lambda^2 - 2\lambda - 3 = 0$ .....(1)

To prove that A satisfies the equation (1) i.e., $A^2 - 2A - 3I = 0$

$$A^2 = A.A = \begin{bmatrix} 1 & 2 \\ 2 & 1 \end{bmatrix}\begin{bmatrix} 1 & 2 \\ 2 & 1 \end{bmatrix}$$

i.e., $$A^2 = \begin{bmatrix} 1+4 & 2+2 \\ 2+2 & 4+1 \end{bmatrix} = \begin{bmatrix} 5 & 4 \\ 4 & 5 \end{bmatrix}$$

Now, $$A^2 - 2A - 3I = \begin{bmatrix} 5 & 4 \\ 4 & 5 \end{bmatrix} - 2\begin{bmatrix} 1 & 2 \\ 2 & 1 \end{bmatrix} - 3\begin{bmatrix} 1 & 0 \\ 0 & 1 \end{bmatrix}$$

$$= \begin{bmatrix} 5 & 4 \\ 4 & 5 \end{bmatrix} + \begin{bmatrix} -2 & -4 \\ -4 & -2 \end{bmatrix} + \begin{bmatrix} -3 & 0 \\ 0 & -3 \end{bmatrix}$$

$$= \begin{bmatrix} 5-2-3 & 4-4+0 \\ 4-4+0 & 5-2-3 \end{bmatrix} = \begin{bmatrix} 0 & 0 \\ 0 & 0 \end{bmatrix} = 0$$

$\therefore$ $A^2 - 2A - 3I = 0$ which means that A satisfies the equation (1).

Note: Since A satisfies (1) $A^2 - 2A - 3I = 0$ .....(2)

Multiply both sides of (2) by A^{-1},

$$A^2 A^{-1} - 2A.A^{-1} - 3I\,A^{-1} = 0$$

$$AI - 2I - 3A^{-1} = 0$$

$\therefore$ $$3A^{-1} = A - 2I = \begin{bmatrix} 1 & 2 \\ 2 & 1 \end{bmatrix} - 2\begin{bmatrix} 1 & 0 \\ 0 & 1 \end{bmatrix} = \begin{bmatrix} -1 & 2 \\ 2 & -1 \end{bmatrix}$$

$\therefore$ $$A^{-1} = \frac{1}{3}\begin{bmatrix} -1 & 2 \\ 2 & -1 \end{bmatrix}$$

2. Find the characteristic equation of the matrix $\begin{bmatrix} 1 & -2 \\ 3 & 4 \end{bmatrix}$ and hence find the inverse of the matrix.

$$A = \begin{bmatrix} 1 & -2 \\ 3 & 4 \end{bmatrix}$$

$$A - \lambda I = \begin{bmatrix} 1 & -2 \\ 3 & 4 \end{bmatrix} - \lambda \begin{bmatrix} 1 & 0 \\ 0 & 1 \end{bmatrix} = \begin{bmatrix} 1-\lambda & -2 \\ 3 & 4-\lambda \end{bmatrix}$$

Characteristic equation is $|A - \lambda I| = 0$

i.e., $\begin{vmatrix} 1-\lambda & -2 \\ 3 & 4-\lambda \end{vmatrix} = 0$ i.e., $(1 - \lambda)(4 - \lambda) + 6 = 0$

i.e., $4 - 5\lambda + \lambda^2 + 6 = 0$

i.e., $\lambda^2 - 5\lambda + 10 = 0$ .....(1)

(1) is the characteristic equation of the given matrix. By Cayley – Hamilton, theorem, A satisfies the equation (1).

$\therefore \quad A^2 - 5A + 10\,I = 0$

Multiply by A^{-1},

$$A^2 A^{-1} - 5A.A^{-1} + 10I\,A^{-1} = 0$$

i.e., $AI - 5I + 10\,A^{-1} = 0$

i.e., $A - 5I + 10\,A^{-1} = 0$

$$\therefore \quad 10A^{-1} = 5I - A = \begin{bmatrix} 5 & 0 \\ 0 & 5 \end{bmatrix} - \begin{bmatrix} 1 & -2 \\ 3 & 4 \end{bmatrix} = \begin{bmatrix} 4 & 2 \\ -3 & 1 \end{bmatrix}$$

$$\therefore \quad A^{-1} = \frac{1}{10}\begin{bmatrix} 4 & 2 \\ -3 & 1 \end{bmatrix}$$

3. Verify that the matrix $A=\begin{bmatrix}1 & 0 & -1\\ 1 & 2 & 1\\ 2 & 2 & 3\end{bmatrix}$ satisfies its characteristic equation. Hence find A^{-1}

$$A=\begin{bmatrix}1 & 0 & -1\\ 1 & 2 & 1\\ 2 & 2 & 3\end{bmatrix}$$

$$|A-\lambda I|=\begin{bmatrix}1-\lambda & 0 & -1\\ 1 & 2-\lambda & 1\\ 2 & 2 & 3-\lambda\end{bmatrix}$$

The characteristic equation is $|A-\lambda I|=0$

i.e., $$\begin{bmatrix}1-\lambda & 0 & -1\\ 1 & 2-\lambda & 1\\ 2 & 2 & 3-\lambda\end{bmatrix}=0$$

i.e., $(1-\lambda)\,[(2-\lambda)\,(3-\lambda)-2]-1\,[2-2\,(2-\lambda)\,]=0$

i.e., $(1-\lambda)\,[6-5\lambda+\lambda^2-2\,]-1\,[2-4+2\,\lambda]=0$

i.e., $4(1-\lambda)-5\lambda\,(\,1-\lambda\,)+1\,(1+\lambda)\lambda^2+2-2\lambda=0$

i.e, $4-4\lambda-5\lambda+5\lambda^2+\lambda^2-\lambda^3+2-2\lambda=0$

i.e., $-\lambda^3+6\lambda^2-11\lambda+6=0$

i.e., $\lambda^3-6\lambda^2+11\lambda-6=0$ .....(1)

Now, to prove that A satisfies the equation (1)

i.e., $A^3-6A^2+11\,A-6I=0$

$$A^2=\begin{pmatrix}1 & 0 & -1\\ 1 & 2 & 1\\ 2 & 2 & 3\end{pmatrix}\begin{pmatrix}1 & 0 & -1\\ 1 & 2 & 1\\ 2 & 2 & 3\end{pmatrix}$$

$$=\begin{pmatrix}1+0-2 & 0+0-2 & -1+0-3\\ 1+2+2 & 0+4+2 & -1+2+3\\ 2+2+6 & 0+4+6 & -2+2+9\end{pmatrix}=\begin{pmatrix}-1 & -2 & -4\\ 5 & 6 & 4\\ 10 & 10 & 9\end{pmatrix}$$

$$A^3 = \begin{pmatrix} -1 & -2 & -4 \\ 5 & 6 & 4 \\ 10 & 10 & 9 \end{pmatrix} \begin{pmatrix} 1 & 0 & -1 \\ 1 & 2 & 1 \\ 2 & 2 & 3 \end{pmatrix}$$

$$= \begin{pmatrix} -1-2-8 & 0-4-8 & 1-2-12 \\ 5+6+8 & 0+12+8 & -5+6+12 \\ 10+10+18 & 0+20+18 & -10+10+27 \end{pmatrix} = \begin{pmatrix} -11 & -12 & -13 \\ 19 & 20 & 13 \\ 38 & 38 & 27 \end{pmatrix}$$

$A^3 - 6A^2 + 11A - 6I$

$$= \begin{pmatrix} -11 & -12 & -13 \\ 19 & 20 & 13 \\ 38 & 38 & 27 \end{pmatrix} - 6 \begin{pmatrix} -1 & -2 & -4 \\ 5 & 6 & 4 \\ 10 & 10 & 9 \end{pmatrix} + 11 \begin{pmatrix} 1 & 0 & -1 \\ 1 & 2 & 1 \\ 2 & 2 & 3 \end{pmatrix} - 6 \begin{pmatrix} 1 & 0 & 0 \\ 0 & 1 & 0 \\ 0 & 0 & 1 \end{pmatrix}$$

$$= \begin{pmatrix} -11 & -12 & -13 \\ 19 & 20 & 13 \\ 38 & 38 & 27 \end{pmatrix} + \begin{pmatrix} +6 & +12 & +24 \\ -30 & -36 & -24 \\ -60 & -60 & -54 \end{pmatrix} + \begin{pmatrix} 11 & 0 & -11 \\ 11 & 22 & 11 \\ 22 & 22 & 33 \end{pmatrix} + \begin{pmatrix} -6 & 0 & 0 \\ 0 & -6 & 0 \\ 0 & 0 & -6 \end{pmatrix}$$

$$= \begin{pmatrix} 0 & 0 & 0 \\ 0 & 0 & 0 \\ 0 & 0 & 0 \end{pmatrix} = 0$$

$\therefore \quad A^3 - 6A^2 + 11A - 6I = 0$ .....(2)

Multiply (2) by A^{-1}, we get

$$A^2 - 6A + 11I - 6A^{-1} = 0$$

$\therefore \quad A^{-1} = \frac{1}{6}\left[A^2 - 6A + 11A\right]$

$$= \frac{1}{6}\left[\begin{pmatrix} -1 & -2 & -4 \\ 5 & 6 & 4 \\ 10 & 10 & 9 \end{pmatrix} - 6 \begin{pmatrix} 1 & 0 & -1 \\ 1 & 2 & 1 \\ 2 & 2 & 3 \end{pmatrix} + 11 \begin{pmatrix} 1 & 0 & 0 \\ 0 & 1 & 0 \\ 0 & 0 & 1 \end{pmatrix}\right]$$

$$= \frac{1}{6}\begin{pmatrix} 4 & -2 & 2 \\ -1 & 5 & -2 \\ -2 & -2 & 2 \end{pmatrix}$$

$$A^{-1} = \begin{pmatrix} \frac{2}{3} & \frac{-1}{3} & \frac{1}{3} \\ \frac{-1}{6} & \frac{5}{6} & \frac{-1}{3} \\ \frac{-1}{3} & \frac{-1}{3} & \frac{1}{3} \end{pmatrix}$$

4. Find the inverse of $A = \begin{bmatrix} 5 & -2 \\ 3 & 1 \end{bmatrix}$ using Cayley-Hamilton theorem

$$A - \lambda I = \begin{bmatrix} 5 & -2 \\ 3 & 1 \end{bmatrix} - \lambda \begin{bmatrix} 1 & 0 \\ 0 & 1 \end{bmatrix} = \begin{bmatrix} 5-\lambda & -2 \\ 3 & 1-\lambda \end{bmatrix}$$

The characteristic equation is $|A - \lambda I| = 0$

i.e, $\begin{bmatrix} 5-\lambda & -2 \\ 3 & 1-\lambda \end{bmatrix} = 0$

i.e, $(5 - \lambda)(1 - \lambda) + 6 = 0$

i.e., $5 - \lambda - 5\lambda + \lambda^2 + 6 = 0$

i.e., $\lambda^2 + 6\lambda + 11 = 0$ ..... (1)

(1) is the characteristic equation of the given matrix.

By Cayley-Hamilaton, A satisfies the equaton (1)

i.e., $A^2 - 6A + 11I = 0$

Multiply by A^{-1}, $A^2A^{-1} - 6A\,A^{-1} + 11I\,A^{-1} = 0$

i.e., $A - 6I + 11\,A^{-1} = 0$

i.e. $11A^{-1} = 6I - A = \begin{bmatrix} 6 & 0 \\ 0 & 6 \end{bmatrix} - \begin{bmatrix} 5 & -2 \\ 3 & 1 \end{bmatrix} = \begin{bmatrix} 1 & 2 \\ -3 & 5 \end{bmatrix}$

$\therefore$ $A^{-1} = \frac{1}{11}\begin{bmatrix} 1 & 2 \\ -3 & 5 \end{bmatrix}$

5. Verify Cayley-Hamilton theorem for the matrix $A = \begin{bmatrix} 2 & -1 \\ -1 & 2 \end{bmatrix}$

The characteristic equation of A is $|A - \lambda I| = 0$

i.e., $\begin{vmatrix} 2-\lambda & -1 \\ -1 & 2-\lambda \end{vmatrix} = 0$

i.e., $(2 - \lambda)^2 - 1 = 0$

i.e., $\lambda^2 - 4\lambda + 4 - 1 = 0$

i.e., $\lambda^2 - 4\lambda + 3 = 0$

Consider $A^2 - 4A + 3I = \begin{bmatrix} 2 & -1 \\ -1 & 2 \end{bmatrix}\begin{bmatrix} 2 & -1 \\ -1 & 2 \end{bmatrix} - 4\begin{bmatrix} 2 & -1 \\ -1 & 2 \end{bmatrix} + 3\begin{bmatrix} 1 & 0 \\ 0 & 1 \end{bmatrix}$

$$= \begin{bmatrix} 5 & -4 \\ -4 & 5 \end{bmatrix} - \begin{bmatrix} 8 & -4 \\ -4 & 8 \end{bmatrix} + \begin{bmatrix} 3 & 0 \\ 0 & 3 \end{bmatrix}$$

$$= \begin{bmatrix} -3 & 0 \\ 0 & -3 \end{bmatrix} + \begin{bmatrix} 3 & 0 \\ 0 & 3 \end{bmatrix} = \begin{bmatrix} 0 & 0 \\ 0 & 0 \end{bmatrix} = 0$$

$\therefore\ A^2 - 4A + 3I = 0$

Hence, the Cayley-Hamiliton is verified.

6. Find the inverse of the matrix $A = \begin{bmatrix} 1 & 3 \\ 2 & -1 \end{bmatrix}$ using Cayley – Hamilton theorem.

The characteristic equation of A is $|A - \lambda I| = 0$

i.e., $\begin{vmatrix} 1-\lambda & 3 \\ 2 & -1-\lambda \end{vmatrix} = 0$

i.e., $(1 - \lambda)(-1 - \lambda) - 6 = 0$

i.e., $\lambda^2 - 1 - 6 = 0$

i.e., $\lambda^2 - 7 = 0$

By Cayley – Hamilton theorem, $A^2 - 7I = 0$

Multiply throughout by A^{-1}, we get

$A - 7\ A^{-1} = 0$

$\therefore\ A^{-1} = \frac{1}{7}A$

$$= \frac{1}{7}\begin{bmatrix} 1 & 3 \\ 2 & -1 \end{bmatrix} = \begin{bmatrix} \frac{1}{7} & \frac{3}{7} \\ \frac{2}{7} & \frac{-1}{7} \end{bmatrix}$$

7. Find the inverse of the matrix $A = \begin{bmatrix} -3 & 2 \\ -5 & 1 \end{bmatrix}$ using Cayley–Hamiltion theorem.

The characteristic equation of A is $|A - \lambda I| = 0$

i.e., $$\begin{vmatrix} -3-\lambda & 2 \\ -5 & 1-\lambda \end{vmatrix} = 0$$

i.e., $$(-3-\lambda)(1-\lambda) + 10 = 0$$

$$\lambda^2 + 2\lambda + 7 = 0$$

By Cayley Hamilton theorem, we get

$$A^2 + 2A + 7I = 0$$

Multiply through by A^{-1}, we get

$$A + 2I + 7A^{-1} = 0$$

$$= \frac{1}{7}\left[\begin{pmatrix} 3 & -2 \\ 5 & -1 \end{pmatrix} - \begin{pmatrix} 2 & 0 \\ 0 & 2 \end{pmatrix}\right] = \frac{1}{7}\begin{bmatrix} 1 & -2 \\ 5 & -3 \end{bmatrix}$$

$$= \begin{bmatrix} \frac{1}{7} & \frac{-2}{7} \\ \frac{5}{7} & \frac{-3}{7} \end{bmatrix}$$

8. Find the inverse of $A = \begin{bmatrix} 2 & 3 \\ 2 & 5 \end{bmatrix}$ using Cayley-Hamilton theorem.

The characteristic of A is $|A - \lambda I| = 0$

i.e, $$\begin{vmatrix} 2-\lambda & 3 \\ 2 & 5-\lambda \end{vmatrix} = 0$$

i.e, $(2-\lambda)(5-\lambda) - 6 = 0$

i.e., $\lambda^2 - 7\lambda + 4 = 0$

By Cayley-Hamilton theorem, we get

$$A^2 - 7A + 4I = 0$$

Multiply throughout by A^{-1}, we get

$$A - 7I + 4A^{-1} = 0$$

$$A^{-1} = \frac{1}{4}[7I - A]$$

$$= \frac{1}{4}\left[\begin{pmatrix} 7 & 0 \\ 0 & 7 \end{pmatrix} - \begin{pmatrix} 2 & 3 \\ 2 & 5 \end{pmatrix}\right] = \frac{1}{4}\begin{pmatrix} 5 & -3 \\ -2 & 2 \end{pmatrix}$$

$$\therefore \quad A^{-1} = \begin{pmatrix} \frac{5}{4} & \frac{-3}{4} \\ \frac{-1}{2} & \frac{1}{2} \end{pmatrix}$$

9. Verify Cayley – Hamilton theorem for the matrix $A = \begin{bmatrix} 1 & 3 \\ 4 & 7 \end{bmatrix}$

The characteristic equation of A is $|A - \lambda I| = 0$

i.e., $\begin{vmatrix} 1-\lambda & 3 \\ 4 & 7-\lambda \end{vmatrix} = 0$

i.e., $(1 - \lambda)(7 - \lambda) - 12 = 0$

i.e., $\lambda^2 - 8\lambda - 5 = 0$

Consider $A^2 - 8A - 5I = \begin{bmatrix} 1 & 3 \\ 4 & 7 \end{bmatrix}\begin{bmatrix} 1 & 3 \\ 4 & 7 \end{bmatrix} - 8\begin{bmatrix} 1 & 3 \\ 4 & 7 \end{bmatrix} - 5\begin{bmatrix} 1 & 0 \\ 0 & 1 \end{bmatrix}$

$$= \begin{bmatrix} 13 & 24 \\ 32 & 61 \end{bmatrix} - \begin{bmatrix} 8 & 24 \\ 32 & 56 \end{bmatrix} - \begin{bmatrix} 5 & 0 \\ 0 & 5 \end{bmatrix}$$

$$= \begin{bmatrix} 5 & 0 \\ 0 & 5 \end{bmatrix} - \begin{bmatrix} 5 & 0 \\ 0 & 5 \end{bmatrix} = \begin{bmatrix} 0 & 0 \\ 0 & 0 \end{bmatrix}$$

$\therefore\ A^2 - 8A - 5I = 0$

Hence, The Cayley – Hamilton theorem is verified.

10. Find A^{-1} using Cayley – Hamilton theorem if $A = \begin{bmatrix} 2 & 4 \\ 7 & 3 \end{bmatrix}$

The characteristic of A is $|A - \lambda I| = 0$

i.e, $\begin{vmatrix} 2-\lambda & 4 \\ 7 & 3-\lambda \end{vmatrix} = 0$

i.e, $(2-\lambda)(3-\lambda)-28=0$

i.e., $\lambda^2-5\lambda-22=0$

By Cayley – Hamilton theorem, we get

$$A^2-5A-22I=0$$

Multiply throughout by A^{-1}, we get

$$A-5I-22A^{-1}=0$$

$$\therefore \quad A^{-1}=\frac{1}{22}[A-5I]$$

$$=\frac{1}{22}\left[\begin{pmatrix}2 & 4\\ 7 & 3\end{pmatrix}-\begin{pmatrix}5 & 0\\ 0 & 5\end{pmatrix}\right]$$

$$=\frac{1}{22}\begin{bmatrix}-3 & 4\\ 7 & -2\end{bmatrix}=\begin{bmatrix}\frac{-3}{22} & \frac{2}{11}\\ \frac{7}{22} & \frac{-1}{11}\end{bmatrix}$$

11. Find the Eigen values of the matrix $\begin{bmatrix}1 & 3\\ 2 & -4\end{bmatrix}$

Eigen values are given by $\begin{vmatrix}1-\lambda & 3\\ 2 & -4-\lambda\end{vmatrix}=0$

$(1-\lambda)(-4-\lambda)-6=0$

$\lambda^2+3\lambda-4-6=0$

$\lambda^2+3\lambda-10=0$

$(\lambda+5)(\lambda-2)=0$

$\therefore\ \lambda=-5,\ 2$

$\therefore$ Eigen values are – 5, 2

12. Find the characteristic roots of the matrix $\begin{bmatrix}1 & 3\\ 4 & 2\end{bmatrix}$ (April 2003)

The characteristic equation of A is $|A-\lambda I|=0$

i.e., $\begin{vmatrix}1-\lambda & 3\\ 4 & 2-\lambda\end{vmatrix}=0$

i.e., $(1-\lambda)(2-\lambda)-12=0$

i.e., $\lambda^2-3\lambda-10=0$

$\therefore$ $\lambda=\dfrac{3\pm\sqrt{9+40}}{2}=\dfrac{3\pm 7}{2}$

$\therefore$ $\lambda=5,-2$

13. If $A=\begin{bmatrix}4 & 2\\ 2 & 1\end{bmatrix}$, use Cayley – Hamilton theorem to find A^4.

The characteristic of A is $\begin{vmatrix}4-\lambda & 2\\ 2 & 1-\lambda\end{vmatrix}=0$

i.e., $(4-\lambda)(1-\lambda)-4=0$

i.e., $\lambda^2-5\lambda=0$

By Cayley – Hamilton theorem, we have

$A^2-5A=0 \quad \text{or } A^2=5A$

$\therefore$ $A^4=25A^2=25\times 5A=125A$

$\therefore$ $A^4=\begin{bmatrix}500 & 250\\ 250 & 125\end{bmatrix}$

14. Use Cayley – Hamilton theorem to find the value of

$$A^6-A^4+A^3+5A^2-4A+6I \text{ if } A=\begin{bmatrix}1 & -1\\ 2 & 1\end{bmatrix}$$

The characteristic of A is $\begin{vmatrix}1-\lambda & -1\\ 2 & 1-\lambda\end{vmatrix}=0$

i.e., $(1-\lambda)^2+2=0$

i.e., $\lambda^2-2\lambda+3=0$

By Cayley – Hamilton theorem, we have

$A^2-2A+3I=0$

Given expression $=A^6-A^4+A^3+5A^2-4A+6I$

$=(A^6-2A^4+3A^3)+(A^4-2A^3+3A^2)+2(A^2-2A+3I)$

$=A^3(A^2-2A+3I)+A^2(A^2-2A+3I)+2(A^2-2A+3I)$

$=A^3.O+A^2.O+2.O=O$

Exercise 3.5

I Find the characteristic equation and characteristic roots of each of the following matrices.

1. $\begin{bmatrix} 1 & 2 \\ 3 & 4 \end{bmatrix}$ 2. $\begin{bmatrix} -1 & 2 \\ 2 & 4 \end{bmatrix}$ 3. $\begin{bmatrix} 2 & -3 & 0 \\ 3 & 1 & 3 \\ -3 & 2 & -1 \end{bmatrix}$

II Verify Cayley – Hamilton theorem for each of the following matrices and find inverses.

1. $\begin{bmatrix} 1 & 2 \\ 3 & 4 \end{bmatrix}$ 2. $\begin{bmatrix} 3 & -1 & 2 \\ 1 & 2 & 2 \\ 2 & 0 & 5 \end{bmatrix}$

III 1. If $A = \begin{bmatrix} 2 & 1 \\ -2 & -1 \end{bmatrix}$ find A^6 using Cayley – Hamilton theorem.

2. If $A = \begin{bmatrix} 1 & 2 \\ 3 & 4 \end{bmatrix}$, find the value of $A^5 - 5A^4 - 10A^2 - 3A$ using Cayley –Hamilton theorem.

Answers

I 1. $\lambda^2 - 4\lambda - 5 = 0, \lambda = -1, 5$

2. $\lambda^2 - 3\lambda - 2 = 0, \lambda = 5, -2$

3. $\lambda^3 - 2\lambda^2 + 2\lambda - 4 = 0, \ \lambda = 2 \pm i\sqrt{2}$

II 1. $\frac{1}{2}\begin{bmatrix} -4 & 2 \\ 3 & -1 \end{bmatrix}$ 2. $\frac{1}{8}\begin{bmatrix} -4 & 2 \\ 2 & 1 \end{bmatrix}$ 3. $\frac{1}{23}\begin{bmatrix} -10 & 5 & -6 \\ -1 & 11 & -4 \\ -4 & -2 & 7 \end{bmatrix}$

III 1. $\begin{bmatrix} 2 & 1 \\ -2 & -1 \end{bmatrix}$ 2. $\begin{bmatrix} 1 & 2 \\ 3 & 4 \end{bmatrix}$

3.10 APPLICATION OF MATRICES IN SOLVING PHARMACOKINETICS EQUATIONS

1. Two Compartmental Model Equation

In a Two compartmental model equation, distribution and elimination of drug in the body are given by the differential equations as shown below

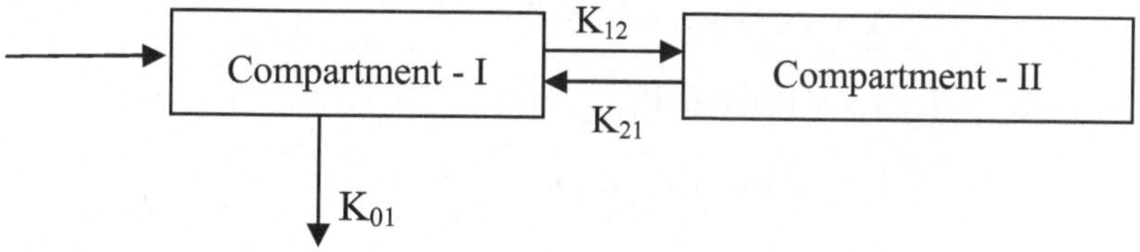

$$\frac{dx_1}{dt} = k_{21}x_2 - k_{12}x_1 - k_{01}x_1$$

$$\frac{dx_2}{dt} = k_{12}x_1 - k_{21}x_2$$

Applying the Laplace transform both side of the differential equation, can be transformed into Linear equations

$$L\{x^1{}_1\} = k_{21}L\{x_2\} - k_{12}L\{x_1\} - k_{01}L\{x_1\}$$

$$L\{x^1{}_2\} = k_{12}L\{x_1\} - k_{21}L\{x_2\}$$

$$S\overline{x}_1 - x_1(0) = k_{12}\overline{x}_2 - k_{01}\overline{x}_1$$

$$S\overline{x}_2 - x_2(0) = k_{12}\overline{x}_1 - \overline{x}_2$$

$$(S + k_{12} + k_{01})\overline{x}_1 - k_{21}\overline{x}_2 = \overline{x}_1(0) \quad \text{..... (1)}$$

$$-k_{12}\overline{x}_1 + (S + k_{21})\overline{x}_2 = 0 \quad \text{..... (2)}$$

Apply Crammer's Rule to solve equation 1 and 2 to find the value of $\overline{x}_1$

$$\Delta = \begin{vmatrix} (s + k_{12} + k_{01}) & -k_{21} \\ -k_{12} & s + k_{21} \end{vmatrix} = (s + k_{12} + k_{01})(s + k_{21}) - (k_{21}k_{12})$$

$$\Delta_1 = \begin{vmatrix} \text{Dose} & -k_{21} \\ 0 & s + k_{21} \end{vmatrix} = (\text{Dose})(s + k_{21}) - 0$$

$$\Delta_2 = \begin{vmatrix} s + k_{12} + k_{10} & \text{Dose} \\ -k_{12} & 0 \end{vmatrix}$$

$$\overline{x}_1 = \frac{\Delta_1}{\Delta} = \frac{(\text{Dose})(s+k_{21})-0}{(s+k_{12}+k_{10})(s+k_{21})-(k_{21}k_{12})}$$

$$\overline{x}_1 = \frac{\Delta_1}{\Delta} = \frac{(\text{Dose})(s+k_{21})}{(s^2+s(k_{12}+k_{10}+k_{21})+k_{10}k_{21})}$$

$$\overline{x}_1 = \frac{\Delta_1}{\Delta} = \frac{(\text{Dose})(s+k_{21})}{(s^2+s(a+b)+ab)}$$

Put $(k_{12}+k_{10}+k_{21}) = a+b$ and $k_{10}k_{21} = ab$

$$\overline{x}_1 = \frac{\Delta_1}{\Delta} = \frac{(\text{Dose})(s+k_{21})}{(s+a)(s+b)}$$

2. Three Compartmental Model Equation

In a three compartmental model equations distribution and elimination of drug in the body is given by the differential equations as shown below:

$K_{12}K_{13}$

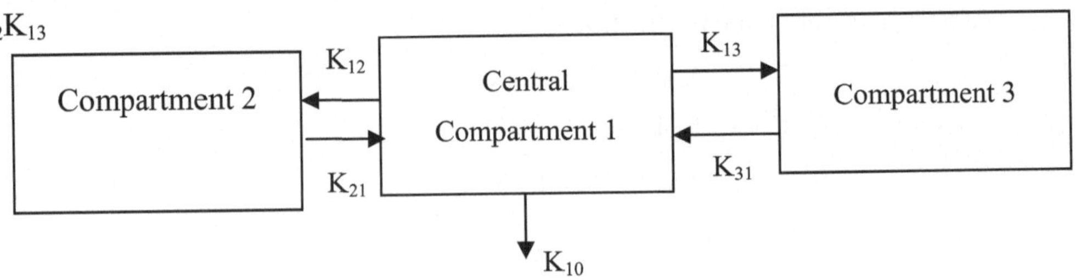

$$\frac{dx_1}{dt} = k_{21}x_2 + k_{31}x_3 - k_{12}x_1 - k_{13}x1 - k_{10}x_1$$

$$\frac{dx_2}{dt} = k_{12}x_1 - k_{21}x_2$$

$$\frac{dx_3}{dt} = k_{13}x_1 - k_{31}x_3$$

Applying the Laplace transform both side of the differential equation, can be transformed into Linear equations

$L\{x'_1\} = k_{21}L\{x_2\} + k_{31}L\{x_3\} \; - k_{12}L\{x_1\} - k_{13}\{x_3\} \; - k_{10}L\{x_1\}$

$L\{x'_2\} = k_{12}L\{x_1\} \; - \; k_{21}L\{x_2\}$

$L\{x'_3\} = k_{13}L\{x_1\} \; - \; k_{31}L\{x_3\}$

$Sx_1 - x_1(0) = k_{21}x_2 + k_{31}x_3 - k_{12}x_1 - k_{13}x_1 - k_{10}x_1$

$Sx_2 - x_2(0) = k_{12}x_1 - k_{21}x_2$

$Sx_3 - x_3(0) = k_{13}x_1 - k_{31}x_3$

$Sx_1 - x_1(0) = k_{21}x_2 + k_{31}x_3 - (k_{12} - k_{13} - k_{10})\,x_1$ ..... (1)

$Sx_2 - x_2(0) = k_{12}x_1 - k_{21}x_2$ ..... (2)

$Sx_3 - x_3(0) = k_{13}x_1 - k_{31}x_3$ ..... (3)

Apply Crammer's Rule to solve systems of linear equations 1, 2 and 3 to find the value of x_1

$$\Delta = \begin{bmatrix} s + k_{12} + k_{13} + k_{10} & -k_{21} & -k_{31} \\ -k_{12} & s + k_{21} & 0 \\ -k_{13} & 0 & s + k_{31} \end{bmatrix}$$

$$\Delta_1 = \begin{bmatrix} 1 & -k_{12} & -k_{13} \\ 0 & s + k_{21} & 0 \\ 0 & 0 & s + k_{31} \end{bmatrix}$$

$$\Delta_2 = \begin{bmatrix} s + k_{12} + k_{13} + k_{10} & 1 & -k_{13} \\ -k_{12} & 0 & 0 \\ -k_{13}0 & 0 & s + k_{31} \end{bmatrix}$$

$$\Delta_3 = \begin{bmatrix} s + k_{12} + k_{13} + k_{10} & -k_{13} & 1 \\ -k_{12} & 0 & 0 \\ -k_{13}0 & s + k_{31} & 0 \end{bmatrix}$$

$$X_1 = \frac{\Delta_1}{\Delta}$$

The value of determinant

$$\Delta_1 = 1((s + k_{21})(s + k_{31}) - 0) - k_{21}(0\text{–}0) - k_{31}(0\text{–}0)$$
$$= (s + k_{21})\,(s + k_{31})$$

The value of determinant

$$\Delta = (s + k_{12} + k_{13} + k_{10})((s + k_{21})(s + k_{31}) - 0) + k_{21}((-k_{12})(s + k_{31}) - 0)$$
$$- k_{31}(0 + k_{13}(s + k_{21}))$$

$$\Delta = (s + k_{12} + k_{13} + k_{10})\,((s^2 + s\,k_{21} + s\,k_{31} + k_{21}k_{31}) - 0)$$
$$+ k_{21}((-sk_{12} + k_{31}) - 0) - k_{31}(0 + k_{13}(s + k_{21}))$$

$$\Delta = s^3 + s^2(k_{10} + k_{12} + k_{13} + k_{21} + k_{31}) + s(k_{10}k_{21} + k_{13}k_{21} +$$
$$k_{10}k_{31} + k_{21}k_{31} + k_{31}k_{12}) + k_{21}k_{31}k_{10}$$

$$\Delta = s^3 + s^2(a + b + c) + s(ab + bc + ca) + abc$$

$$X_1 = \frac{\Delta_1}{\Delta}$$

$$X_1 = \frac{(s + k_{21})(s + k_{31})}{s^3 + s^2(a + b + c) + s(ab + bc + ca) + abc}$$

$$X_1 = \frac{(s + k_{21})(s + k_{31})}{(s + a)(s + b)(s + c)}$$

3. There are two families A and B and there are 4 men, 6 women and 2 children in family A and 2 men, 2 women and 4 children in family B. The recommended daily allowance for calories is: Man 2400, Women 1900, child 1800 and Protein for man 55 gm, women 45 gm and child 33 gm. Represent the above information by matrices. Using matrix multiplication, calculate the total requirement of calories and proteins for each of the two families.

***Solution*:** The members of the two families can be represented by the 2×3 matrix

$$\begin{matrix} & M & W & C \end{matrix}$$
$$D = \begin{pmatrix} 4 & 6 & 2 \\ 2 & 2 & 4 \end{pmatrix}$$

Calories and Proteins recommended for each member can written in a 3×2 matrix as

$$\begin{bmatrix} X \\ Y \\ Z \end{bmatrix} = \begin{bmatrix} 1 \\ 3 \\ 5 \end{bmatrix}$$

Multiply matrices D and E to calculate required amount of calories and Proteins for each family

$$DE = \begin{pmatrix} 4 & 6 & 2 \\ 2 & 2 & 4 \end{pmatrix} \begin{pmatrix} 2400 & 55 \\ 1900 & 45 \\ 1800 & 33 \end{pmatrix}$$

Calories Proteins

$$= \begin{matrix} A \\ B \end{matrix}\begin{pmatrix} 24600 & 556 \\ 15800 & 332 \end{pmatrix}$$

4. The following matrix gives the number of units of three Products P, Q and R that can be processed per hour on three machines A, B and C:

$$\begin{matrix} & \begin{matrix} A & B & C \end{matrix} \\ \begin{matrix} P \\ Q \\ R \end{matrix} & \begin{bmatrix} 10 & 12 & 15 \\ 13 & 11 & 20 \\ 16 & 18 & 14 \end{bmatrix} \end{matrix}$$

Determine, by using matrix algebra, how many units of each product can be produced, if the number of hours available on machine A, B and C are 54, 46 and 48 respectively

***Solution*:** The number of hours available for the machines A, B and C to manufacture the items P, Q and R represented in matrix as

$$\begin{matrix} P \\ Q \\ R \end{matrix}\begin{bmatrix} 54 \\ 46 \\ 48 \end{bmatrix}$$

The number of units of each product that can be produced can be written as

$$\begin{bmatrix} 10 & 12 & 15 \\ 13 & 11 & 20 \\ 16 & 18 & 14 \end{bmatrix}\begin{bmatrix} 54 \\ 46 \\ 48 \end{bmatrix} = \begin{bmatrix} P \\ Q \\ R \end{bmatrix}$$

$$10 \times 54 + 12 \times 46 + 15 \times 28 = P$$

$$13 \times 54 + 11 \times 46 + 20 \times 48 = Q$$

$$16 \times 54 + 18 \times 46 + 14 \times 48 = R$$

$$540 + 552 + 420 = P$$

$$702 + 506 + 960 = Q$$

$$864 + 828 + 672 = R$$

$$1512 = P$$

$$2168 = Q$$

$$2364 = R$$

The Product P = 1512 Units, Q = 2168 and R = 2364 units

5. The total number of units of three Products P = 9, Q = 52 R = 0 that are processed by three machines A, B and C is given by the matrix

$$\begin{array}{c} \\ P \\ Q \\ R \end{array}\begin{array}{c} \begin{array}{ccc} A & B & C \end{array} \\ \begin{bmatrix} 1 & 1 & 1 \\ 2 & 5 & 7 \\ 2 & 1 & -1 \end{bmatrix} \end{array}$$

Determine, the time taken by each machines to process the product P, Q and R.

***Solution*:** Let X, Y and Z be the time taken by the machines A, B and C to process the product P, Q and R

The number of units of each product that can be produced can be written as

$$\begin{bmatrix} 1 & 1 & 1 \\ 2 & 5 & 7 \\ 2 & 1 & -1 \end{bmatrix}\begin{bmatrix} X \\ Y \\ Z \end{bmatrix} = \begin{bmatrix} 9 \\ 52 \\ 0 \end{bmatrix}$$

$$X + Y + Z = 9$$

$$2X + 5Y + 7Z = 52$$

$$2X + Y - Z = 0$$

Solve these three equation by Crammer's Rule

$$\Delta = \begin{bmatrix} 1 & 1 & 1 \\ 2 & 5 & 7 \\ 2 & 1 & -1 \end{bmatrix}$$

$$= 1(-5-7) - 1(-2-14) + 1(2-10) = -12 + 16 - 8 = -4$$

$$\Delta_1 = \begin{bmatrix} 9 & 1 & 1 \\ 52 & 5 & 7 \\ 0 & 1 & -1 \end{bmatrix}$$

$$= 9(-5-7) - 1(-52-0) + 1(52-0) = -108 + 52 + 52 = -4$$

$$\Delta_2 = \begin{bmatrix} 1 & 9 & 1 \\ 2 & 52 & 7 \\ 2 & 0 & -1 \end{bmatrix}$$

$$= 1(-52 - 0) - 9(-2 - 14) + 1(0 - 104)$$

$$= -52 + 144 - 104 = -12$$

$$\Delta_3 = \begin{bmatrix} 1 & 1 & 9 \\ 2 & 5 & 52 \\ 2 & 1 & 0 \end{bmatrix}$$

$$= 1(0 - 52) - 1(0 - 104) + 9(2 - 10) = -52 + 104 - 72 = -20$$

$$X = \frac{-4}{-4} = 1 \qquad Y = \frac{-12}{-4} = 3 \qquad Z = \frac{-20}{-4} = 5$$

$$\begin{bmatrix} X \\ Y \\ Z \end{bmatrix} = \begin{bmatrix} 1 \\ 3 \\ 5 \end{bmatrix}$$

6. The total weight of ingredient present in drug P = 500mg, drug Q = 300 mg and drug R = 400mg. The amount of ingredient that present are given in a matrix as shown below. Calculate individual amount of ingredient present in each drug.

$$\begin{array}{c} \\ P \\ Q \\ R \end{array} \begin{array}{c} \begin{array}{ccc} A & B & C \end{array} \\ \begin{bmatrix} 2 & 2 & 1 \\ 1 & 1 & 1 \\ 2 & 1 & 1 \end{bmatrix} \end{array}$$

Solution:

Let X, Y and Z be the Price of ingredients A, B and C

The above mentioned data can be written as

$$\begin{bmatrix} 2 & 2 & 1 \\ 1 & 1 & 1 \\ 2 & 1 & 1 \end{bmatrix} \begin{bmatrix} X \\ Y \\ Z \end{bmatrix} = \begin{bmatrix} 500 \\ 300 \\ 400 \end{bmatrix}$$

$$2X + 2Y + Z = 500$$

$$X + Y + Z = 300$$

$$2X + Y + Z = 400$$

Solve these three equation by Crammer's Rule

$$\Delta = \begin{bmatrix} 2 & 2 & 1 \\ 1 & 1 & 1 \\ 2 & 1 & 1 \end{bmatrix} = 2(1-1) - 2(1-2) + 1(1-2) = 1$$

$$\Delta_1 = \begin{bmatrix} 500 & 2 & 1 \\ 300 & 1 & 1 \\ 400 & 1 & 1 \end{bmatrix}$$

$$= 500(1-1) - 2(300-400) + 1(300-400)$$

$$= 0 + 200 - 100 = 100$$

$$\Delta_2 = \begin{bmatrix} 2 & 500 & 1 \\ 1 & 300 & 1 \\ 2 & 400 & 1 \end{bmatrix}$$

$$= 2(300-400) - 500(1-2) + 1(400-300)$$

$$= -200 + 500 - 100 = 200$$

$$\Delta_3 = \begin{bmatrix} 2 & 2 & 500 \\ 1 & 1 & 300 \\ 2 & 1 & 400 \end{bmatrix}$$

$$= 2(400-300) - 2(400-600) + 500(1-2)$$

$$= -200 + 800 - 500 = 100$$

$$X = \frac{100}{1} = 100 \qquad Y = \frac{200}{1} = 200 \qquad Z = \frac{100}{1} = 100$$

7. The stability of a pharmaceutical formulation obtained by using 2^2 factorial design is as listed below. Calculate coefficient of each factor by applying matrix method and form a polynomial or linear or regression equation

Levels	Factor ↓	Low	High
1.	Concentration (X_1)	3 gm	6 gms
2.	Temperature (X_2)	6 °C	12 °C

Combination	X_1	X_2	Y (Stability)
1	3	6	7
a	6	6	11
b	3	12	9
ab	6	12	10

***Solution*:** These four combinations can be written in the form of matrix as

$$X = \begin{bmatrix} 1 & 3 & 6 \\ 1 & 6 & 6 \\ 1 & 3 & 12 \\ 1 & 6 & 12 \end{bmatrix} \quad \beta = \begin{bmatrix} b \\ b_1 \\ b_2 \\ b_2 \end{bmatrix} \quad Y = \begin{bmatrix} 7 \\ 11 \\ 9 \\ 10 \end{bmatrix}$$

Obtain the transpose matrix of X and it is denoted as X^T

$$X^T = \begin{bmatrix} 1 & 1 & 1 & 1 \\ 3 & 6 & 3 & 6 \\ 6 & 6 & 12 & 12 \end{bmatrix}$$

$$\text{Then the Product of } X^T X = \begin{bmatrix} 1 & 1 & 1 & 1 \\ 3 & 6 & 3 & 6 \\ 6 & 6 & 12 & 12 \end{bmatrix} \begin{bmatrix} 1 & 3 & 6 \\ 1 & 6 & 6 \\ 1 & 3 & 12 \\ 1 & 6 & 12 \end{bmatrix}$$

$$= \begin{bmatrix} 4 & 18 & 36 \\ 18 & 90 & 162 \\ 36 & 162 & 360 \end{bmatrix}$$

$$\text{Cofactor Matrix of is } X^T X = \begin{bmatrix} 6156 & -648 & -324 \\ -648 & 144 & 0 \\ -324 & 0 & 36 \end{bmatrix}$$

The value of the determinant $X^T X = 4 \times 6156 + 18 \times (-648) + 36 \times (-324)$

$\Delta = 1296$

$$\text{Adj } X^TX = \begin{bmatrix} 6156 & -648 & -324 \\ -648 & 144 & 0 \\ -324 & 0 & 36 \end{bmatrix}$$

$$(X^TX)^{-1} = \frac{1}{1296}\begin{bmatrix} 6156 & -648 & -324 \\ -648 & 144 & 0 \\ -324 & 0 & 36 \end{bmatrix}$$

$$= \begin{bmatrix} 4.75 & -0.5 & -0.25 \\ -0.5 & 0.11 & 0 \\ -0.25 & 0 & 0.02 \end{bmatrix}$$

$$X^Ty = \begin{bmatrix} 1 & 1 & 1 & 1 \\ 3 & 6 & 3 & 6 \\ 6 & 6 & 12 & 12 \end{bmatrix}\begin{bmatrix} 7 \\ 11 \\ 9 \\ 10 \end{bmatrix}$$

$$= \begin{bmatrix} 37 \\ 174 \\ 336 \end{bmatrix}$$

The least squares estimates of $\beta = (X^TX)^{-1}X^Ty$

$$\begin{bmatrix} b \\ b_1 \\ b_2 \end{bmatrix} = \begin{bmatrix} 4.75 & -0.5 & -0.25 \\ -0.5 & 0.11 & 0 \\ -0.25 & 0 & 0.02 \end{bmatrix}\begin{bmatrix} 37 \\ 174 \\ 336 \end{bmatrix}$$

$$\begin{bmatrix} b \\ b_1 \\ b_2 \end{bmatrix} = \begin{bmatrix} 4.75 \\ -0.64 \\ -2.53 \end{bmatrix}$$

Then the least square fit is $Y = b + b_1X_1 + b_2X_2$

$$Y = 4.75 - 0.64X_1 - 2.53X_2$$

8. A pharmaceutical formulation prepared and yield obtained for one factor with different levels is as listed below. Calculate coefficient of single factor by applying matrix method and form linear or a polynomial or regression equation and Calculate the Predicted values.

Combination	X(Factor)	Y (Yield)
1	5	3
2	8	4
3	7	5
4	6	2
5	4	1

***Solution*:** These four combinations can be written in the form of matrix as

$$X = \begin{bmatrix} 1 & 5 \\ 1 & 8 \\ 1 & 7 \\ 1 & 6 \\ 1 & 4 \end{bmatrix} \quad \beta = \begin{bmatrix} a \\ b \end{bmatrix} \quad Y = \begin{bmatrix} 3 \\ 4 \\ 5 \\ 2 \\ 1 \end{bmatrix}$$

Obtain the transpose matrix of X and it is denoted as X^T

$$X^T = \begin{bmatrix} 1 & 1 & 1 & 1 & 1 \\ 5 & 8 & 7 & 6 & 4 \end{bmatrix}$$

Then the Product of $X^TX = \begin{bmatrix} 1 & 1 & 1 & 1 & 1 \\ 5 & 8 & 7 & 6 & 4 \end{bmatrix} \begin{bmatrix} 1 & 5 \\ 1 & 8 \\ 1 & 7 \\ 1 & 6 \\ 1 & 4 \end{bmatrix}$

$$\begin{bmatrix} 5 & 30 \\ 30 & 190 \end{bmatrix}$$

Cofactor Matrix of is $X^TX = \begin{bmatrix} 190 & -30 \\ -30 & 5 \end{bmatrix}$

The value of the determinant $X^TX = 5 \times 190 - (-30 \times -30) = 950 - 900$

$$= 50$$

$$\Delta = 50$$

$$\text{Adj } (X^TX) = \begin{bmatrix} 190 & -30 \\ -30 & 5 \end{bmatrix}$$

$$(X^TX)^{-1} = \frac{1}{50}\begin{bmatrix} 190 & -30 \\ -30 & 5 \end{bmatrix}$$

$$X^Ty = \begin{bmatrix} 1 & 1 & 1 & 1 & 1 \\ 5 & 8 & 7 & 6 & 4 \end{bmatrix}\begin{bmatrix} 3 \\ 4 \\ 5 \\ 2 \\ 1 \end{bmatrix}$$

$$= \begin{bmatrix} 15 \\ 98 \end{bmatrix}$$

The least squares estimates of $\beta = (X^T X)^{-1} X^T Y$

$$= \frac{1}{50}\begin{bmatrix} 190 & -30 \\ -30 & 5 \end{bmatrix}\begin{bmatrix} 15 \\ 98 \end{bmatrix}$$

$$\beta = \begin{bmatrix} a \\ b \end{bmatrix}\begin{bmatrix} -1.8 \\ 0.8 \end{bmatrix}$$

Then the least square fit is $Y = a + bX$

$Y = -1.8 + 0.8X$

Tria(RUNS)	**X**	**Predicted Values $Y = -1.8+0.8X$**
1	5	2.2
2	8	4.6
3	7	3.8
4	6	3
5	4	1.4

9. Quantitative structure activity relationship (QSAR) correlates measurable or Calculatable Physical or molecular properties to some specific biological activity in terms of an mathematical equation.

   Once a valid QSAR has been determined, it should be possible to predict the biological activity of related drug candidates before their synthesis and biological screening.

To correlate the Physioco_chemical Properties of drug likely compounds with biological activity, we will use statistical analysis or tools to analyse the data.

We can use linear regression or multilinear regression depending upon the number of Physio-chemical parameters to be determined

Example of a QSAR....

m –X	P – Y	π	$\sigma+$	$E_{S(meta)}$	$Log(1/C)_a$
H	H	0.00	0.00	1.24	7.46
F	H	0.13	0.35	0.78	7.52
H	F	0.15	– 0.07	1.24	8.16
Cl	H	0.76	0.40	0.27	8.16
Cl	F	0.91	0.33	0.27	8.19
Br	H	.94	0.41	0.08	8.30
I	H	1.15	0.36	– 0.16	8.40
Me	H	0.51	– 0.07	0.00	8.46
Br	F	1.09	0.34	0.08	8.57
H	Cl	0.70	0.11	1.24	8.68
Me	F	0.66	– 0.14	0.00	8.82
H	Br	1.02	0.15	1.24	8.89
Cl	Cl	1.46	0.51	0.27	8.89
Br	Cl	1.64	0.52	0.08	8.92
Me	Cl	1.21	0.04	0.00	8.96
Cl	Br	1.78	0.55	0.27	9.00
Me	Br	1.53	0.08	0.00	9.22
H	I	1.26	0.14	1.24	9.25
H	Me	0.52	– 0.31	1.24	9.30
Me	Me	1.03	– 0.38	0.00	9.30
Br	Br	1.96	0.56	0.08	9.35
Br	Me	1.46	0.10	0.08	9.52

***Solution*:** The set of given values can be written in the form Matrix X as

$$X = \begin{bmatrix} 1 & 0 & 0 & 1.24 \\ 1 & 0.13 & 0.35 & 0.78 \\ 1 & 0.15 & -0.07 & 1.24 \\ 1 & 0.76 & 0.4 & 0.27 \\ 1 & 0.91 & 0.33 & 0.27 \\ 1 & 0.94 & 0.41 & 0.08 \\ 1 & 1.15 & 0.36 & -0.16 \\ 1 & 0.51 & -0.07 & 0 \\ 1 & 1.09 & 0.34 & 0.08 \\ 1 & 0.7 & 0.11 & 1.24 \\ 1 & 0.66 & -0.14 & 0 \\ 1 & 1.02 & 0.15 & 1.24 \\ 1 & 1.46 & 0.51 & 0.27 \\ 1 & 1.64 & 0.52 & 0.08 \\ 1 & 1.21 & 0.04 & 0 \\ 1 & 1.78 & 0.55 & 0.27 \\ 1 & 1.53 & 0.08 & 0 \\ 1 & 1.26 & 0.14 & 1.24 \\ 1 & 0.52 & -0.31 & 1.24 \\ 1 & 1.03 & -0.38 & 0 \\ 1 & 1.96 & 0.56 & 0.08 \\ 1 & 1.46 & 0.1 & 0.08 \end{bmatrix}$$

$$Y = \begin{bmatrix} 7.46 \\ 7.52 \\ 8.16 \\ 8.16 \\ 8.19 \\ 8.3 \\ 8.4 \\ 8.46 \\ 8.57 \\ 8.68 \\ 8.82 \\ 8.89 \\ 8.89 \\ 8.92 \\ 8.96 \\ 9 \\ 9.22 \\ 9.25 \\ 9.3 \\ 9.3 \\ 9.35 \\ 9.52 \end{bmatrix}$$

Then Obtain the transpose of the Matrix X, written as X^T, $X^T X$, $(X^T X)^{-1}$ and the Produt of,

$$(X^T X)^{-1} X^T Y \text{ then}$$

$$F = (X^T X)^{-1} X^T Y$$

$b_0 = 7.61906$, $b_1 = 1.258964$, $b_2 = -1.45961$ $b_3 = 0.20792$

$Y = 7.61906 + 1.25864\,A - 1.45965\,B + 0.25792\,C$ is the required regression equation to find the predicted values.

CHAPTER 4

ANALYTICAL GEOMETRY

4.1 INTRODUCTION

Analytical Geometry is the study of geometry using algebraic methods. During 17th century a well known French mathematician **Rene Descartes** (1596-1650) thought of using algebra in geometry and developed the subject which we now call Algebraic Geometry or Co-ordinate or Analytical Geometry. It was shown that every point in a plane can be represented by an ordered pair (x, y) of real numbers uniquely and conversely for every ordered pair of real numbers there exists a point in the plane. Thus each geometrical figure can be associated with an algebraic equation in x and y and its properties can be studied with the help of algebraic equation. Analytical geometry also plays very important role in solving few problems of Pharmokinetics.

4.2 CARTESIAN RECTANGULAR CO-ORDINATE SYSTEM

In Algebra, one can see how a real number can be represented by a point on the number line. Every real number can be represented by a point on the number line *l* and conversely every point on *l* represents some real number.

Every ordered pair of real numbers can be represented by a point in a plane with reference to two fixed lines, called reference axes. The axes of reference may be perpendicular (rectangular) or may be inclined at an angle θ (oblique). However, we consider the reference axes as always perpendicular.

XOX' and YOY' are two fixed lines at right angles, intersecting at O. The point O is called the origin and the two lines are called the axes of reference or co-ordinate axes. XOX' is called as x-axis and YOY' is called as y-axis.

Let P be any point in the plane. Draw PM $\perp$ X-axis and PN $\perp$ to Y-axis. Take OM = NP = x, ON = MP = y. The x and y are called the Cartesian rectangular co-ordinates of the point P. x is called the x-co-ordinate (or abscissa) and y is called y–co–ordinate (or ordinate) of the point P. we write P = (x, y) to mention the fact that the co-ordinates of the point P are x and y. Note that the x-co-ordinate of the point P is the distance of P from the y-axis and the Y-co-ordinate is its distance from the X-axis. The co-ordinates of M are (x, 0) and co-ordinates of N (0, y) i.e., M ≡ (x, 0), N ≡ (0, y). For any point on the X-axis, the y co-ordinate is 0 i.e., (y = 0) and for any point on the Y-axis the x-co-ordinate is 0 i.e., (x = 0). The co-ordinates of the origin O are (0, 0) i.e., O ≡ (0, 0).

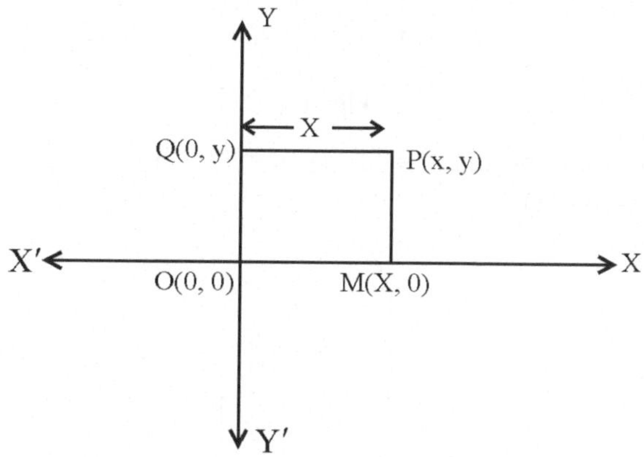

Fig. 4.1

4.2.1 Signs of the Coordinates

The x-coordinate is positive or negative according as the point is to right or to left of Y-axis. The y-coordinate is positive or negative according as the point is above or below X-axis. The two reference axes XOX′ and YOY′ divide the plane into four parts (quadrants). The signs of the coordinates are marked in the Fig. 4.2.

I quadrant (XOY)	:	x is positive, y is positive
II quadrant (X^IOY)	:	x is negative, y is positive
III quadrant (X^IOY^I)	:	x is negative, y is negative
IV quadrant (XOY^I)	:	x is positive, y is negative

The arrow marks on x, y axes indicate that they are the positive directions of x and y axes

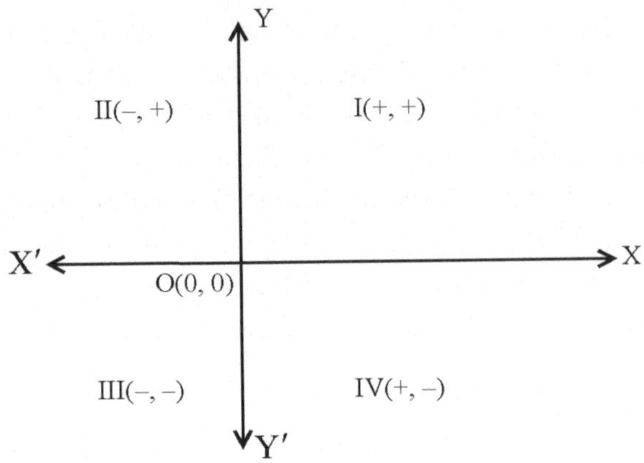

Fig. 4.2

***Example* 1:** Mark the points A ≡ (3, 4), B ≡ (5, –3), C ≡ (–2, 4), D ≡ (–5, –6), E ≡ (0, –3)

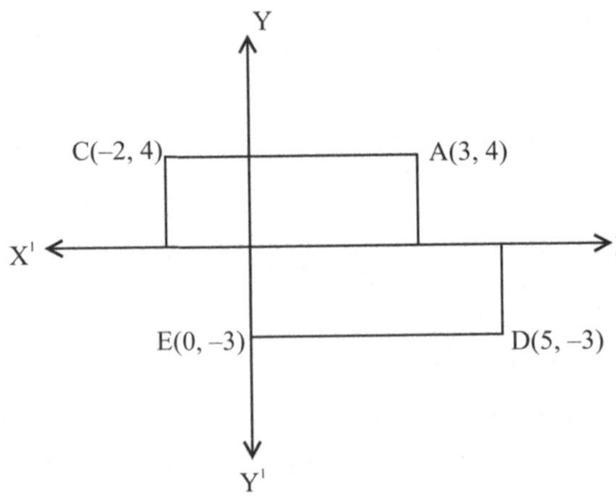

Fig. 4.3

***Example* 2:** Mark the points A ≡ (3, 5) and B ≡ (–1, 6). What is the reflection of A in the x-axis? What is the reflection of B in the y-axis?

Mark A ≡ (3, 5) and B ≡ (–1, 6). Draw AM ⊥ to X-axis and produce AM to A' such that AM = MA'. Then A' is the Reflection of A in the x-axis. From the figure $A' \equiv (3, -5)$. Draw BN ⊥ to y-axis and produce it to B' such that $BN = NB^1$. Then B^1 is the reflection of b in y-axis. $B' \equiv (1, 6)$. Note that the reflection of P(x, y) in x-axis is P(x, –y) and the reflection in y-axis is P(–x, y).

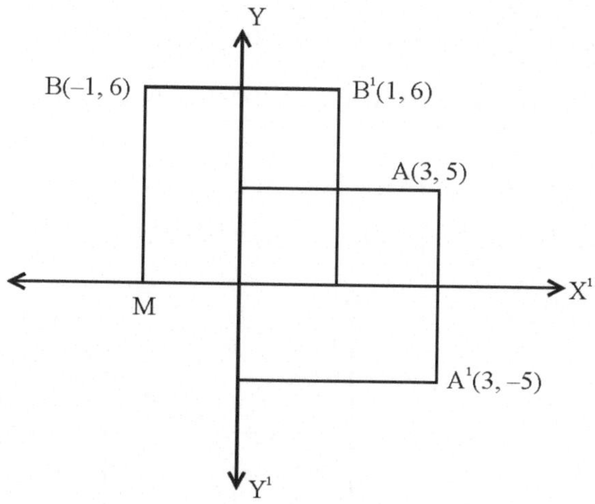

Fig. 4.4

4.2.2 Distance Formula

(i) Distance of a point P(x, y) from the origin O = (0, 0)

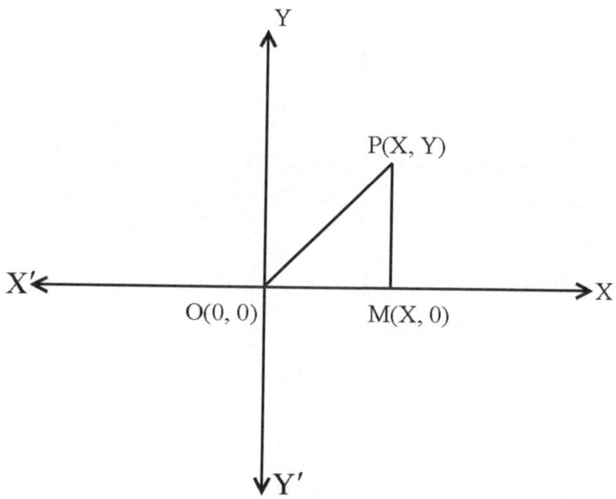

Fig. 4.5

Let P be a point and its co-ordinates are (x, y). Draw PM ⊥ to X-axis and join OP. Then OM = x, MP = y.

From the Δ OPM, $OP^2 = OM^2 + MP^2 = x^2 + y^2$

$$\therefore \qquad OP = \sqrt{x^2 + y^2}$$

That is, distance of a point P(x, y) from the origin is given by $\sqrt{x^2 + y^2}$

The result holds good whatever may be the quadrant in which the point P lies.

For example: The distance of P(3, –4) from the origin is

(ii) Distance between the points (x_1, y_1) and (x_2, y_2)

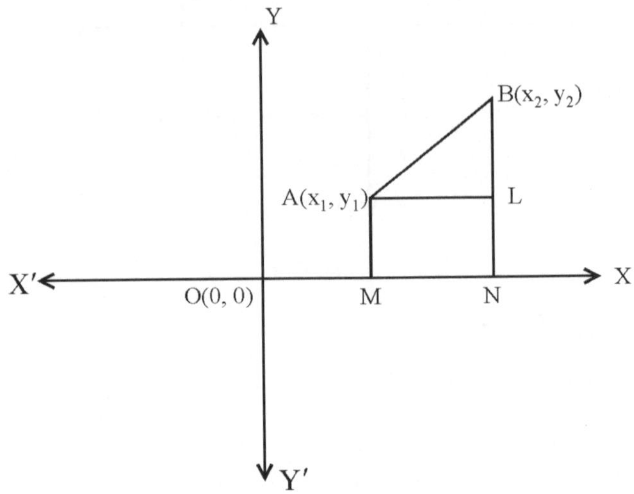

Fig. 4.6

Let A and B be the points (x_1, y_1) and (x_2, y_2) respectively, join AB. Draw AM and BN perpendicular to X-axis. Draw AL ⊥ to BN. Then $OM = x_1$, $MA = y_1$, $ON = x_2$, $NB = y_2$.

Here $AL = MN = ON - OM = (x_2 - x_1)$

and $BL = BN - LN = BN - AM = (y_2 - y_1)$

So from the Δ ABL, we have $AB^2 = AL^2 + BL^2$

i.e., $AB^2 = (x_2 - x_1)^2 + (y_2 - y_1)^2$

$$\therefore \quad AB = \sqrt{(x_2 - x_1)^2 + (y_2 - y_1)^2}$$

Hence the distance between the points (x_1, y_1) and (x_2, y_2)

$$d = \sqrt{(x_2 - x_1)^2 + (y_2 - y_1)^2}$$

This is known as the distance formula

Note: (i) Putting $x_1 = 0$, $y_1 = 0$ we get the distance of the point (x_2, y_2) from the origin i.e., $\sqrt{x_2^2 + y_2^2}$

Worked Examples

1. Find distance between the points A(–3, 1) and B = (3, 2).

$$AB = \sqrt{(x_2 - x_1)^2 + (y_2 - y_1)^2}$$

$$= \sqrt{(3+3)^2 + (2-12)^2} = \sqrt{36+1} = \sqrt{37}$$

2. If the distance between (a, 2) and (3, 4) is a $2\sqrt{2}$ find a.

Distance $= \sqrt{(3-a)^2 + (4-2)^2} = 2\sqrt{2}$

i.e., $\sqrt{9-6a+a^2+4} = 2\sqrt{2}$ Squaring both sides

$13 - 6a + a^2 = 8$

i.e., $a^2 - 6a + 5 = 0$

i.e., $(a - 5)(a - 1) = 0$

∴ $a = 1$ or $a = 5$

3. Show that the points A(2, –4) B(4, –2) C(7, 1) are collinear

$$AB = \sqrt{(4-2)^2 + (-2+4)^2} = \sqrt{4+4} = \sqrt{8} = 2\sqrt{2}$$

$$BC = \sqrt{(7-4)^2 + (1+2)^2} = \sqrt{9+9} = \sqrt{18} = 3\sqrt{2}$$

$$AC = \sqrt{(7-2)^2 + (1+4)^2} = \sqrt{25+25} = \sqrt{50} = 5\sqrt{2}$$

∴ A, B, C are collinear

Now AB + BC = $5\sqrt{2}$ = AC

4. Prove that the points (–2, 5), (3, –4), (7, 10) form a right angled isosceles triangle.

Take A = (–2, 5) B = (3, –4) C = (7, 10)

$$AB = \sqrt{(3\times 2)^2 + (-4-5)^2} = \sqrt{25+81} = \sqrt{106}$$

$$BC = \sqrt{(7-3)^2 + (10+4)^2} = \sqrt{16+196} = \sqrt{212}$$

$$AC = \sqrt{(7+2)^2 + (10-5)^2} = \sqrt{81+25} = \sqrt{106}$$

Now $AB^2 + AC^2 = BC^2$ and AB = AC = $\sqrt{106}$

∴ ABC is a right angled isosceles triangle

5. Prove that (7, 9), (3, –7), (–3, 3) form an isosceles triangle.

   Take A = (7, 9) B = (3, –7) C = (–3, 3)

$$AB = \sqrt{(3-7)^2 + (-7-9)^2} = \sqrt{16+256} = \sqrt{272}$$

$$BC = \sqrt{(-3-3)^2 + (3+7)^2} = \sqrt{36+100} = \sqrt{136}$$

$$AC = \sqrt{(-3-7)^2 + (3-9)^2} = \sqrt{100+36} = \sqrt{136}$$

$$AC = BC$$

$\therefore$ Triangle is isosceles

6. Show that the points (2, 4) (2, 6) $(2+\sqrt{3}, 5)$ are the vertices of an equilateral triangle.

   Take A = (2, 4) B = (2, 6) C = $(2+\sqrt{3}, 5)$

$$AB = \sqrt{(2-2)^2 + (6-4)^2} = \sqrt{0+4} = 2$$

$$BC = \sqrt{(\sqrt{3})^2 + (5-6)^2} = \sqrt{3+1} = 2$$

$$AC = \sqrt{(\sqrt{3})^2 + (5-4)^2} = \sqrt{3+1} = 2$$

$$AB = BC = AC = 2$$

$\therefore$ ΔABC, is equilateral

7. Prove that the points (–3, 1) (–6, –7) (3, –9) and (6, –1) are the vertices of a parallelogram.

   Take A = (–3, 1) B = (–6, –7) C = (3, –9), D = (6, –1)

$$AB = \sqrt{(-6+3)^2 + (-7-1)^2} = \sqrt{9+64} = \sqrt{73}$$

$$BC = \sqrt{(3+6)^2 + (-9+7)^2} = \sqrt{81+4} = \sqrt{85}$$

$$CD = \sqrt{(6-3)^2 + (-1\times 9)^2} = \sqrt{9+64} = \sqrt{73}$$

$$AD = \sqrt{(6+3)^2 + (-1-1)^2} = \sqrt{81+4} = \sqrt{85}$$

$\therefore$ $AB = CD = \sqrt{73}$ and $BC = AD = \sqrt{85}$

This means that the opposite sides are equal $\therefore$ ABCD is a parallelogram

8. Prove that the points (8, 4) (5, 7) (–1, 1) and (2, 2) form a rectangle

Take A = (8, 4) B = (5, 7) C = (–1, 1) D = (2, –2)

$$AB = \sqrt{(5-8)^2 + (7-4)^2} = \sqrt{3^2 + 3^2} = \sqrt{18}$$

$$BC = \sqrt{(-1-5)^2 + (1-7)^2} = \sqrt{36+36} = \sqrt{72}$$

$$CD = \sqrt{(2+1)^2 + (-2-1)^2} = \sqrt{9+9} = \sqrt{18}$$

$$AD = \sqrt{(2-8)^2 + (-2-4)^2} = \sqrt{36+36} = \sqrt{72}$$

$$AC = \sqrt{(-1-8)^2 + (1-4)^2} = \sqrt{81+9} = \sqrt{90}$$

$$BD = \sqrt{(2-5)^2 + (-2-7)^2} = \sqrt{9+81} = \sqrt{90}$$

Now AB = CD = $\sqrt{81}$, BC = AD = $\sqrt{72}$

∴ Opposite sides are equal. Further AC = BD = $\sqrt{90}$

i.e., the diagonals are also equal

∴ ABCD is a rectangle

Note: A quadrilateral in which the opposite sides are equal is a parallelogram. Further if the diagonals are also equal then the quadrilateral is a rectangle. Similarly a quadrilateral in which all the sides are equal is a rhombus. Further if the diagonals are equal then it is a square. In a parallelogram and rhombus the diagonals are not necessarily equal.

9. Show that (3, 2), (7, 6), (–1, 2), (–5, –6) are the vertices of a rhombus

Take A = (3, –2) B = (7, 6) C = (–1, 2) D = (–5, –6)

$$AB = \sqrt{(7-3)^2 + (6-2)^2} = \sqrt{16+64} = \sqrt{80}$$

$$BC = \sqrt{(-1-7)^2 + (2-6)^2} = \sqrt{64+16} = \sqrt{80}$$

$$CD = \sqrt{(-5+1)^2 + (-6-2)^2} = \sqrt{16+64} = \sqrt{80}$$

$$AD = \sqrt{(-5-3)^2 + (-6+2)^2} = \sqrt{64+16} = \sqrt{80}$$

AB = BC = CD = AD = $\sqrt{80}$. All the sides are equal

∴ ABCD is a rhombus

10. Show that the points (4, 1), (1, 6), (–4, 3) and (–1, –2) form a square

Take A = (4, 1) B = (1, 6) C = (–4, 3) D = (–1, –2)

$$AB = \sqrt{(1-4)^2 + (6-1)^2} = \sqrt{9+25} = \sqrt{34}$$

$$BC = \sqrt{(-4-1)^2 + (3-6)^2} = \sqrt{25+9} = \sqrt{34}$$

$$CD = \sqrt{(-1+4)^2 + (-2-3)^2} = \sqrt{9+25} = \sqrt{34}$$

$$AD = \sqrt{(-1-4)^2 + (-2-1)^2} = \sqrt{25+9} = \sqrt{34}$$

$$AC = \sqrt{(-4-4)^2 + (3-1)^2} = \sqrt{64+4} = \sqrt{68}$$

$$BD = \sqrt{(-1-1)^2 + (-2-6)^2} = \sqrt{4+64} = \sqrt{68}$$

AB = BC = CD = AD = $\sqrt{34}$ and AC = BD = $\sqrt{68}$

∴ All the sides are equal and the diagonals are also equal

∴ ABCD is a square

Exercise 4.1

1. Find the distance between the following pair of points.

   (i) (3, 6) and B(–2, 5) (ii) (2, –2) and (4, 3)

2. Find the images of the point (7, –8) in x and y-axis.
3. Show that the points (–2, 3), (–6, 4) and (–10, 5) lie on the same line.
4. Prove that the points (1, 5), (–7, 9) and (–10, –17) are the vertices of a right angled triangle.
5. Prove that the points (1, 3), (3, –1), (–5, –5) are the vertices of right angled triangle.
6. Show that the points (4, 1), (3, 4), (2, 1) form an isosceles triangle.
7. Prove that (3, 2), (7, 4) and $(5+\sqrt{3}, 3-2\sqrt{3})$ are the vertices of an equilateral triangles.
8. Given A = (2, 3), B = (6, 5), C = (2, 1) and D = (–6, –7). Show that ABCD is rhombus of area 48 sq. units.
9. Show that the points (0, –1), (2, 1), (0, 3) and (–2, 1) form a square.
10. Show that (0, –1), (2, 1) (0, 3) and (–2, 1) are the vertices of a square.

11. Show that the point S(4, 3) is the centre of the circle passing through the points A(9, 3), B(7, –1), C(–1, 3). What is the radius of the circle ?
12. Show that (11, 2) is the circumcentre of the triangle whose vertices are (1, 2), (5, –6), (3, 4).
13. Find the co-ordinates of the circumcentre of the triangle whose vertices are (1, 1), (2, –1) and (3, 2).
14. For a point P, the abscissa = ordinate. If the distance of P from (1, 3) is 10, what are the co-ordinate of P ?
15. If the point (x, y) is equidistance from (a, 0) and (2a, a) show that $x + y - 2a = 0$.
16. If two vertices of an equilateral triangle are (1, –1) and $(-\sqrt{3}, -\sqrt{3})$. Find the co-ordinates of the third vertex.
17. P(x, 0) is such that it is equidistant from (–4, 6) and (14, 2). Find x.

Answers

1. (i) $\sqrt{26}$ (ii) $\sqrt{29}$ 2. (7, 8), (–7, –8) 13. $\left(\frac{5}{2}, \frac{1}{2}\right)$

14. (–5, –5) or (9, 9) 16. $(2-\sqrt{3}, -2-\sqrt{3})$ 17. $\frac{37}{9}$

4.2.3 Section Formula

Co–ordinates of a point dividing a given line in a given ratio m : n

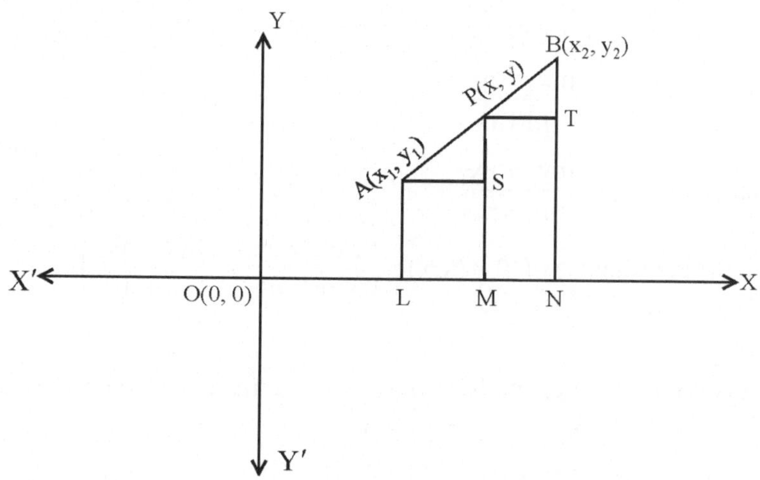

Fig. 4.7

Let A and B be any two points (x_1, y_1) and (x_2, y_2) respectively. Let $P = (x, y)$ be any which divide AB internally in the ratio m : n. That is $\frac{AP}{PB} = \frac{m}{n}$

We are given the co-ordinates of A and B and the ratio m : n. We have to find the co-ordinates of P, i.e., x and y.

Draw AL, PM, BN ⊥ to x-axis, AS ⊥ PM and PT ⊥ BN.

$$OL = x_1, LA = y_1, ON = x_2, BN = y_2, OM = x, PM = y$$

The triangles ASP and PTB are similar

(because $\hat{ASP} = \hat{PTB} = 90°; \hat{PAS} = \hat{BPT}$ (corresponding angles)

$$\therefore \quad \frac{AS}{PT} = \frac{SP}{TB} = \frac{AP}{PB} \qquad \text{..... (1)}$$

Now $AS = LM = OM - OL = x - x_1$; $SP = PM - SM = PM - AL = y - y_1$

$$PT = MN = ON - OM = x_2 - x; \; TB = BN - TN = BN - PM = y_2 - y$$

and $$\frac{AP}{PB} = \frac{m}{n}$$

So from (1), we get $\frac{x - x_1}{x_2 - x} = \frac{y - y_1}{y_2 - y} = \frac{m}{n}$

Taking, $\frac{x - x_1}{x_2 - x} = \frac{m}{n}$, we get

$$nx - nx_1 = mx_2 - mx$$

or $$x(m + n) = mx_2 + nx_1$$

$$\therefore \quad x = \frac{mx_2 + nx_1}{m + n}$$

Similarly, $$y = \frac{my_2 + ny_1}{m + n}$$

Hence the coordinates of $P \equiv (x, y) = \left(\frac{mx_2 + nx_1}{m + n}, \frac{my_2 + ny_1}{m + n}\right)$ .....(2)

Note:

(i) If Q divides AB externally in the ratio m:n, the coordinates of Q are

$$\left(\frac{mx_2 - nx_1}{m - n}, \frac{my_2 - ny_1}{m - n}\right) \qquad \text{..... (3)}$$

(2) and (3) are called section formulae

(ii) The following scheme may be adopted while applying the formulae to the problems.

Internal division:

$$P \equiv \left(\frac{mx_2 + nx_1}{m+n}, \frac{my_2 + ny_1}{m+n} \right)$$

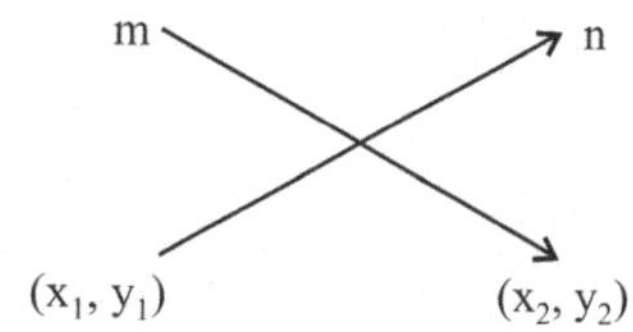

External division:

$$Q \equiv \left(\frac{mx_2 - nx_1}{m-n}, \frac{my_2 - ny_1}{m-n} \right)$$

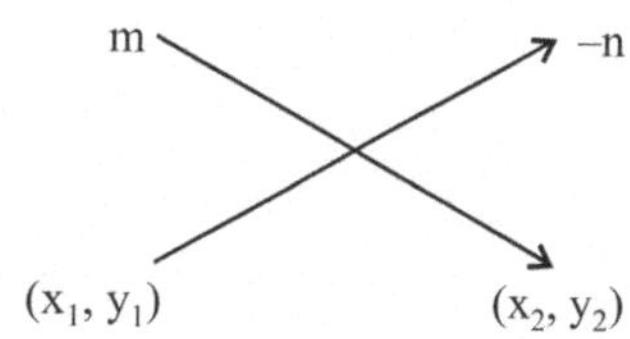

(iii) *Mid-point formula*: If p is the mid point of the line joining $A(x_1, y_1)$ and $B(x_2, y_2)$ then m:n = 1:1 and so the co-ordinates of P are $\left(\frac{x_1 + x_2}{2}, \frac{y_1 + y_2}{2} \right)$

(iv) *Centroid of a triangle*: To find the co-ordinates of the centroid of a triangle whose vertices are (x_1, y_1), (x_2, y_2), (x_3, y_3)

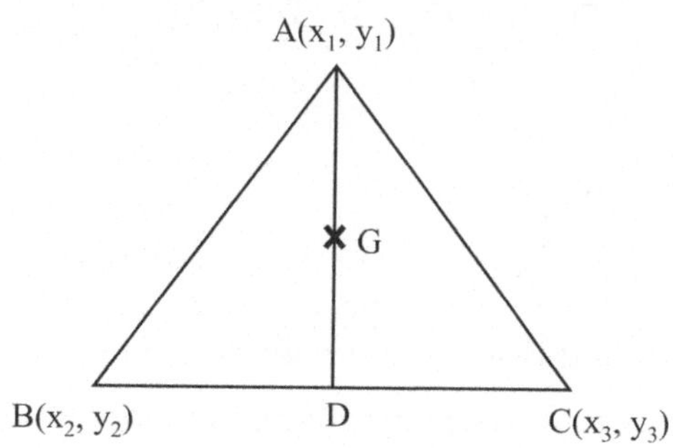

Fig. 4.8

Let ABC be the triangle formed by the given points. Let D be the mid-point of BC. The centriod G lies on AD and divides it in the ratio 2 : 1

Now, $D = \left(\frac{x_2 + x_3}{2}, \frac{y_2 + y_3}{2} \right)$ Since G divides AD internally in the ratio 2:1, we have

$$G \equiv \left(\frac{2\left(\frac{x_2 + x_3}{2}\right) + 1.x_1}{2+1}, \frac{2\left(\frac{x_2 + y_2}{2}\right) + 1.\, y_1}{2+1} \right)$$

$$G \equiv \left(\frac{x_2 + x_3 + x_1}{3}, \frac{y_2 + y_3 + y_1}{3} \right)$$

i.e.,
$$G \equiv \left(\frac{x_1 + x_2 + x_3}{3}, \frac{y_1 + y_2 + y_3}{3} \right)$$

Worked Examples

1. Find the co-ordinates of the point which divides the joining the points A(2, 7) and B(–1, –3) internally in the ratio 2:1.

   Let the point P divide AB internally in the ratio 2:1, then

$$P \equiv \left(\frac{mx_2 + nx_1}{m+n}, \frac{my_2 + ny_1}{m+n} \right)$$

$$= \left(\frac{2(-1) + 1(2)}{2+1}, \frac{2(-3) + 1(7)}{2+1} \right)$$

$$= \left(0, \frac{1}{3} \right)$$

2. Find the co-ordinates of the point which divides the line joining the points A(–1, –2) and B(4, 6) externally in the ratio 5:3

   Let the point P divide AB externally in the ratio 5:3

$$P \equiv \left(\frac{mx_2 - nx_1}{m-n}, \frac{my_2 - ny_1}{m-n} \right)$$

$$= \left(\frac{5(4) - 3(-1)}{5-3}, \frac{5(6) - 3(-2)}{5-3} \right) = \left(\frac{23}{2}, 18 \right)$$

3. Find the co-ordinates of the points of trisection of the line joining the points (5, –6) and (–3, 4).

   Take A = (5, –6), B(–3, 4). Let P and Q divide AB into 3 equal parts. Then P and Q are the points of trisection of AB. Now P divides AB internally in the ratio 1:2 and Q divides AB internally in the ratio 2 : 1.

$$P = \left(\frac{-3+10}{1+2}, \frac{4-12}{1+2}\right)$$

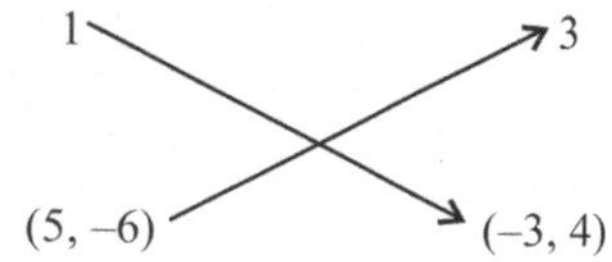

$$= \left(\frac{7}{3}, \frac{-8}{3}\right)$$

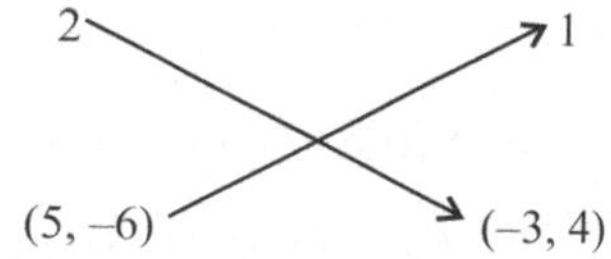

$$Q = \left(\frac{-6+5}{3}, \frac{8-6}{3}\right) = \left(\frac{-1}{3}, \frac{2}{3}\right)$$

so the points of trisection are $\left(\frac{7}{3}, \frac{-8}{3}\right)$ and $\left(\frac{-1}{3}, \frac{2}{3}\right)$

4. Find the ratio which the point (–5, 2) divides the line joining the points (–7, 1) and (3, 6).

   Let (–5, 2) divide the joins of (–7, 1) and (3, 6) in the ration r:1.

$$(-5, 2) = \left(\frac{3r-7}{r+1}, \frac{6r+1}{r+1}\right)$$

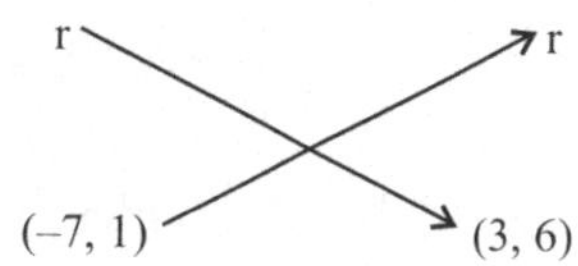

$$\therefore \quad \frac{3r-7}{r+1} = 5, \ \frac{6r+1}{r+1} = 2$$

i.e., $3r - 7 = -5r - 5$

i.e., $8r = 2$

$\therefore\ r = \frac{1}{4}$ we get the same value if we take the other equation.

$\therefore$ The point (–5, 2) divides the line joining the points (–7, 1) and (3, 6) internally in the ratio of 1 : 4

5. Find what ratios in which the line joining the points (–2, 1) and (3, 4) is cut by the co-ordinate axes.

   Take A = (–2, 1) B = (3, 4)

   Let AB cut the axis at P(x, 0) and y-axis at Q(0, y). Let P divide AB in the ratio r : 1

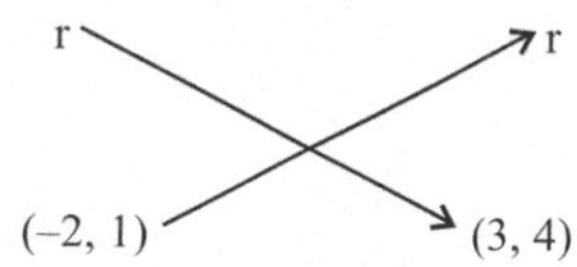

$$P = \left(\frac{3r-2}{r+1}, \frac{4r+1}{r+1}\right) = (x, 0)$$

$$\therefore \quad \frac{3r-2}{r+1} = x \qquad \text{..... (1)}$$

$$\frac{4r+1}{r+1} = 0 \qquad \text{..... (2)}$$

From (2), $4r + 1 = 0 \therefore r = \frac{-1}{4}$. The negative sign indicates that P divides AB externally in the ratio 1 : 4

Let Q divide AB in the ratio k : 1

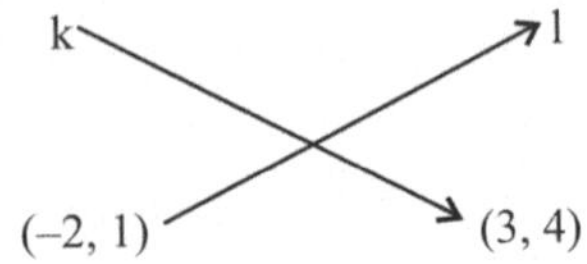

$$Q = \left(\frac{3k-2}{k+1}, \frac{4k+1}{k+1}\right) = (0, y)$$

$$\therefore \quad \frac{3k-2}{k+1} = 0$$

$\therefore$ i.e., $3k - 2 = 0$

$$k = \frac{2}{3}$$

So Q divides AB internally in the ratio 3:2. Hence the x-axis cuts the lines externally in the ratio 1:4 and y-axis cuts the line internally in the ratio 2:3.

6. Three vertices of a rectangle are (2, 1) (–4, –1) (–2, –3). Find the co-ordinates of the fourth vertex.

Take D = (x, y) and E be the intersection of the diagonals.

E is the middle point of AC

$$= \left(\frac{2-2}{2}, \frac{1-3}{2}\right) = (0, -1)$$

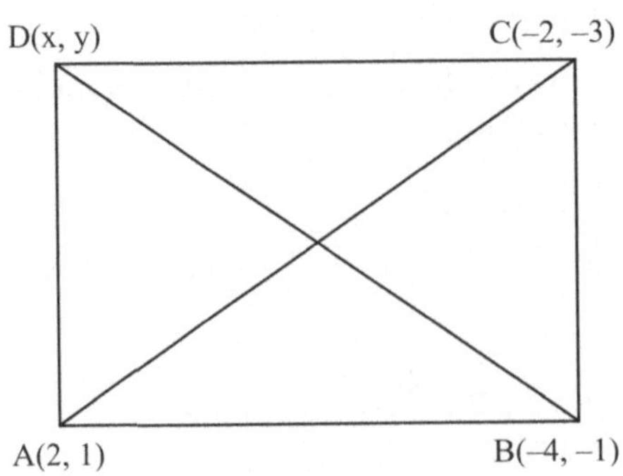

Fig. 4.9

E is also the mid-point of BD

$\therefore \quad E = \left(\frac{x-4}{2}, \frac{y-1}{2}\right) = (0, -1)$

$\therefore \quad x - 4 = 0, y - 1 = -2$

$x = 4 \quad y = -1$

$\therefore \quad D = (4, -1)$

7. Using the mid-point formula show that (–7, –3) (–10, –1) (–1, –13) (2, –15) are the vertices of a parallelogram.

Take A = (–7, –3), B = (–10, –1), C = (–1, –13), D = (2, –15)

$$\text{Middle point of } AC = \left(\frac{-7-1}{2}, \frac{-3-13}{2}\right) = (-4, -8)$$

$$\text{Middle point of } BD = \left(\frac{-10+2}{2}, \frac{-1-15}{2}\right) = (-4, -8)$$

Thus the middle points of the diagonals AC and BD are the same. As the diagonals bisect each other in ABCD, ABCD is a parallelogram.

8. Find the centroid of the triangle formed by the points (1, 6), (7, 1) and (1, 5)

$$\text{Centroid } G = \left(\frac{1+7+1}{3}, \frac{6+1+5}{3}\right) = (3, 4)$$

9. Find the centroid of the triangle formed by the points (2, 1), (5, 2), (–1, 3).

$$\text{Centroid } = \left(\frac{x_1+x_2+x_3}{3}, \frac{y_1+y_2+y_3}{3}\right)$$

$$= \left(\frac{2+5-1}{3}, \frac{1+2+3}{3}\right) = (2, 2)$$

10. The centroid of a triangle is (2, 7) and the two vertices are (4, 8) and (–2, 6). Find the third vertex.

Take the third vertex as (x, y)

$$\text{Then} \quad (2, 7) = \left(\frac{4-2+x}{3}, \frac{8+6+y}{3}\right)$$

$$(2,\ 7) = \left(\frac{2+x}{3},\ \frac{14+y}{3}\right)$$

$\therefore\ 2 + x = 6 \qquad 14 + y = 21$

$x = 4 \qquad y = 7$

$\therefore$ Third vertex = (4, 7)

11. The middle points of the sides of a triangle are (–1, –2) (6, 1) and (3, 5). Find the co-ordinates of the vertices.

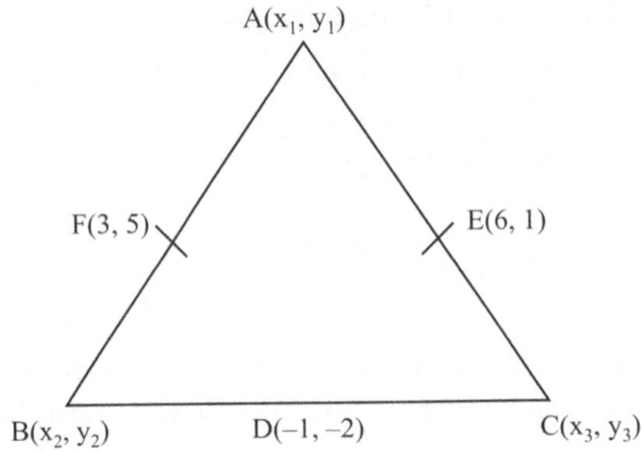

Fig. 4.10

Let D, E, F be the middle point of BC, CA, and AB

D = (–1, –2) E = (6, 1)

F = (3, 5) take A = (x_1, y_1)

B = (x_2, y_2) C = (x_3, y_3)

D is the middle point of BC

$$\therefore \qquad (-1,\ -2) = \left(\frac{x_2 + x_3}{2},\ \frac{y_2 + y_3}{2}\right)$$

$\therefore\ x_2 + x_3 = -2$ ..... (1)

$\therefore\ y_2 + y_3 = -4$ ..... (2)

E is the mid-point of CA

$$\therefore \qquad (6,\ 1) = \left(\frac{x_1 + x_3}{2},\ \frac{y_1 + y_3}{2}\right)$$

$\therefore\ x_2 + x_3 = 12$ ..... (3)

$\therefore\ y_2 + y_3 = 2$ ..... (4)

F is the middle point of AB

$$\therefore \qquad (3,\ 5) = \left(\frac{x_2 + x_3}{2},\ \frac{y_2 + y_3}{2}\right)$$

$\therefore\ x_2 + x_1 = 6$ ..... (5)

$\therefore\ y_2 + y_1 = 10$ ..... (6)

Taking (1) + (3) + (5), $2(x_1 + x_2 + x_3) = 16$

$\therefore \qquad x_1 + x_2 + x_3 = 8$ ..... (7)

(7) – (1) $\Rightarrow x_1 = 10$

(7) – (3) $\Rightarrow x_2 = -4$

(7) – (5) $\Rightarrow x_3 = 2$

Taking (2) + (4) + (6), $2(y_1 + y_2 + y_3) = 8$

$\therefore\ y_1 + y_2 + y_3 = 4$ ..... (8)

(8) – (2) $\Rightarrow y_1 = 8$

(8) – (4) $\Rightarrow y_2 = 2$

(8) – (6) $\Rightarrow y_3 = -6$

$\therefore\ A = (x_1, y_1) = (10, 8)\ B = (x_2, y_2) = (-4, 2)$

$C = (x_3, y_3) = (2, -6)$

Exercise 4.2

1. Find the co-ordinates of the point dividing AB in given ratio in each of the following cases:

(i)	$A \equiv (2, 5)$,	$B \equiv (-3, 8)$;	(ii) 4 : 5 internally
(iii)	$A \equiv (-7, 1)$,	$B \equiv (3, 6)$;	(iv) 3 : 2 externally
(v)	$A \equiv (0, 0)$	$B \equiv (8, 10)$;	(vi) 2 : 1 externally
(vii)	$A \equiv (-1, -4)$,	$B \equiv (8, 6)$;	(viii) 5 : 7 internally

2. The line joining the points A(10, 12) and B(– 6, 6) is divided into 3 equal parts at P and Q. Find the co-ordinates of P and Q.

3. Find the points which divide the line joining the points (8, 12) and (12, 8) into four equal parts.

4. Find the co-ordinates of the middle points of the sides of the ΔABC where $A \equiv (4, 6)$, $B \equiv (6, 8)$ and $C \equiv (10, 6)$.

5. D, E, F are the middle points of BC, CA, AB of the triangle formed by A(–4, 5), B(8, 3) and C(0, –7). Find the lengths of the medians AD, BE, CF.

6. ABCD is a parallelogram in which $A \equiv (-6, -7)$, $B \equiv (3, -9)$ and $C \equiv (6, -1)$. Find the co-ordinates of D.

7. Find the ratio in which the point P(–1, 4) divide the line joining the points A(–7, 1) and B(3, 6).

8. Find the ratio in which x-axis divides the line segment joining the points (–2, 6) and (4, –2).

9. Find the ratios in which the axes of co-ordinates divide the lines joining the points (3, 5) and (–2, 7). Find also the co-ordinates of the points of section.

10. Find in what ratios the line joining the points (7, –3) and (–6, 1) is cut by the co-ordinates axes.

11. ABCD is a parallelogram in which A and B are respectively (2, 5) and (3, 1). If the point of intersection of the diagonals is (4, 4), find the co-ordinates of C and D.

12. Find the centroid of the triangle formed by the points (4, 8), (–2, 6) and (4, 7).

Answers

1. (i) $\left(-\frac{2}{9}, \frac{57}{9}\right)$ (ii) (23, 16) (iii) (16, 20) (iv) $\left(\frac{11}{4}, \frac{1}{6}\right)$
2. $\left(\frac{14}{3}, 10\right)$
3. (9, 11), (10, 10), (11, 9)
4. (8, 7), (7, 6), (5, 7)
5. $\sqrt{113}$, $\sqrt{116}$, $5\sqrt{5}$
6. (–3. 1)
7. 3:2, Internally
8. 3:1. Internally
9. 5:7, Externally, 3:2 Internally
10. 3:1, Internally, 7 : 6 Internally
11. (6, 3) (5, 7)
12. (2, 7)

4.3 STRAIGHT LINE

4.3.1 Slope or Gradient of a Straight Line

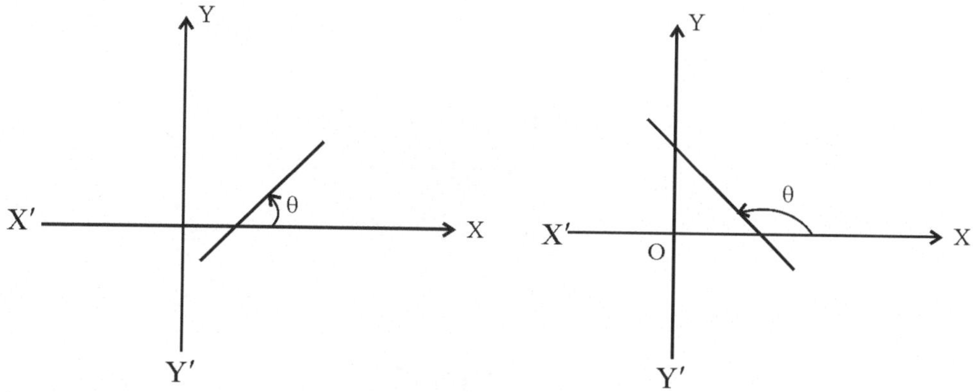

Fig. 4.11

If a straight line makes an angle θ with the positive direction of the X–axis then tan θ is called as slope or gradient of the straight line. The angle 'θ' is called the inclination of the line to the X-axis. The angle θ is measured from the positive direction of the X–axis in the anticlockwise direction as shown in the above figures. For example, if a straight line makes an angle 45° with the positive direction of the X–axis, its slope is tan 45° or equal to 1. If a straight line makes an angle 120° with the positive direction of x – axis then its slope is $\tan 120^\circ = \tan(180^\circ - 60^\circ) = -\tan 60^\circ = -\sqrt{3}$.

Note: (i) The slope or gradient of a line is positive or negative according to the inclination 'θ' of the line of the x-axis is acute or obtuse.

(ii) If a straight line is || to X-axis then θ = 0. ∴ tan θ = 0. So the slope of the line is 0 and conversely. In particular, the slope of the X-axis is zero.

(iii) If a straight line is ⊥ to X-axis then $\theta = 90^0$, $\tan\theta = \tan 90^0 = \infty$.

So the slope of the line is infinite and conversely. In particular, the slope of Y–axis is infinite.

4.3.2 Conditions for Parallelism and Perpendicularity of Two Lines

Let AB and CD be two parallel lines. If AB is inclined at an angle θ to the axis, then CD is also inclined with angle θ to the x-axis. So the slope of AB = tanθ = the slope of CD.

Hence if two lines are parallel, then their slopes are equal and conversely.

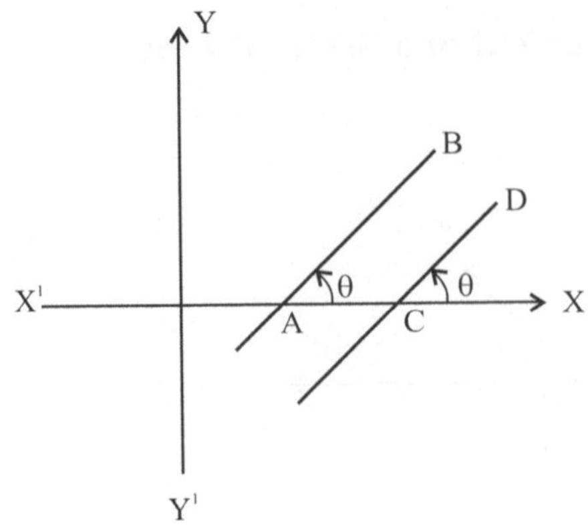

Fig. 4.12

AB and AC are perpendicular lines as shown in the figure. Let AB be inclined at an angle θ to the X–axis. Then AC is inclined at an angle 90 + θ to the X–axis. Now the slope of AB = tan θ.

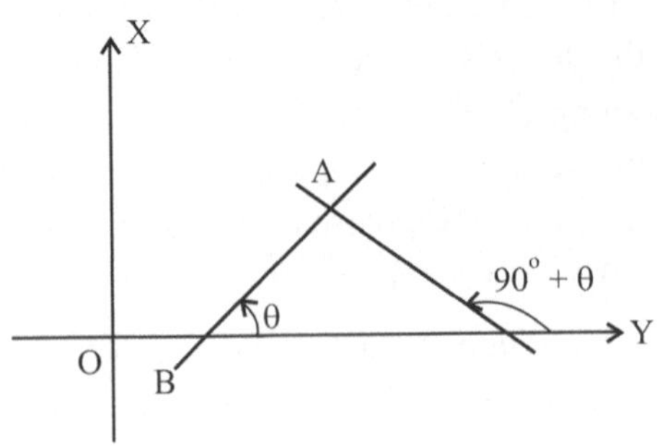

Fig. 4.13

The slope of AC is = tan (90 + θ) = – cot θ.

∴ (Slope of AB) (Slope of AC) = (tan θ) (– cot θ) = –1

Thus, if two lines are perpendicular then the product of their slopes is –1 and conversely.

Note: If we take the slope of two lines as m_1 and m_2 then the lines are parallel if $m_1 = m_2$ and they are perpendicular if $m_1m_2 = -1$.

4.3.3 Slope of a Line Joining Two Points

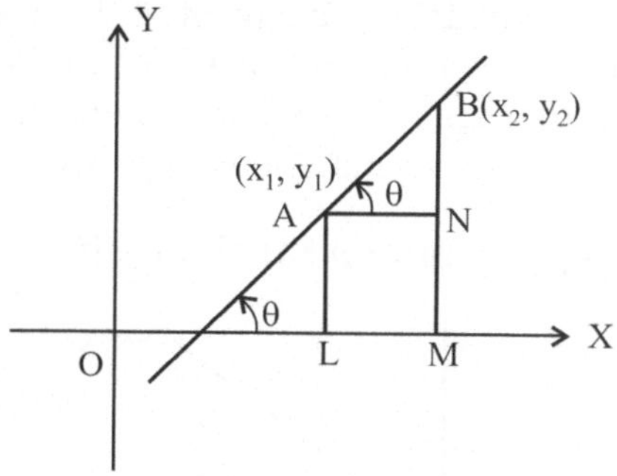

Fig. 4.14

Let A and B be the points (x_1, y_1) and (x_2, y_2) respectively. Let AB be inclined at an angle θ to the x-axis. Draw AL, BM ⊥ to X-axis and AN ⊥ to BM. $OL = x_1$, $AL = y_1$, $OM = x_2$, $BM = y_2$

Since AN is || to x-axis, $B\hat{A}N = \theta$

The slope of AB $= \tan\theta = \frac{AN}{AB} = \frac{BM - NM}{LM} = \frac{BM - AL}{OM - OL} = \frac{y_2 - y_1}{x_2 - x_1}$

∴ The slope of the line joining the two points (x_1, y_1) and (x_2, y_2) is $\frac{y_2 - y_1}{x_2 - x_1}$

For example, if A ≡ (3, –4) and B≡ (–1, 5) the slope of AB $= \frac{y_2 - y_1}{x_2 - x_1} = \frac{5-(-4)}{-1-3} = \frac{9}{-4} = -\frac{9}{4}$

Intercepts on x and y axes

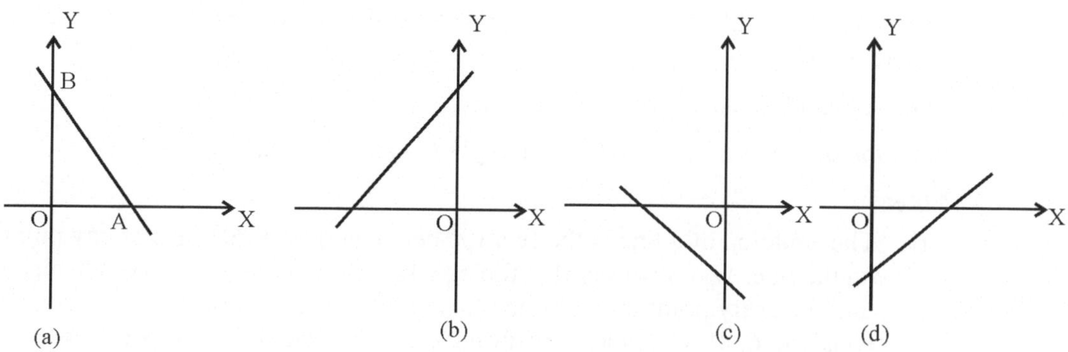

Fig. 4.15

In figure if a straight line cuts the x-axis at A and Y-axis at B, OA is called the X-intercept and OB is called the y-intercept of the line. Here in Fig. 4.15(a), both intercepts OA, OB are positive. In Fig.4.15(b), x-intercept is negative and y-intercept is positive. In Fig.4.15 (c) both intercepts are negative and in Fig.4.15 (d), x-intercept is positive and Y-intercept is negative.

4.3.4 Slope-Intercept form of a Straight Line

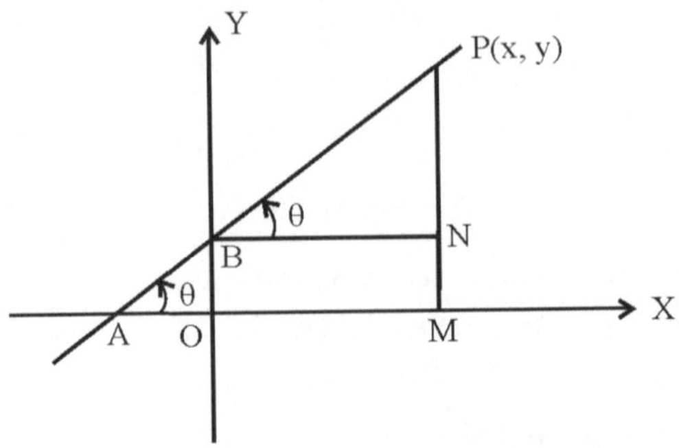

Let the line cut the x-axis at A and Y-axis at B and be inclined at an angle θ to x-axis. Slope of the line = tan θ = m (given)

$$OB = y - \text{intercept} = c \text{ (given)}$$

Let P(x, y) be any point on the line. Drawn PM ⊥ to X-axis and BN ⊥ to PM. From the triangle BPN we have

$$\tan\theta = \frac{PN}{BN} \quad \text{i.e., } m = \frac{PM - NM}{OM} \quad \text{i.e., } m = \frac{PM - OB}{OM}$$

$$\text{i.e., } \quad m = \frac{y - c}{x} \text{ or } mx = y - c \text{ or } y = mx + c$$

This is the equation of the straight line whose slope is m and

Example: A straight line is inclined at 135° to the X-axis and is Y-intercept is 6. Find its equation.

Here m = tan θ = tan 135° = – 1; c = 6

Equation of the line is, y = mx + c i.e, y = (–1) x + 6 i.e., x + y = 6

Note:

(i) The equation of a line is the relation between the coordinates of any point on the line. When we say that the equation of a line is $x + y = 6$, we mean that for every point on that line the sum of x and y co-ordinates is always equal to 6. If you take any point on this line, the x co-ordinate + y co-ordinate of that point is 6 and conversely if there is a point whose x co-ordinate + y co-ordinate is 6 then that point is on the line. For example (4, 2) is a point on the line because 4 + 2 = 6. (–5, 11) is a point on the lines because –5 + 11 = 6, (3, 2) is not a point on the line because $3 + 2 \neq 6$. Further if (x_1, y_1) is a point on the line, then we can write $x_1 + y_1 = 6$.

(ii) If c = 0 the line passes through O. That is y = mx is the equation of a line passing through the origin and having the slope m.

4.3.5 Point–Slope Form

Equation of a straight line passing through a given point (x_1, y_1) and having a given slope m.

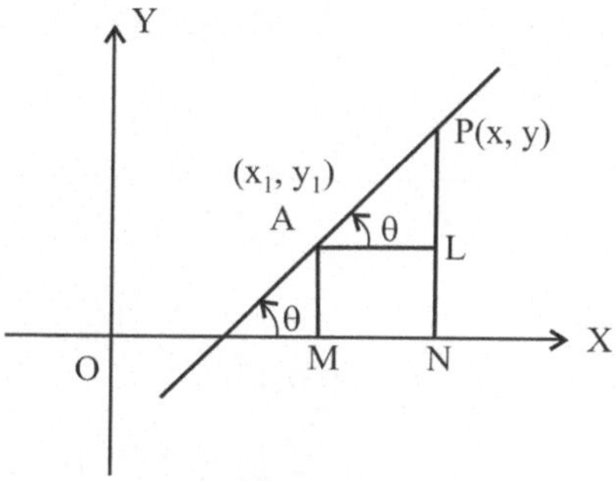

Fig. 4.16

Let the straight line pass through the point $A(x_1, y_1)$ and be inclined at an angle θ to the line is tan θ = m (given). Let P(x, y) be any point on the line. Draw AM, PN ⊥ to x-axis and AL ⊥ to PN.

$$OM = x_1,\ AM = y_1,\ ON = x,\ PN = y.\ P\hat{A}L = \theta \text{ (because AL } \| \text{ to x-axis)}$$

From the triangle APL, $\tan\theta = \dfrac{PL}{AL}$

i.e., $m = \dfrac{PN - LN}{MN}$ i.e., $m = \dfrac{PN - AM}{ON - OM}$ i.e., $m = \dfrac{y - y_1}{x - x_1}$

$\therefore$ $y - y_1 = m(x - x_1)$

Hence the equation of the line passing through the points (x_1, y_1) and having the slope m is $y - y_1 = m(x - x_1)$

Example: A straight line is inclined to the x-axis at an angle $\frac{\pi}{3}$ and passes through the point (–2, 3). Find its equation.

$$(x_1, y_1) \equiv (-2, 3);\ m = \tan(\pi/3) = \sqrt{3}$$

Equation of the line is $y - y_1 = m(x - x_1)$

$$y - 3 = \sqrt{3}(x + 2) \text{ i.e., } x\sqrt{3} - y + 3 3 + 2\sqrt{3} = 0$$

4.4 TWO POINT FORM

4.4.1 Equation of a Straight Line Passing through Two Points

Let the straight line pass through the points $A(x_1, y_1)$ an $B(x_2, y_2)$. Let $P(x, y)$ be any point on the line AB.

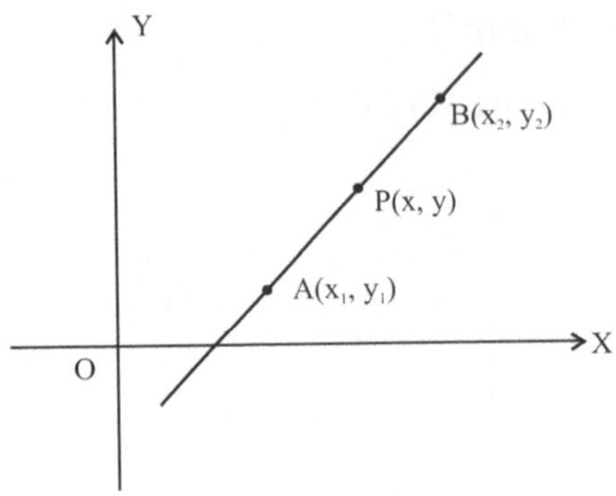

Fig. 4.17

$$\text{Slope of AP} = \frac{y - y_1}{x - x_1}; \qquad \text{Slope of AB} = \frac{y_2 - y_1}{x_2 - x_1}$$

Since A, P, B lie on the same line, slope of AP = slope of AB

i.e.,
$$\frac{y - y_1}{x - x_1} = \frac{y_2 - y_1}{x_2 - x_1}$$

Hence the equation of the line passing through the points (x_1, y_1) and (x_2, y_2) is

$$\frac{y - y_1}{x - x_1} = \frac{y_2 - y_1}{x_2 - x_1}$$

$$(y - y_1) = \left(\frac{y_2 - y_1}{x_2 - x_1}\right)(x - x_1)$$

Example

1. Find the equation of the straight line which passes through the points (2, – 3) and (5, 6).

Solution: $(x_1, y_1) = (2, -3)$; $(x_2, y_2) = (5, 6)$

Equation of the lines is

i.e., $\frac{y+3}{x-2} = \frac{6+3}{5-2}$ i.e., $\frac{y+3}{x-2} = \frac{9}{3}$ i.e., $\frac{y+3}{x-2} = \frac{3}{1}$

$$3x - 6 = y + 3; \; 3x - y - 9 = 0$$

4.4.2 Intercept Form

Equation of a straight line whose x and y intercepts are given

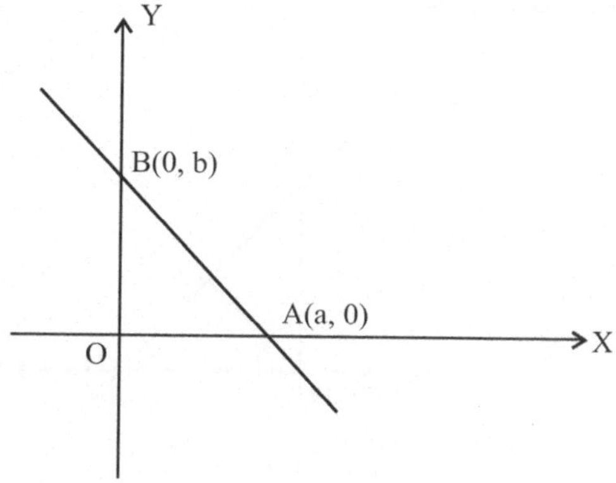

Fig. 4.18

Let the straight line cut the X-axis at A and Y-axis at B.

OA = x – intercept = a

OB = y – intercept = b

$\therefore$ A ≡ (a, 0); B≡(0, b)

Using two-point form, the equation of AB is $\frac{y-y_1}{x-x_1}=\frac{y_2-y_1}{x_2-x_1}$

i.e., $\frac{y-0}{x-a}=\frac{b-0}{o-a}$ i.e., $\frac{y}{x-a}=\frac{b}{-a}$

$$bx - ab = -ay;\ bx + ay = ab(\div by\, ab)\ \frac{x}{a}+\frac{y}{b}=1$$

$\therefore$ The equation of the straight line when x and y intercepts are a, b respectively is $\frac{x}{a}+\frac{y}{b}=1$

Example: A straight line cut off positive intercepts 3 and 5 on x and y axes repectively. Find its equation.

Here a = 3, b = 5. $\therefore$ Equation of the line is $\frac{x}{a}+\frac{y}{b}=1$

i.e., $\frac{x}{3}+\frac{y}{5}=1$ or $5x+3y=15$

4.4.3 Normal Form

Equation of a straight line for which the length of ⊥ from the origin is p and α is the inclination of the ⊥ to X-axis

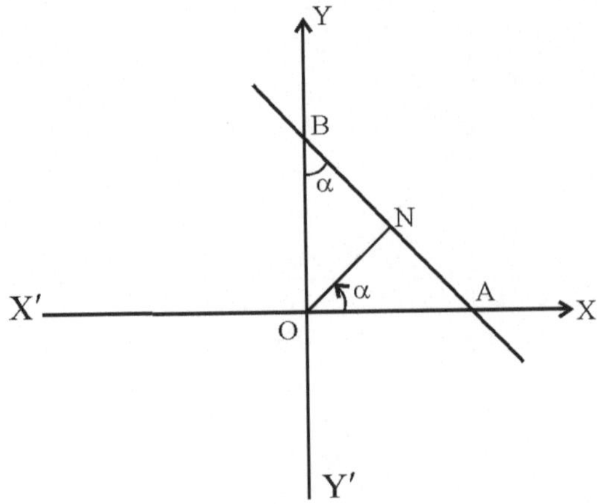

Fig. 4.19

Let the line cut the X-axis at A and Y-axis at B.

Draw ON ⊥ to AB.

ON = p Take $X\hat{O}N = \alpha$ Then $B\hat{O}N = 90^0 - \alpha$

∴ OBN = α

From the Δ OAN, $\cos\alpha = \frac{ON}{OA} = \frac{P}{OA}$

∴ $OA \cos\alpha = p$

or $$OA = \frac{p}{\cos\alpha}.$$

From the Δ OBN, $\sin\alpha = \frac{ON}{OB} = \frac{p}{OB}$

∴ $OB \sin\alpha = p$ ..... (2)

Since OA and OB are x and y intercepts of the lines equation of the line is

$$\frac{x}{OA} + \frac{y}{OB} = 1$$

i.e., $$\frac{x\cos\alpha}{p} + \frac{y\sin\alpha}{p} = 1$$

i.e., $x \cos \alpha + y \sin \alpha = p$

This is the equation of the line where p is the length of ⊥ from the origin to the line and α is the angle between the perpendicular and the positive direction of x-axis

Note: α is always measured from the positive direction of X-axis, in the anticlockwise direction.

Example: The length of ⊥ from the origin to a line is $5\sqrt{2}$ and the perpendicular is inclined at an angle $\frac{3\pi}{4}$ to the X-axis. What is the equation of line?

Here $p = 5\sqrt{2}, \quad \alpha = \frac{3\pi}{4}$

Equation of the line $x \cos\alpha + y \sin\alpha = p$

$$x \cos\frac{3\pi}{4} + y \sin\frac{3\pi}{4} = 5\sqrt{2} \text{ or } x\left(-\frac{1}{\sqrt{2}}\right) + y\left(\frac{1}{\sqrt{2}}\right) = 5\sqrt{2}$$

$$-x + y = 10 \quad \text{or} \quad x - y + 10 = 0$$

General Equation of a Line

The general first degree equation ax + by + c = 0, where a, b, c are constants (not all of them 0 at the same time) always represents a straight line.

$$ax + by + c = 0 \qquad .....(1)$$

(1) represents some locus and we have to prove that the locus is a straight line. Let $A(x_1, y_1)$ and $B(x_2, y_2)$ be points on the locus represented by (1). So we have,

$$ax_1 + by_1 + c = 0; \; ax_2 + by_2 + c = 0 \qquad .....(2)$$

Let $P(x_3, y_3)$ be the point which divides AB internally (or externally) in the ratio r : 1

Then $$P(x_3, y_3) \equiv \left[\frac{rx_2 + 1.x_1}{r+1}, \frac{ry_2 + 1.y_1}{r+1}\right]$$

So we have, $$x_3 = \frac{rx_2 + x_1}{r+1}, \; y_3 = \frac{ry_2 + y_1}{r+1}$$

Substitute $x = x_3$, $y = y_3$ in the LHS of (1). Then,

LHS of (1) = $ax_3 + by_3 + c$

$$= a\left(\frac{rx_2 + x_1}{r+1}\right) + b\left(\frac{ry_2 + y_1}{r+1}\right) + c$$

$$= \frac{arx_2 + ax_1 + bry_2 + by_1 + cr + c}{r+1}$$

$$= \frac{r(0) + 0}{r+1} = 0 \qquad \text{[using (2)]}$$

This means the point $P(x_3, y_3)$ lies on the locus (1). But $P(x_3, y_3)$ is any point on the line AB. So every point on the line AB lies on the locus (1). Therefore, the locus (1) should be the equation of the line AB. Thus the equation $ax + by + c = 0$ represents straight line.

Note:

(i) If a, b, c are all non–zero constants, then we can write.

$ax + by + c = 0$ as $by = ax - c$ or $y = \frac{ax}{b} - \frac{c}{b}$ which is of the form

$y = mx + c$ where $m = -\frac{a}{b}$ and y – intercepts is $\frac{-c}{b}$

$\therefore$ Slope of the line $ax + by + c = 0$ is $\frac{-c}{b}$ i.e., $\frac{-\text{coefficient of x}}{\text{coefficient of y}}$

For example slope of $\frac{x}{4} + \frac{4}{3} = 1$ is $= \frac{\frac{-1}{4}}{\frac{1}{3}} = \frac{-3}{4}$

(ii) If $a \neq 0$, $b \neq 0$, $c \neq 0$, then the equation (1) becomes $ax + by = 0$ or $y = \frac{-a}{b}x$ which is a straight line passing through the origin and having the slope $\frac{-a}{b}$

(iii) If $a = 0$, $b \neq 0$, $c \neq 0$, then the equation (1) becomes $by + c = 0$ or $y = \frac{-c}{b}$ which is a straight line parallel to x-axis

(iv) If $a \neq 0$, $b = 0$, $c \neq 0$, then the equation (1) becomes $ax + c = 0$ or $x = \frac{-c}{a}$ which is a straight line parallel to y-axis.

(v) If $a = 0$, $b \neq 0$, $c = 0$, Then the equation (1) is $by = 0$ or $y = 0$ which is the axis.

(vi) If $a \neq 0$, $b \neq 0$, $c = 0$, then the equation (1) is $ax = 0$ or $x = 0$, which is the y-axis.

Exercise 4.3

1. If (x, 2) is a point on the join of (2, 5) and (–1, 4), find x.
2. If A = (2, 3), B = (–2, 4), C = (1, 6), D = (2, 10), Show that AB $\perp$ CD
3. Find the equation of the line cutting off the intercept –6 on the Y-axis and inclined at an angle 60^0 to the X-axis
4. Find the equation of the straight line passing through the point A = (3, 2) and B = (4, 5)
5. Find the equation of the straight line making an angle 120° with the positive direction of X-axis and passing through (–1, 2)
6. Find the equation of the straight line cutting off intercepts which are in the ratio 3:5 and passing through (4, –3)
7. ABC is a triangle formed by the points A = (4, 8), B = (2, 4) and C = (6, 6). Find the equations of the lines (i) passing through A and Parallel to BC (ii) passing through B and Perpendicular to AC
8. Prove that the middle point of the join of (3, –1) and (5, 11) lies on the line joining the points (–1, –2) and (4, 5).
9. Show that the $3x + 4y - 7 = 0$ and $6x + 8y + 3 = 0$ are parallel to each other.
10. Show that the lines $6x - 10y + 3 = 0$ and $2x - y + 1 = 0$ are perpendicular to each other
11. If the lines $6x - 10y + 3 = 0$ and $kx - 5y + 8 = 0$ are parallel, find the value of k.
12. Find the equations of the straight lines passing through (–1, –5) and respectively parallel and perpendicular to the line $2x + 3y - 5 = 0$
13. Find the equation of the line given that $p = 5$, $\alpha = 60^0$
14. Find the equation of the line given that $p = 6$, $\alpha = 150^0$

Answers

1. -7,

3. $Y = \sqrt{3}x - 6$

4. $3x - y - 8 = 0$

5. $\sqrt{3}x + y - 2 + \sqrt{3}$

6. $5x + 3y = 11$

7. $x - 2y + 12 = 0, x - y + 2 = 0$

11. $k = 3$

12. $2x + 3y + 17 = 0$ & $3x - 2y - 7 = 0$

13. $x + \sqrt{3}y = 0$

14. $x - \sqrt{3}y + 3 = 0$

4.5 APPLICATION IN PHARMACY

1. The slope of straight line is used to know the rate of change of concentration or to calculate the elimation rate constant of a drug between time intervals t_1 and t_2, where the corresponding concentrations are measured as $\log c_1$ and $\log c_2$, when the elimination of Pharmacokinetics Parameters in IV bolus method is written in the form of $\log(C) = \log(C_0) - \frac{K_e t}{2.303}$ when it is tansformed from natural Logarithms to Common logarithms.

   The Equation can written as $\log(C) = -\frac{K_e t}{2.303} + \log(C_0)$ and it can be compared with equation of the straight Y = mX + C, where m is slope and C is intercept

Time	Con	Log(C)
1	8	0.9031
2	6.3	0.7993
3	4.9	0.6902
4	4	0.6021
5	3.2	0.5051
6	2.5	0.3979

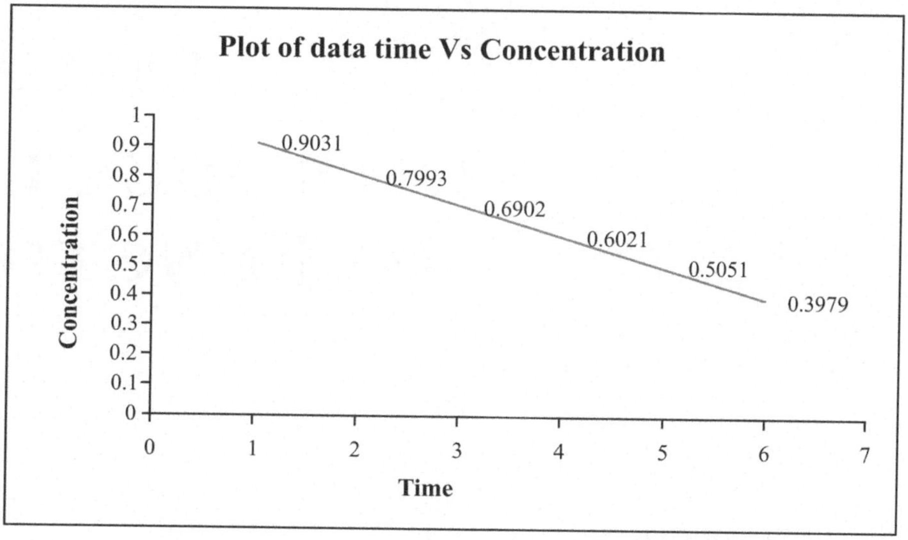

Fig. 4.20

Slope = – 0.1091/2.303

Equate slope with $-\frac{K_e}{2.303}$

$-K_e = (-0.1091)$

The Elimination rate constant $K_e = 0.1091$

CHAPTER 5

INTRODUCTION TO FUNCTIONS

5.1 INTRODUCTION

Function: A function, in mathematics, is a rule that assigns each element of a set to an element of the same or of another set.

Real Valued Function: The function that assign to each real number, from some set of real numbers, to another set of real numbers. Such functions are called as real-valued function. This will be called as simply a function.

Example: If $y = x^2$

$$A = \{1, 2, 3, 4, 5, 6\}$$

$$B = \{1, 4, 9, 16, 25, 36\}$$

The rule that assigns one number to another may be of any nature. For example, we may want to assign every number to its square.

We write this function in the form as $X \rightarrow Y$, where $Y = X^2$. Here X is called as independent variable (representing the number to which we assign to another variable) and Y is called as dependent (which represents the number assigned to the first one) variable.

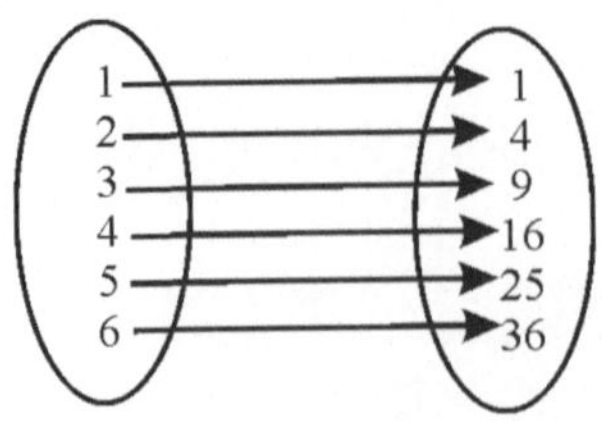

The Set of numbers to which other numbers are assigned is called the **Domain of Definition** of a function.

5.2 CLASSIFICATION REAL VALUED FUNCTIONS

1. **Algebraic functions:** Any real valued function which involves different powers of x, which are connected by the four fundamental operations of arithmetic (+, –, ×, ÷) and the constant quantities are called as algebraic function.

   Example: $f(x) = x^2$, $f(x) = x^3 + 5x^2 - 3x + 1$, $f(x) = \frac{x+1}{x^3 - 1}$

2. **Transcendental functions:** A function which is not algebraic is called a transcendental function. They are classified as:

   (a) Trigonometric functions

   (b) Logarithmic functions and

   (c) Exponential function.

   (a) ***Trigonometric functions***: The function of the type y = sin(x), y = cos(x), y = tan(x), y = cosec(x), y = sec(x) and y = cot(x) are called as trigonometric functions.

   (b) ***Logarithmic functions***: A function of the form $y = \log_a x$ is called as logarithmic function, and a is a positive number not equal to 1.

   When x = 1, y = 0. When x > 1, the logarithmic function increases without any bound (i.e., tends to ∞) and similarly it increases negatively without any bound (i.e., tends to –∞) when 0 < x < 1. The graph of logarithm function is as shown below.

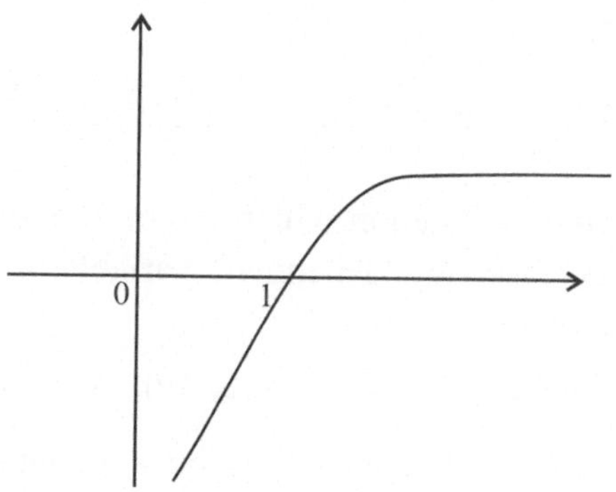

(c) ***Exponential functions***: A function of the form $y = a^x$ or $y = e^x$ is called as exponential function, a and e are positive real numbers

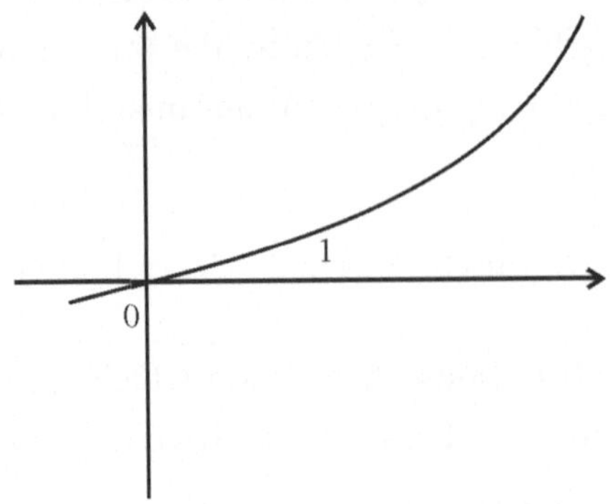

5.3 TYPES OF REAL VALUED FUNCTIONS

1. ***Even functions***: A function $Y = f(x)$ is called as even function of x, if for all values of x,

$$f(-x) = f(x)$$

Example: $y = \cos(x), \quad y = x^2$

2. ***Odd functions***: A function $y = f(x)$ is called as odd function of x if for all values of x,

$$f(-x) = -f(x)$$

Example: $y = \sin(x), \quad y = x^3$

3. ***Explicit functions***: A function in which the dependent variable y is expresses uniquely in terms of the independent variable x is called as explicit function.

Example: $Y = x^2, \; Y = x^3 + 5x^2 - 3x + 1, \; f(x) = \dfrac{x+1}{x^3 - 1}$

4. ***Implicit functions***: A function which is not explicit is called as implicit function. In this case, the dependent variable y cannot be expressed uniquely in term of x.

Example: $x^2 + y^2 = 25, \; a^x + b^y + \cos x = 0, \quad x^3 + y^3 + 3xy(x + y) = 0$

5. ***Parametric functions***: Let $Y = f(x)$ be a given function. If both the independent variable x and the dependent variable y can be expressed in

terms of a third variable θ is called as parametric form of the function, θ is called the parameter.

Example: If $y=\sqrt{1-x^2}$, $x = \cos(\theta)$, $y = \sin(\theta)$ will satisfy the function $y=\sqrt{1-x^2}$.

5.4 LIMITS AND CONTINUITY

Introduction

The concept of real valued functions has already been introduced in chapter. In this chapter, we develop two important fundamental concepts of calculus viz. the limit and the continuity of a function which distinguish calculus from algebra and trigonometry. We use limits to describe the way a function $f:R \to R$ varies. Some functional vary continuously i.e., a small change in x produce a small change in f(x). Some functions have values that jump or vary erratically. We are familiar with drawing graph of a function. In doing so, we plot function values in a graph sheet and the plotted points are connected with an unbroken curve assuming that we are working with a continuous function but this is not always true. During 1920s, the physicists discovered that in many practical situations the corresponding function varies in a discrete passion and not continuously. For example, the vibrating atoms in a hydrogen molecule can oscillate only at discrete energy levels and heated atoms emit light at discrete frequencies and not in continuous spectra. Because of these reasons, the concept of continuity has attained a great importance.

5.4.1 Limit of a Function

We first try to understand the intuitive idea of limit of a function by considering the following example.

Consider the function $f(x)=\dfrac{x^2-1}{x-1}$. This function is defined at all real values of x except at x = 1. Because at x = 1, $f(1)=\dfrac{0}{0}$ which is neither equal to 1 nor equal to ∞ and is a meaningless expression. Such an expression is called an indeterminate in mathematics. In this case, we say that the function is not defined at x = 1. Our aim is to know the behavior of the function near 1 i.e., value of the function f(x) at x which is slightly greater than or slightly less than 1. This can be seen from the following tables.

For $\quad x \neq 1, \quad f(x) = \dfrac{x^2 - 1}{x - 1} = \dfrac{(x-1)(x+1)}{(x-1)} = x + 1$

Table 1

For $\quad x < 1$

Value of x is increasing and approaching 1 ↓ 1

x	f(x)
.9	1.9
.99	1.99
.999	1.999
.9999	1.9999
-	-
-	-
-	-
-	-
-	-
-	-
-	-
-	-
-	-

Value of f(x) is increasing and approaching 2 ↓ 2

Table 2

For $x > 1$

Value of x is decreasing and approaching 1 ↓ 1

x	f(x)
1.1	2.1
1.01	2.01
1.001	2.001
1.0001	2.0001
1.00001	2.00001
-	-
-	-
-	-
-	-
-	-
-	-
-	-
-	-

Value of f(x) is decreasing and approaching 2 ↓ 2

From the above tables, we conclude that when x approaches the value 1, the function f(x) approaches the value 2. This situation can be represented on the real number line as follows.

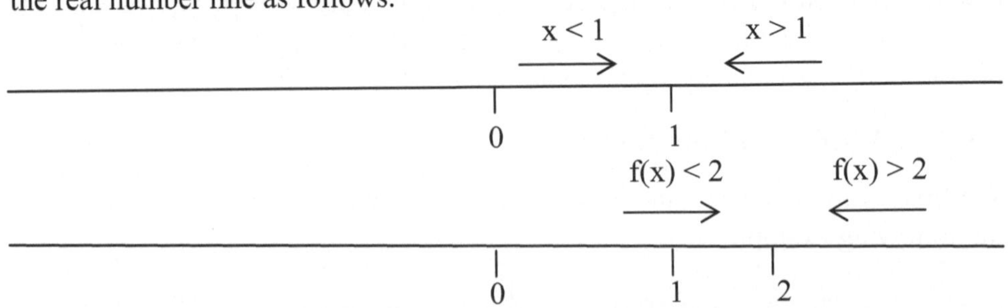

The value 2 to which the function f(x) approaches as x approaches 1 is called the limit of the function. Even though the function f(x) assumes the indeterminate form $\frac{0}{0}$ at x = 1, we can find a well defined value to which the function f(x) approaches. In this case, we write $\lim\limits_{x \to 1} f(x) = 2$. We read this as "limit of the function f(x) as x tends to 1 is equal to 2". From the above example, $\lim\limits_{x \to x_0} f(x) = 1$ means informally when x is sufficiently close to x_0, f(x)

gets close to *l*. To give formal definition of the limit of a function, we need the meaning of an interval and the inequality $|x - x_0| < m$.

5.4.2 Interval

Let a and b be two real numbers represented on the real number line as shown in the figure. Then the set of all real numbers [note that there are infinitely many real numbers between a and b]

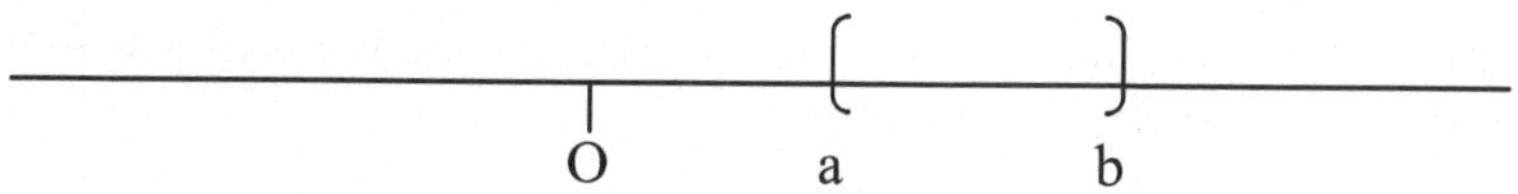

which lies between a and b on the number line is called an open interval if a and b are excluded from the set. This set is denoted by (a, b). a and b are called end points of the interval. If a and b are included in the set then the set is called a closed interval denoted by [a, b]. If a is excluded from the set and b is included in the set, then it is called – half open closed interval denoted by (a, b]. Similarly we can define (a, b) which is called half – closed – open interval. The open interval (a, b) is equivalent to the double inequality $a < x < b$ which means all real numbers x lying between a and b.

Meaning of $| x - x_0 | < m$

We defined the modules of x i.e. $|x|$ as follows,

$$|x| = x \quad \text{if } x \geq 0$$

$$= -x \quad \text{if } < 0$$

$$\therefore \quad |x - x_0| = x - x_0 \text{ if } x - x_0 \geq 0 \text{ or } x \geq x_0$$

$$= -(x - x_0) \text{ if } x - x_0 < 0 \text{ or } x < x_0$$

Hence the inequality $|x - x_0| < m$ can be split as $x - x_0 < m$ and $-(x - x_0) < m$

i.e., $x_0 - m < x < x_0 + m$

Combining the two inequalities, we get,

$$x_0 - m < x < x_0 + m$$

which means that x belongs to the interval $(x_0 - m, x_0 + m)$

$\therefore \; |x - x_0| < m \Rightarrow x \in (x_0 - m, x_0 + m)$ which is an open interval with x_0 as mid-point. We can represent this graphically as follows.

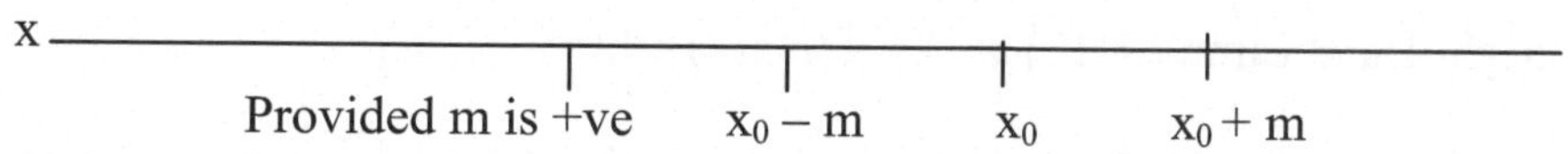

Hence if we say x is sufficiently close to x_0, then it means that x belongs to an open interval with x_0 as mid-point.

Definition of Limit of a Function (∈ - δ Definition) : A function f(x) is said to tend to the limit l as x tends to x_0, if given ∈ > 0, however small it may be there exists a δ > 0 such that $|f(x) - l| < \in$ when $|x - x_0| < \delta$

The above definition of limit of a function simply says that when x is very close to x_0, the function f(x) is very close to l. In this case, we write $\lim_{x \to x_0} f(x) = 1$

***Note*:** suppose a function f(x) is defined at x = x_0, then the limit of the function is the value of the function i.e., $f(x_0)$ itself. Later we will see that the function is continuous at such. For example,

$$\lim_{x \leftarrow 2} \frac{x^2 - 1}{x - 1} = \frac{4 - 1}{2 - 1} = 3$$

Left Hand and Right Hand Limits

Suppose the function f(x) tends to the limit l_1 as x tends to x_0 from values which are greater than x_0. That is, on the number lines, x is tending to x_0 from right side of x_0 as shown in the figure.

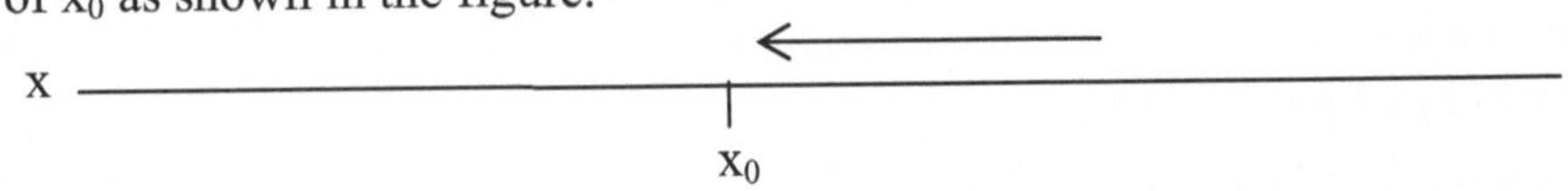

This limit is called the right hand limit of the function denoted by $\lim_{x \to x_0 + 0} f(x) = l_1$

If the function f(x) tends to the limit l_2 as x tends to x_0 from values which are less than x_0. That is on the number line, x is tending to x_0 from left side of x_0 as shown in the figure.

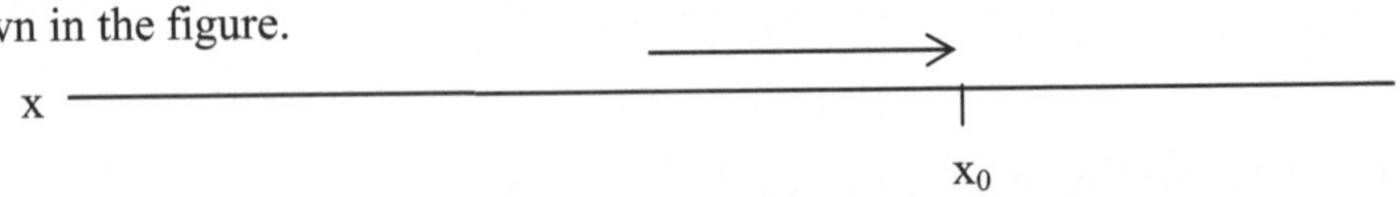

this limit is called the left hand limit of the function denoted by $\lim_{x \to x_0 + 0} f(x) = l_2$.

If $l_1 = l_2$, then we say that the $\lim_{x \to x_0} f(x)$ exists.

For example, consider the function $f(x) = \begin{cases} x + 1 & \text{if } x \leq 0 \\ x + 2 & \text{if } x > 0 \end{cases}$

Left Hand Limit (LHL) at $0 = \lim_{x \to 0-0} f(x) = \lim_{x \to 0} x + 1 = 1$

Right Hand Limit (RHL) at $0 = \lim_{x \to 0+0} f(x) = \lim_{x \to 0} x + 2 = 2$

In this case, both LHL and RHL exists but $\lim_{x \to 0} f(x)$ does not exist. $(\because 1 \neq 2)$

Consider the function f(x) = $f(x)=\begin{cases}3x+1 \text{ if } x\geq 2\\ 4x-1 \text{ if } x<2\end{cases}$

In this case, LHL at $2=\lim\limits_{x\to 2-0} f(x)=\lim\limits_{x\to 2} 4x-1=7$

RHL at $2=\lim\limits_{x\to 2+0} f(x)=\lim\limits_{x\to 2} 3x+1=7$

Here, both LHL and RHL at 2 exist and $\lim\limits_{x\to 0} f(x)$ also exists

$(\because \text{LHL} = \text{RHL} = 7)$

We now state some important properties of limits of functions (Algebra of limits) which we use in finding limits of given functions.

Let $\lim\limits_{x\to a} f(x)=l, \lim\limits_{x\to a} g(x)=m$

1. *Sum rule*: $\lim\limits_{x\to a}[f(x)+g(x)]=l+m$
2. *Difference rule*: $\lim\limits_{x\to a}[f(x)-g(x)]=l-m$
3. *Product rule*: $\lim\limits_{x\to a}[f(x).g(x)]=lm$
4. *Constant multiple rule*: $\lim\limits_{x\to a}[cf(x)]=cl$, where c is a constant
5. *Quotient rule*: $\lim\limits_{x\to a}\frac{f(x)}{g(x)}=\frac{1}{m}$ where $m\neq 0$
6. *Power rule*: $\lim\limits_{x\to a}[f(x)]^{\frac{m}{n}}=l^{\frac{m}{n}}$ where m and n are integers, provide $l^{\frac{m}{n}}$ is a real number.

To evaluate the limit of a function at a given point, we use some standard limits. Let us state and prove three such standard limits.

Show that $\lim\limits_{x®a}\frac{x^n-a^n}{x-a}=na^{n-1}$, where n is any rational number.

Case 1: Let n be a positive integer

Using the formula

$$(x^n-a^n)=(x-a)(x^{n-1}+x^{n-2}.\ a+x^{n-3}.\ a^2+...+a^{n-1})$$

$$\lim_{x\to a}\left(\frac{x^n-a^n}{x-a}\right)=\lim_{x\to a}\left[\frac{(x-a)(x^{n-1}+x^{n-2}.a+x^{n-3}.a^2+...+a^{n-1}}{(x-a)}\right]$$

$$=\lim_{x\to a}\left[(x^{n-1}+x^{n-2}.\ a+x^{n-3}.\ a^2+...+a^{n-1}\right]$$

$$=a^{n-1}+a^{n-2}.\ a+a^{n-3}.\ a^2+...+a^{n-1}$$

$$=a^{n-1}+a^{n-1}.\ a+a^{n-1}+...+a^{n-1}$$

$$=na^{n-1}(\because \text{there are n terms})$$

$$\therefore \qquad \lim_{x\to a}\left(\frac{x^n-a^n}{x-1}\right)=n.a^{n-1} \text{ when n is a positive integer.}$$

Case 2: Let n be a negative integer

Take n = – m where m is a positive integer

$$\text{Now, } \therefore \lim_{x\to a}\left(\frac{x^n-a^n}{x-a}\right)=\lim_{x\to a}\left(\frac{x^{-m}-a^{-m}}{x-a}\right)(\because n=-m)$$

$$=\lim_{x\to a}\left[\frac{\frac{1}{x^m}-\frac{1}{a^m}}{x-a}\right]=\lim_{x\to a}\left[\frac{1}{x^m a^m}\left(\frac{a^m-x^m}{x-a}\right)\right]$$

$$=\lim_{x\to a}\left[\frac{-1}{x^m a^m}\left(\frac{x^m-a^n}{x-a}\right)\right]$$

$$=\frac{-1}{a^m a^m}.m.a^{m-1} \text{ (Using case 1)}$$

$$=\frac{-m.a^{m-1}}{a^{2m}}=-m.a^{m-1-2m}=-m.a^{-m-1}=n.a^{n-1}(\because -m=n)$$

$$\therefore \qquad \lim_{x\to a}\left(\frac{x^n-a^n}{x-a}\right)=n.a^{n-1} \text{ when n is a negative integer}$$

Case 3: Let n be a fraction (positive or negative)

Take $n=\frac{p}{q}$ where q is a positive integer and p is any integer.

Now $\therefore \quad \lim_{x\to a}\left(\frac{x^n - a^n}{x - a}\right) = \lim_{x\to a}\left(\frac{x^{\frac{p}{q}} - a^{\frac{p}{q}}}{x - a}\right)$ .....(1)

Take $x = y^q$ and $a = c^q$, then $x^{p/q} = (y^q)^{p/q} = y^p$ and $a^{p/q} = (c^q)^{p/q} = c^p$

Further when $x \rightarrow a$, $y^p \rightarrow c^p$ i.e., $y \rightarrow c$ So, (1) becomes

$$\lim_{x\to a}\left(\frac{x^{\frac{p}{q}} - a^{\frac{p}{q}}}{x - a}\right) = \lim_{x\to c}\left[\frac{y^p - c^p}{y^q - c^q}\right]$$

$$= \lim_{y\to c}\left[\frac{\left(\frac{y^p - c^p}{y - c}\right)}{\left(\frac{y^q - c^q}{y - c}\right)}\right] \quad .....(2)$$

by dividing both Nr and Dr by $(y - c)$

$$\frac{\lim_{y\to c}\left(\frac{y^p - c^p}{y - c}\right)}{\lim_{y\to c}\left(\frac{y^q - c^q}{y - c}\right)} = \frac{pc^{p-1}}{qc^{q-1}} \text{ by cases (1) and (2)}$$

$$= \left(\frac{p}{q}\right)c^{(p-q)}$$

$$= \left(\frac{p}{q}\right)(a^{1/q})^{(p-q)} \qquad \because c^q = a \Rightarrow c \Rightarrow a^{1/q}$$

$$= \frac{p}{q}a^{\frac{p-q}{q}}$$

$$= \left(\frac{p}{q}\right)a^{(p/q-1)} = n.a^{n-1} \qquad \left(\because \frac{p}{q} = n\right)$$

$$\therefore \quad \lim_{x\to a}\left(\frac{x^n - a^n}{x - a}\right) = n.a^{n-1} \text{ where n is a fraction}$$

Hence for all rational values of n,

$$\therefore \quad \lim_{x\to a}\left(\frac{x^n - a^n}{x - a}\right) = n.a^{n-1}$$

Worked Examples

1. Evaluate $\lim\limits_{x\to 5}\dfrac{x^2-25}{x-5}$

Given limit $=\lim\limits_{x\to 5}\dfrac{x^2-5^2}{x-5}=2.5^{2-1}=2\times 5=10$

2. Evaluate $\lim\limits_{x\to 2}\dfrac{x^3+8}{x+2}$

Given limit $=\lim\limits_{x\to 2}\dfrac{x^3-(-2)^3}{x-(-2)}=3(-2)^{3-1}$

$=3(-2)^2$

$=3\times 4=12$

3. Evaluate $\lim\limits_{x\to 3}\dfrac{x-3}{\sqrt[3]{x}-\sqrt[3]{3}}$

Given limit $=\lim\limits_{x\to 3}\dfrac{\frac{1}{x^{1/3}-3^{1/3}}}{x-3}=\dfrac{1}{\frac{1}{3}\times 3^{\frac{1}{3}-1}}=\dfrac{3}{3^{\frac{-2}{3}}}$

$=3.3^{2/3}=3^{5/3}$

4. Evaluate $\lim\limits_{x\to a}\dfrac{x^{\frac{5}{8}}-a^{\frac{5}{8}}}{x^{\frac{1}{3}}-a^{\frac{1}{3}}}$

$=\dfrac{\frac{5}{8}a^{5/8-1}}{\frac{1}{3}a^{1/3-1}}=\dfrac{15a^{-3/8}}{8a^{-2/3}}=\dfrac{15}{8}a^{-3/8+2/3}$

$=\dfrac{15}{8}a^{7/24}$

5. Evaluate $\lim_{x\to 2}\left[\dfrac{\dfrac{1}{x^3}-\dfrac{1}{8}}{x-2}\right]$

$$\text{given limit} = \lim_{x\to 2}\frac{-1}{8x^3}\left[\frac{x^3-8}{x-2}\right]$$

$$= -\frac{1}{8\times 2^3}\left[3\times 2^{3-1}\right] = \frac{1}{64}\times 12 = -\frac{3}{16}$$

Exponential Limits

1. $\lim_{n\to\infty}\left(1+\dfrac{1}{n}\right)^n = e$

2. $\lim_{n\to\infty}(1+x)^{\frac{1}{x}} = e \;(\text{as } n\to\infty,\, x\to 0)$

CHAPTER 6

DIFFERENTIATION

6.1 INTRODUCTION

Differentiation is the process of finding the derivative of a function. The derivative of a function measures the rate at which a function changes. The concept of derivative is one of the most important ideas in calculus. The derivatives of functions are widely used in science, economics, computer science, Pharmacy and in medicine. In this chapter we study the techniques of finding derivatives of functions.

6.2 DERIVATIVE OF A FUNCTION

Consider a function $y = x^2 + 3$, let the value of x be 1 then $y = 1^2 + 3 = 4$

Suppose x is changed from 1 to 1.1. Then $y = (1.1)^2 + 3 = 4.21$

Increase in the value of y is $4.21 - 4 = 0.21$

These small changes in the values of x and y are called increments. The increment in x or the small change in x and y is written as Δx and Δy. In the above example, $\Delta x = 0.1$, $\Delta y = 0.21$. The ratio of the increments is

$$\frac{\Delta y}{\Delta x} = \frac{0.21}{0.1} = 2.1$$

Similarly, when $x = 0.9$, $y = 3.81$ so that $\Delta y = -0.19$

$$\therefore \quad \frac{\Delta y}{\Delta x} = \frac{-0.19}{-0.1} = 1.9$$

When Δx is made sufficiently small (positive or negative) $\frac{\Delta y}{\Delta x}$ tends to the value 2. This value is called the derivative of y w.r.t. x when x = 1. So, the derivative of a function can be defined as follows:

Consider y = f(x) where f(x) is a continuous function. If x is changed to x + Δx, where Δx is a small quantity then y changes to y + Δy, Δy being very small. Δx is a small change is x and Δy is the corresponding small change in y. Δx and Δy are called increments in x and y respectively.

Now $y = f(x),\ y + \Delta y = f(x + \Delta x)$

$\therefore \quad \Delta y = f(x + \Delta x) - y = f(x + \Delta x) - f(x)$

Dividing by Δx, $\frac{\Delta y}{\Delta x} = \frac{f(x+\Delta x) - f(x)}{\Delta x}$. This is called an incrementary ratio.

Taking limits on both sides as Δ x → 0.

$$\lim_{\Delta x \to 0}\left(\frac{\Delta y}{\Delta x}\right) = \lim_{\Delta x \to 0}\left[\frac{f(x+\Delta x) - f(x)}{\Delta x}\right]$$

If this limit exists, then it is called the derivative of y w.r.t. x or differential coefficient of y w.r.t x and it is written as $\frac{dy}{dx}$.

Thus $$\lim_{\Delta x \to 0}\left(\frac{\Delta y}{\Delta x}\right) = \frac{dy}{dx}$$

$$\therefore \quad \frac{dy}{dx} = \lim_{\Delta x \to 0}\left[\frac{f(x+\Delta x) - f(x)}{\Delta x}\right] \quad .....(1)$$

writing Δx= h,

$$\frac{dy}{dx} = \lim_{h \to 0}\left[\frac{f(x+h) - f(x)}{h}\right] \quad .....(2)$$

The process of finding the derivative of a function f(x) by using eq.(6.1) or eq.(6.2) is known as finding the derivative of a **function from first principles.**

Note: (i) Δx, Δy may be positive or negative.

(ii) $\frac{dy}{dx}$ is also denoted by $\frac{d}{dx}(y)$, y_1, y', D y or $f'(x)$

6.2.1 Right and Left Hand Derivatives

The right hand derivatives of f(x) at x = a is defined as

$$R\ f'(x) = \lim_{h \to 0+0}\left[\frac{(f(a+h) - f(a)}{h}\right] \text{ provided this limit exists.}$$

In this case h tends to 0 through the positive values.

The left hand derivative of f(x) at x = a is defined as

$$L f'(a) = \lim_{h \to 0-0} \left[\frac{(f(a-h) - f(a)}{-h} \right]$$ provided this limit exists. Hence h tends to 0 through the negative values.

A function f(x) is said to be differentiable at x = a if

$$f'(a) = \lim_{h \to 0} \left[\frac{(f(a+h) - f(a)}{h} \right] \text{ exists.}$$

This implies $R\ f'(a) = L\ f'(a)$

i.e., $$\lim_{h \to 0+0} \left[\frac{(f(a+h) - f(a)}{h} \right] = \lim_{h \to 0+0} \left[\frac{(f(a-h) - f(a)}{-h} \right] = f'(a)$$

In both definitions h is always positive.

Example: Consider the function $f(x) = x^2 \sin\left(\frac{1}{x}\right)$ for $x \neq 0$ and f(0) = 0.

Find out whether the derivative of f(x) exists at x = 0

$$R f'(0) = \lim_{h \to 0+0} \left[\frac{(f(0+h) - f(0)}{h} \right]$$

$$= \lim_{h \to 0+0} \left[\frac{h^2 \sin\left(\frac{1}{h}\right) - (0)}{h} \right]$$

Since f(0 + h) = f(h)

$$= h^2 \sin\left(\frac{1}{h}\right)$$

$$= \lim_{h \to 0+0} \left[h \sin\left(\frac{1}{h}\right) \right] \qquad \text{as} \qquad h \to 0, \frac{1}{h} \to \infty$$

$$= 0 \times \text{a finite quantity}$$

$$= 0$$

But $\sin\left(\frac{1}{h}\right)$ lies between –1 and +1

$$\therefore\ R f'(0) = 0$$

$$L f'(a) = \lim_{h\to 0-0}\left[\frac{(f(0-h)-f(0)}{-h}\right]$$

$$= \lim_{h\to 0+0}\left[\frac{-h^2\sin\left(\frac{1}{h}\right)-(0)}{-h}\right]$$

$$= \lim_{h\to 0+0}\left[h\sin\left(\frac{1}{h}\right)\right] = 0$$

$\therefore$ $R\ f(0) = L f'(0) = 0$

$\therefore$ The given function is differentiable at x = 0

Differentiability Implies Continuity

Or

If a function f(x) is differentiable at x = a then f(x) is continuous at x = a.

Given: f(x) is differentiable at x = a

To prove that: f(x) is continuous at x = a

Proof: By data $f'(x)$ exists

$$\lim_{h\to 0}\left[\frac{(f(a+h)-f(a)}{h}\right] = f'(a) \text{ exists} \qquad .....(1)$$

Now $$f(a+h)-f(a) = \frac{f(a+h)-f(a)}{h}.h$$

Taking limits on both sides as $h \to 0$, we get

$$\lim_{h\to 0}\left[f(a+h)-f(a) = \lim_{h\to 0} f'(a).h = 0\right] \quad \text{[using eq.(6.3)]}$$

$\therefore$ $$\lim_{h\to 0} f(a+h) = f(a)$$

Put a + h = x then

$\therefore$ $$\lim_{x\to a} f(x) = f(a)$$

$\therefore$ f(x) is continuous at x = a

When $h \to 0$ $x \to a$

The converse of the above proposition is not true. That is continuity does not imply differentiability. This is illustrated by the following example.

Take f(x) = | x |

$$= \begin{cases} x & \text{if } x > 0 \\ 0 & \text{if } x = 0 \\ -x & \text{if } x < 0 \end{cases}$$

$$\lim_{x \to 0+0} f(x) = \lim_{x \to 0+0} (x) = 0, \quad \lim_{x \to 0-0} = f(x) = \lim_{x \to 0-0} (-x) = 0$$

$$\therefore \lim_{x \to 0+0} f(x) = \lim_{x \to 0-0} f(x) = 0 = f(0)$$

∴ f(x) is continuous at x = 0

$$R f'(0) = \lim_{h \to 0+0} \left[\frac{(f(0+h) - f(0)}{h} \right]$$

$$\lim_{h \to 0+0} \left[\frac{(h-0)}{h} \right] = 1$$

$$Lf'(a) = \lim_{h \to 0-0} \left[\frac{(f(0-h) - f(0)}{-h} \right]$$

Since f(0 – h) = f(–h)

= – (–h) = h

$$= \lim_{h \to 0-0} \left[\frac{(h-0)}{-h} \right] = -1$$

$$\therefore R\ f'(0) \neq L\ f'(0)$$

∴ The function f(x) = |x| is not differentiable at x = 0 even though it is continuous at that point.

Example: The amount drug that excreted through urine for a fixed period of time as listed below. Find the rate of change of excretion of drug with respect to time.

Time (t hr)	**Drug Excreted (X_u) mg**	**Change in Time Δt**	**Change in Excretion ΔX_u**	$\frac{\Delta t}{\Delta X_u}$ **or** $\frac{dt}{dx_u}$
0	0	1	4.0	4.0
1	4.0	1	3.8	3.8
2	7.8	1	3.5	3.5
3	11.3	1	9.1	3.0
6	20.4	3	13.5	2.2
12	33.9	6	14.7	1.2

6.3 DERIVATIVE OF A CONSTANT

Take y = c where c is a constant

Since y = c is a constant function, the change in x will not cause a change in y in other words, $\Delta y = 0$

$$\therefore \quad \frac{\Delta y}{\Delta x} = \frac{0}{\Delta x} = 0$$

$$\lim_{\Delta x \to 0}\left(\frac{\Delta y}{\Delta x}\right) = 0 \qquad \text{i.e., } \frac{dy}{dx} = 0$$

$$\therefore \quad \frac{d}{dx}(\text{constant}) = 0$$

∴ The derivative of a constant is zero

Examples: $\frac{d}{dx}(2) = 0,\ \frac{d}{dx}\left(\frac{-5}{2}\right) = 0,\ \frac{d}{dx}(a) = 0$ if a is a constant

6.3.1 Derivative of a Product of a Constant and a Function

Take y = c u where c is a constant and u is a function of x. Change x to $x + \Delta x$, let u change to $u + \Delta u$ and y change to $y + \Delta y$

$$y + \Delta y = c\,(u + \Delta u);\ \ \Delta y = c\,(u + \Delta u) - y$$

$$\Delta y = c\,(u + \Delta u) - cu;\ \Delta y = c\,.\,\Delta u$$

$$\frac{\Delta y}{\Delta x} = c\frac{\Delta u}{\Delta x}$$

Taking limits as $\Delta x \to 0$, $\lim_{\Delta x \to 0}\left(\frac{\Delta y}{\Delta x}\right) = \lim_{\Delta x \to 0}\left(c\frac{\Delta u}{\Delta x}\right)$

$$\frac{dy}{dx} = c\frac{du}{dx} \text{ i.e., } \frac{d}{dx}(c\,u) = c.\frac{du}{dx}$$

$$\frac{d}{dx}(\text{consant} \times \text{function}) = \text{consant} \times \frac{d}{dx}(\text{function})$$

6.3.2 Derivative of the Sum or Difference of Two Functions

Let y = u + v where u and v are functions of x

Change x to x + Δx;

let u change to u + Δu; v to v + Δv and y to y + Δy

$$y + \Delta y = (u + \Delta u) + (v + \Delta v)$$

$$\therefore \quad \Delta y = (u + \Delta u) + (v + \Delta v) - (u + v)$$

i.e., $\Delta y = (\Delta u + \Delta v)$

divide by $\Delta x, \dfrac{\Delta y}{\Delta x} = \dfrac{\Delta u}{\Delta x} + \dfrac{\Delta v}{\Delta x}$

Taking limits as $\Delta x \to 0, \ \lim_{\Delta x \to 0}\left(\dfrac{\Delta y}{\Delta x}\right) = \lim_{\Delta x \to 0}\left(\dfrac{\Delta u}{\Delta x} + \dfrac{\Delta v}{\Delta x}\right)$

i.e., $\dfrac{dy}{dx} = \lim_{\Delta x \to 0} \dfrac{\Delta u}{\Delta x} + \lim_{\Delta x \to 0} \dfrac{\Delta y}{\Delta x} = \dfrac{du}{dx} + \dfrac{dv}{dx}$

i.e., $\dfrac{d}{dx}(u + v) = \dfrac{du}{dx} + \dfrac{dv}{dx}$

Similarly, $\dfrac{d}{dx}(u - v) = \dfrac{du}{dx} - \dfrac{dv}{dx}$

In general if u, v, w, … are functions of x then

$$\frac{d}{dx}(u \pm v \pm w \pm \ldots) = \frac{du}{dx} + \frac{du}{dx} + \frac{dw}{dx} + \ldots$$

6.3.3 Derivative of the Product of Two Functions (Product Formula)

Let y = u v where u and v are function of x. Change x to x + Δx, let u change to u + Δu; v to v +Δv and y to y + Δy

Then $y + \Delta y = (u + \Delta u)\ (v + \Delta v)$

$$\therefore \quad \Delta y = (u + \Delta u)\ (v + \Delta v) - y$$

$$\Delta y = u\,v + u.\Delta v + v\,\Delta u + \Delta u\ \Delta v - uv \qquad \text{(since } y = u\,v\text{)}$$

$$\Delta y = u.\Delta v + v.\,\Delta u + \Delta u\,\Delta v$$

Divide by Δx and take limits as $\Delta x \to 0$

$$\lim_{\Delta x \to 0}\left(\frac{\Delta y}{\Delta x}\right) = \lim_{\Delta x \to 0}\left[u.\frac{\Delta v}{\Delta x} + v.\frac{\Delta u}{\Delta x} + \frac{\Delta u.\Delta v}{\Delta x}\right]$$

$$= \lim_{\Delta x \to 0}\left(u.\frac{\Delta v}{\Delta x}\right) + \lim_{\Delta x \to 0}\left(v.\frac{\Delta u}{\Delta x}\right) + \lim_{\Delta x \to 0}\left(\frac{\Delta u \Delta v}{\Delta x}\right)$$

$$= u.\lim_{\Delta x \to 0}\left(\frac{\Delta v}{\Delta x}\right) + v.\lim_{\Delta x \to 0}\left(\frac{\Delta u}{\Delta x}\right) + \lim_{\Delta x \to 0}\frac{\Delta u}{\Delta x}.\lim_{\Delta x \to 0}\Delta v$$

As $\Delta x \to 0$, $\Delta v \to 0$. Hence,

$$\frac{dy}{dx} = u\frac{dv}{dx} + v\frac{du}{dx}$$

i.e.,
$$\frac{d}{dx}(u\ v) = u.\frac{dv}{dx} + v.\frac{du}{dv}$$

Note:

(i) $\frac{dy}{dx} = u\frac{dv}{dx} + v\frac{du}{dx}$ Multiply by $\frac{1}{y}$

$$\frac{1}{y}\frac{dy}{dx} = \frac{v}{y}\frac{du}{dx} + \frac{u}{y}\frac{dv}{dx}$$

i.e.,
$$\frac{1}{y}\frac{dy}{dx} = \frac{u}{u\,v}\frac{dv}{dx} + \frac{v}{u\,v}\frac{du}{dx}$$ (Because $y = u\ v$)

i.e.,
$$\frac{1}{y}\frac{dy}{dx} = \frac{1}{v}\frac{dv}{dx} + \frac{1}{u}\frac{du}{dx}$$

Thus, if $y = u\ v$ where u and v are functions of x then

$$\frac{1}{y}\frac{dy}{dx} = \frac{1}{u}\frac{du}{dx} + \frac{1}{v}\frac{dv}{dx}$$

(ii) The formula can be remembered as follows:

$$\frac{d}{dx}(u\ v) = u.\frac{dv}{dx} + v.\frac{du}{dv}$$

= (first function) $\frac{d}{dx}$ (second function) + (second function).

$\frac{d}{dx}$ (first function)

(iii) If $y = u\ v\ w$ where u, v, w are functions of x then

$$\frac{dy}{dx} = u\,v\frac{dw}{dx} + u\,w\frac{dv}{dx} + v\,w\frac{du}{dx}$$

$y = u\ v\ w$ or $y = (u\ v)w$

Consider u v as first function and w as second function. Apply the product rule

$$\frac{dy}{dx} = \frac{d}{dx}[(u\,v)w]$$

$$= (u\,v)\frac{dw}{dx} + w\frac{d}{dx}(u\,v) = u\,v\frac{dw}{dx} + w\left[u.\frac{dv}{dx} + v\frac{du}{dx}\right]$$

$$= (u\,v)\frac{dw}{dx} + (u\,w)\frac{dv}{dx} + (v\,w)\frac{du}{dx}$$

$$\therefore \quad \frac{d}{dx}(u\,v\,w) = (u\,v)\frac{dw}{dx} + (u\,w)\frac{dv}{dx} + (v\,w)\frac{du}{dx}$$

6.3.4 Derivative of the Quotient of Two Functions (Quotient Formula)

Let $y = \frac{u}{v}$ where u and v are functions of x. Change x to x + Δx; then let u change to u + Δu; v to v + Δv and y to y + Δy.

$$\therefore \quad y + \Delta y = \frac{u + \Delta u}{v + \Delta v}; \quad \Delta y = \frac{u + \Delta u}{v + \Delta v} - y$$

i.e., $$\Delta y = \frac{u + \Delta u}{v + \Delta v} - \frac{u}{v}$$

i.e., $$\Delta y = \frac{v(u + \Delta u) - u(v + \Delta v)}{v(v + \Delta v)}$$

$$= \frac{vu + v\,\Delta u - uv - u\,\Delta v}{v^2 + v\,\Delta v}$$

$$= \frac{v\,\Delta u - u\,\Delta v}{v^2 + v\,\Delta v}$$

Divide by Δx and take limits as Δx → 0

$$\lim_{\Delta x \to 0}\left(\frac{\Delta y}{\Delta x}\right) = \lim_{\Delta x \to 0}\left[\frac{v\frac{\Delta u}{\Delta x} - u.\frac{\Delta v}{\Delta x}}{v^2 + v\,\Delta v}\right]$$

i.e., $$\frac{dy}{dx} = \left[\frac{v\frac{du}{dx} - u.\frac{dv}{dx}}{v^2 + 0}\right]$$ because $\Delta v \to 0$ when $\Delta x \to 0$

$$\therefore \quad \frac{dy}{dx} = \left[\frac{v\frac{du}{dx} - u.\frac{dv}{dx}}{v^2}\right]$$

or $$\frac{d}{dx}\left(\frac{u}{v}\right) = \frac{v\frac{du}{dx} - u.\frac{dv}{dx}}{v^2}$$

This is known as Quotient formula or Quotient rule.

Note: The above formula is remembered as

$$\frac{d}{dx}\left(\frac{u}{v}\right) = \frac{(\text{Denominator})\frac{d}{dx}(\text{Numerator}) - (\text{Numerator})\frac{d}{dx}(\text{Denominator})}{(\text{Denominator})^2}$$

$$= \frac{(\text{Dr})\frac{d}{dx}(\text{Nr}) - (\text{Nr})\frac{d}{dx}(\text{Dr})}{(\text{Dr})^2}$$

6.3.5 Derivative of x^n w.r.t. where n is any Rational Number

$$\frac{d}{dx}(x^n) = n\,x^{n-1}$$

where n is any rational number

Let $y = x^n$

When x changes to $x + \Delta x$, let y change to $y + \Delta y$

$$y + \Delta y = (x + \Delta x)^n; \quad \Delta y = (x + \Delta x)^n - x^n$$

Divide by Δx. $$\frac{\Delta y}{\Delta x} = \frac{(x + \Delta x)^n - x^n}{\Delta x}$$

Taking limits as $\Delta x \to 0$

$$\lim_{\Delta x \to o}\left(\frac{\Delta y}{\Delta x}\right) = \lim_{\Delta x \to 0}\frac{(x+\Delta x)^n - x^n}{\Delta x}$$

$$\frac{dy}{dx} = \lim_{\Delta x \to 0}\left[\frac{(x+\Delta x)^n - x^n}{(x+\Delta x) - x}\right]$$

Put $x + \Delta x = z$; when $\Delta x \to 0$, $z \to x$

$$\lim_{z \to x}\left[\frac{z^n - x^n}{z - x}\right] = n.x^{n-1} \qquad \left[\because \lim_{x \to 0}\left(\frac{x^n - a^n}{x - a}\right) = n\, a^{n-1}\right]$$

$$\therefore \qquad \frac{d}{dx}(x^n) = nx^{n-1}$$

6.3.6 Derivative of e^x

Take $y = e^x$ .....(1)

y change to $y + \Delta y$ when x changes to $x + \Delta x$

$y + \Delta y = e^{x+\Delta x}$ .....(2)

Taking (2) – (1), $\Delta y = e^{x+\Delta x} - e^x$

i.e., $\Delta y = e^x(e^{\Delta x} - 1)$

Divide both sides by Δx

$$\frac{\Delta y}{\Delta x} = \frac{e^x(e^{\Delta x} - 1)}{\Delta x}$$

Taking limits as $\Delta x \to 0$

$$\lim_{\Delta x \to 0}\frac{\Delta y}{\Delta x} = \lim_{\Delta x \to 0}\left[\frac{e^x(e^{\Delta x} - 1)}{\Delta x}\right]$$

$$\therefore \qquad \frac{dy}{dx} = e^x.1$$

since $$\lim_{\Delta x \to 0}\frac{(e^{\Delta x} - 1)}{\Delta x} = 1$$

$$\therefore \qquad \frac{d}{dx}(e^x) = e^x$$

6.3.7 Derivative of $\log_e x$

Take $y = \log_e x$

y change to $y + \Delta y$ when x changes to $x + \Delta x$ .....(1)

$y + \Delta y = \log_e (x + \Delta x)$ .....(2)

(2) – (1) gives, $\Delta y = \log_e (x + \Delta x) - \log_e (x)$

$$\Delta y = \log_e\left(\frac{x+\Delta x}{x}\right) \qquad \text{since } \log m - \text{long } n = \log\left(\frac{m}{n}\right)$$

$$\Delta y = \log_e\left(1+\frac{\Delta x}{x}\right)$$

$$\frac{\Delta y}{\Delta x} = \frac{1}{\Delta x}\log_e\left(1+\frac{\Delta x}{x}\right) = \frac{1}{x}.\frac{x}{\Delta x}\log_e\left(1+\frac{\Delta x}{x}\right)$$

$$\frac{\Delta y}{\Delta x} = \frac{1}{x}\log\left(1+\frac{\Delta x}{x}\right)^{\frac{x}{\Delta x}} \qquad \because \; k \log m = \log m^k$$

$$\lim_{\Delta x\to 0}\left(\frac{\Delta y}{\Delta x}\right) = \lim_{\Delta x\to 0}\left[\frac{1}{x}\log_e\left(1+\frac{\Delta x}{x}\right)^{\frac{x}{\Delta x}}\right]$$

Take $\frac{\Delta x}{x} = X$

Then when $\Delta x \to 0$, $X \to 0$ and $\frac{x}{\Delta x} = \frac{1}{X}$

$$= \lim_{\Delta x\to 0}\left[\frac{1}{x}\log_e(1+X)^{\frac{1}{X}}\right]$$

$$= \frac{1}{x}\log_e e = \frac{1}{x} \qquad \because \; \lim_{\Delta x\to 0}(1+X)^{\frac{1}{X}} = e$$

$$\therefore \qquad \frac{d}{dx}(\log_e x) = \frac{1}{x}$$

6.3.8 Derivative of a^x

Take $y = a^x$ .....(1)

Change x to $x + \Delta x$, let y change to $y + \Delta y$

$y + \Delta y = a^{x+\Delta x}$ ......(2)

eq.(2) – (1) gives, $\Delta y = a^{x+\Delta x} - a^x$

i.e., $\Delta y = a^x(a^{\Delta x} - 1)$

Divide by, $\Delta x, \frac{\Delta y}{\Delta x} = \frac{a^x(a^{\Delta x} - 1)}{\Delta x}$

Taking as $\Delta x \to 0$

$$\lim_{\Delta x \to 0}\left(\frac{\Delta y}{\Delta x}\right) = \lim_{\Delta x \to 0}\left[\frac{ax(a^{\Delta x} - 1)}{\Delta x}\right]$$

$$\frac{dy}{dx} = a^x.\log_e a \qquad \text{since} \quad \lim_{\Delta \to 0}\left(\frac{(a^{\Delta x} - 1)}{\Delta x}\right) = \log_e a$$

$$\therefore \qquad \frac{d}{dx}a^x = a^x.\log_e a$$

6.4 DERIVATIVE OF TRIGONOMETRIC FUNCTIONS FROM FIRST PRINCIPLES

I sin x

Let y = sin x .....(1)

Let x change to x + Δx, y to y + Δy

$$y + \Delta y = \sin(x + \Delta x) \qquad .....(2)$$

eq.(2) – (1) gives $\Delta y = \sin(x + \Delta x) - \sin x$

Use the formula $\sin C - \sin D = 2\cos\left(\frac{C+D}{2}\right)\sin\left(\frac{C-D}{2}\right)$, then

$$\Delta y = 2\cos\left(\frac{x + \Delta x + x}{2}\right)\sin\left(\frac{x + \Delta x - x}{2}\right)$$

$$= 2\cos\left(\frac{2x + \Delta x}{2}\right)\sin\left(\frac{\Delta x}{2}\right)$$

Divide by $\Delta x, \frac{\Delta y}{\Delta x} = \left[\frac{2\cos\left(\frac{2x + \Delta x}{2}\right)\sin\left(\frac{\Delta x}{2}\right)}{\Delta x}\right]$

Taking limits as $\Delta x \to 0$

$$\lim_{\Delta x \to 0}\left(\frac{\Delta y}{\Delta x}\right) = \lim_{\Delta x \to 0}\left[\frac{2\cos\left(\frac{2x+\Delta x}{2}\right)\sin\left(\frac{\Delta x}{2}\right)}{\Delta x}\right]$$

$$\frac{dy}{dx} = \lim_{\Delta x \to 0}\left[\frac{2\cos\left(\frac{2x+\Delta x}{2}\right)\sin\left(\frac{\Delta x}{2}\right)}{2.\frac{\Delta x}{2}}\right]$$

$\therefore$ $$\frac{dy}{dx} = \cos\left(\frac{2x+0}{2}\right).1 = \cos x \quad \text{since} \quad \lim_{\Delta x \to 0}\left[\frac{\sin\left(\frac{\Delta x}{2}\right)}{\left(\frac{\Delta x}{2}\right)}\right] = 1$$

$\therefore$ $$\frac{d}{dx}(\sin x) = \cos x$$

II cos x

Let $y = \cos x$ .....(1)

Let y change to $y + \Delta y$, x to $x + \Delta x$

$y + \Delta y = \cos(x + \Delta x)$ .....(2)

eq.(2) – (1) gives, $\Delta y = \cos(x + \Delta x) - \cos x$

Use the formula $\cos C - \cos D = -2\sin\left(\frac{C+D}{2}\right)\sin\left(\frac{C-D}{2}\right)$, then

$$\Delta y = -2\sin\left(\frac{x+\Delta x+x}{2}\right)\sin\left(\frac{x+\Delta x-x}{2}\right)$$

$$\Delta y = -2\sin\left(\frac{2x+\Delta x}{2}\right)\sin\left(\frac{\Delta x}{2}\right)$$

divide by Δx $$\frac{\Delta y}{\Delta x} = \frac{-2\sin\left(\frac{2x+\Delta x}{2}\right)\sin\left(\frac{\Delta x}{2}\right)}{\Delta x}$$

$$\lim_{\Delta x \to 0}\left(\frac{\Delta y}{\Delta x}\right) = \left[\frac{-2\sin\left(\frac{2x+\Delta x}{2}\right)\sin\left(\frac{\Delta x}{2}\right)}{2.\frac{\Delta x}{2}}\right]$$

$$\frac{dy}{dx} = \frac{-2\sin\left(\frac{2x+0}{2}\right)}{2} = -\sin x$$

$$\therefore \quad \frac{d}{dx}(\cos x) = -\sin x$$

III tan x

Let y = tan x .....(1)

Let y change to y + Δy, x to x + Δx

$y + \Delta y = \tan(x + \Delta x)$ ....(2)

eq.(2) – (1) gives, $\Delta y = \tan(x + \Delta x) - \tan x$

$$\Delta y = \frac{\sin(x+\Delta x)}{\cos(x+\Delta x)} - \frac{\sin x}{\cos x}$$

$$\Delta y = \frac{\sin(x+\Delta x)\cos x - \cos(x+\Delta x)\sin x}{\cos(x+\Delta x)\cos x}$$

Use the formula, sin A cos B – cos A sin B = sin (A – B)

$$\therefore \quad \Delta y = \frac{\sin(x+\Delta x - x)}{\cos(x+\Delta x)\cos x}$$

divide by Δx $\frac{\Delta y}{\Delta x} = \frac{\sin\Delta x}{\Delta x\cos(x+\Delta x)\cos x}$

$$\lim_{\Delta x \to 0}\left(\frac{\Delta y}{\Delta x}\right) = \lim_{\Delta x \leftarrow 0}\left[\frac{\sin\Delta x}{\Delta x.\cos(x+\Delta x)\cos x}\right]$$

$$\frac{dy}{dx} = \frac{1}{\cos(x+0)\cos x} = \frac{1}{\cos^2 x} = \sec^2 x$$

$$\therefore \quad \frac{d}{dx}(\tan x) = \sec^2 x$$

IV cot x

Let y = cot x .....(1)

Let y change to y + Δy, x to x + Δx

$$y + \Delta y = \cot(x + \Delta x) \quad .....(2)$$

eq.(2) – (1) gives, Δy = cot (x + Δx) – cot x

$$\Delta y = \frac{\cos(x+\Delta x)}{\sin(x+\Delta x)} - \frac{\sin x}{\cos x}$$

$$\Delta y = \frac{\cos(x+\Delta x)\sin x - \sin(x+\Delta x)\cos x}{\sin(x+\Delta x)\sin x}$$

$$\Delta y = \frac{-[\sin(x+\Delta x)\cos x - \cos(x+\Delta x)\sin x}{\sin(x+\Delta x)\sin x}$$

$$\therefore \quad \Delta y = \frac{-\sin(x+\Delta x - x)}{\sin((x+\Delta x)\sin x}$$

divide by Δx

$$\frac{\Delta y}{\Delta x} = \frac{-\sin \Delta x}{\Delta x \sin(x+\Delta x)\sin x}$$

$$\lim_{\Delta x \to 0}\left(\frac{\Delta y}{\Delta x}\right) = \lim_{\Delta x \leftarrow 0}\left[\frac{-\sin\Delta x}{\Delta x.\sin(x+\Delta x)\sin x}\right]$$

$$\frac{dy}{dx} = \frac{-1}{\sin(x+0)\sin x} = \frac{-1}{\sin^2 x} = -\mathrm{cosec}^2 x$$

$$\therefore \quad \frac{d}{dx}(\cot x) = -\mathrm{cosec}^2 x$$

V sec x

Let y = sec x .....(1)

Let y change to y + Δy, x to x + Δx

$$y + \Delta y = \sec(x + \Delta x) \quad .....(2)$$

eq. (2) – (1) gives, Δy = sec (x + Δx) – sec x

$$\Delta y = \frac{1}{\cos(x+\Delta x)} - \frac{1}{(\cos x)} \qquad \left(\text{since } \sec\theta = \frac{1}{\cos\theta}\right)$$

$$\Delta y = \frac{\cos x - \cos(x+\Delta x)}{\cos(x+\Delta x)\cos x}$$

Use the formula $\cos C - \cos D = -2\sin\left(\frac{C+D}{2}\right)\sin\left(\frac{C-D}{2}\right)$

$$\Delta y = \frac{-2\sin\left(\frac{x+x+\Delta x}{2}\right)\sin\left(\frac{x-x-\Delta x}{2}\right)}{\cos(x+\Delta x).\cos x}$$

$$\Delta y = \frac{-2\sin\left(\frac{2x+\Delta x}{2}\right)\sin\left(\frac{-\Delta x}{2}\right)}{\cos(x+\Delta x).\cos x}$$

$$\Delta y = \frac{2\sin\left(\frac{2x+\Delta x}{2}\right)\sin\left(\frac{\Delta x}{2}\right)}{\cos(x+\Delta x).\cos x}$$ [since $\sin(-\theta) = -\sin\theta$]

Divide by $\frac{\Delta y}{\Delta x} = \frac{2\sin\left(\frac{2x+\Delta x}{2}\right)\sin\left(\frac{\Delta x}{2}\right)}{\cos(x+\Delta x).\cos x\Delta x}$

$$\lim_{\Delta x\to 0}\left(\frac{\Delta y}{\Delta x}\right) = \lim_{\Delta x\leftarrow 0}\left[\frac{2\sin\left(\frac{2x+\Delta x}{2}\right)\sin\left(\frac{\Delta x}{2}\right)}{\cos(x+\Delta x)\cos x.2.\frac{\Delta x}{2}}\right]$$

$$\frac{dy}{dx} = \frac{\sin\left(\frac{2x+0}{2}\right).1}{\cos(x+0)\cos x} = \frac{\sin x}{\cos x.\cos x} = \tan x.\sec x$$

$\therefore \quad \frac{d}{dx}(\sec x) = \sec x \tan x$

VI cosec x

Let y = cosec x .....(1)

Let y change to $y + \Delta y$, x to $x + \Delta x$

$y + \Delta y = \text{cosec}\,(x + \Delta x)$ .....(2)

eq.(2) – (1) gives, $\Delta y = \text{cosec}\,(x + \Delta x) - \text{cosec}\,x$

$$\Delta y = \frac{1}{\sin(x+\Delta x)} - \frac{1}{(\sin x)}$$ $\left(\text{since } \text{cosec}\theta = \frac{1}{\sin\theta}\right)$

$$\Delta y = \frac{\sin x - \sin(x+\Delta x)}{\sin(x+\Delta x)\sin x}$$

Use the formula $\sin C - \sin D = 2\cos\left(\frac{C+D}{2}\right)\sin\left(\frac{C-D}{2}\right)$

$$\Delta y = \frac{2\cos\left(\frac{x+x+\Delta x}{2}\right)\sin\left(\frac{x-x-\Delta x}{2}\right)}{\sin(x+\Delta x).\sin x}$$

$$\Delta y = \frac{2\cos\left(\frac{2x+\Delta x}{2}\right)\sin\left(\frac{-\Delta x}{2}\right)}{\sin(x+\Delta x).\sin x}$$

$$\Delta y = \frac{-2\cos\left(\frac{2x+\Delta x}{2}\right)\sin\left(\frac{\Delta x}{2}\right)}{\sin(x+\Delta x).\sin x.\Delta x} \qquad [\text{since } \sin(-\theta) = -\sin\theta]$$

$$\lim_{\Delta x\to 0}\left(\frac{\Delta y}{\Delta x}\right) = \lim_{\Delta x\leftarrow 0}\left[\frac{-2\cos\left(\frac{2x+\Delta x}{2}\right)\sin\left(\frac{\Delta x}{2}\right)}{\sin(x+\Delta x)\sin x.2.\frac{\Delta x}{2}}\right]$$

$$\frac{dy}{dx} = \frac{-2\cos\left(\frac{2x+0}{2}\right).1}{\sin(x+0)\sin x.2} = \frac{-\cos x}{\sin x.\sin x} = \frac{-\cos x}{\sin x}.\frac{1}{\sin x}$$

$$= -\cot x \operatorname{cosec} x$$

$$\therefore \qquad \frac{d}{dx}(\operatorname{cosec} x) = -\operatorname{cosec} x \cot x$$

6.5 DIFFERENTIATION OF INVERSE TRIGONOMETRIC FUNCTIONS

Derivative of $\sin^{-1}x$

Take $y = \sin^{-1}x$ then $\sin y = x$

Differentiate w.r.t. x, $\frac{d}{dx}(\sin y) = \frac{d}{dx}(x)$ i.e., $\cos y\frac{dy}{dx} = 1$

$$\therefore \qquad \frac{dy}{dx} = \frac{1}{\cos y} = \frac{1}{\sqrt{1-\sin^2 y}} = \frac{1}{\sqrt{1-x^2}} \qquad (\text{since } \sin y = x)$$

$$\therefore \qquad \frac{d}{dx}(\sin^{-1}x) = \frac{1}{\sqrt{1-x^2}}$$

Derivative of $\cos^{-1}x$

Take $y = \cos^{-1}x$ then $\cos y = x$

Differentiate w.r.t. x, $\frac{d}{dx}(\cos y) = \frac{d}{dx}(x)$ i.e., $-\sin y\frac{dy}{dx} = 1$

$$\therefore \quad \frac{dy}{dx} = \frac{-1}{\sin y} = \frac{-1}{\sqrt{1-\cos^2 y}} = \frac{-1}{\sqrt{1-x^2}} \quad (\text{since } \cos y = x)$$

$$\therefore \quad \frac{d}{dx}(\cos^{-1}x) = \frac{-1}{\sqrt{1-x^2}}$$

Derivative of $\tan^{-1}x$

Take $y = \tan^{-1}x$ then $\tan y = x$

Differentiate w.r.t. x, $\frac{d}{dx}(\tan y) = \frac{d}{dx}(x)$ i.e., $\sec^2 y\frac{dy}{dx} = 1$

$$\therefore \quad \frac{dy}{dx} = \frac{1}{\sec^2 y} = \frac{1}{1+\tan^2 y} = \frac{1}{1+x^2} \quad (\text{since } \tan y = x)$$

$$\therefore \quad \frac{d}{dx}(\tan^{-1}x) = \frac{1}{1+x^2}$$

Derivative of $\sec^{-1}x$

Take $y = \sec^{-1}x$ then $\sec y = x$

Differentiate w.r.t. x, $\frac{d}{dx}(\sec y) = \frac{d}{dx}(x)$ i.e., $\sec y \tan y\frac{dy}{dx} = 1$

$$\therefore \quad \frac{dy}{dx} = \frac{1}{\cos y} = \frac{1}{\sqrt{1-\sin^2 y}} = \frac{1}{\sqrt{1-x^2}} \quad (\text{since } \sin y = x)$$

$$\therefore \quad \frac{dy}{dx} = \frac{1}{\sec y \tan y} = \frac{1}{\sec y\sqrt{\sec^2 y - 1}} = \frac{1}{x\sqrt{x^2-1}}$$

$$\because \quad 1+\tan^2 y = \sec^2 y$$

Hence, $\tan y = \sqrt{\sec^2 y - 1}$

$$\therefore \quad \frac{d}{dx}(\sec^{-1}x) = \frac{1}{x\sqrt{x^2-1}}$$

Similarly,

$$\therefore \quad \frac{d}{dx}(\cot^{-1}x) = \frac{-1}{1+x^2} \quad \text{and} \quad \frac{d}{dx}(\text{cosec}^{-1}x) = \frac{-1}{x\sqrt{x^2-1}}$$

Derivative of $\sin^{-1}x$ w.r.t. x from First Principles

Take $y = \sin^{-1}x$; then $\sin y = x$ .....(1)

$\sin(y + \Delta y) = x + \Delta x$ .....(2)

Where Δy is the change in y for a change Δx in x

eq.(2) – (1) give, $\sin(y + \Delta y) - \sin y = \Delta x$

$$2\cos\left(\frac{y+\Delta y+y}{2}\right)\sin\left(\frac{y+\Delta y-y}{2}\right) = \Delta x$$

$$\left[\because \sin C - \sin D = 2\cos\left(\frac{C+D}{2}\right)\sin\left(\frac{C-D}{2}\right)\right] \text{ divide by } \Delta x$$

$$2\cos\left(\frac{2y+\Delta y}{2}\right)\sin\left(\frac{\Delta y}{2}\right) = \Delta x$$

$$\frac{2\cos\left(\frac{2y+\Delta y}{2}\right)\sin\left(\frac{\Delta y}{2}\right)}{\Delta x} = 1$$

$$\lim_{\Delta x \leftarrow 0}\left[\frac{2\cos\left(\frac{2y+\Delta y}{2}\right)\sin\left(\frac{\Delta y}{2}\right)}{2.\left(\frac{\Delta y}{2}\right)}.\frac{\Delta y}{\Delta x}\right] = 1$$

$$\lim_{\Delta x \leftarrow 0}\left[\frac{2\cos\left(\frac{2y+\Delta y}{2}\right)\sin\left(\frac{\Delta y}{2}\right)}{2.\left(\frac{\Delta y}{2}\right)}\right].\lim_{\Delta x \to 0}\frac{\Delta y}{\Delta x} = 1$$

$$\cos\left(\frac{2y+0}{2}\right).\frac{dy}{dx} = 1 \quad \text{i.e., } \cos y\frac{dy}{dx} = 1$$

$$\frac{dy}{dx} = \frac{1}{\cos y} = \frac{1}{\sqrt{1-\sin^2 y}} = \frac{1}{\sqrt{1-x^2}}$$

Derivative of $\tan^{-1}x$ w.r.t. x from First Principles

Take $y = \tan^{-1}x$; then $\tan y = x$ .....(1)

$$\tan(y + \Delta y) = x + \Delta x \qquad \text{.....(2)}$$

Where Δy is the change in y for a change Δx in x

eq.(2) – (1) give, $\sin(y + \Delta y) - \sin y = \Delta x$

i.e., $$\frac{\sin(y+\Delta y)}{\cos(y+\Delta y)} - \frac{\sin y}{\cos y} = \Delta x$$

i.e, $$\frac{\sin(y+\Delta y)\cos y - \cos(y+\Delta y)\sin y}{\cos(y+\Delta y)\cos y} = \Delta x$$

i.e., $$\frac{\sin(y+\Delta y - y)}{\cos(y+\Delta y)\cos y} = \Delta x$$

i.e., $$\frac{\sin\Delta y}{\cos(y+\Delta y)\cos y} = \Delta x \qquad \text{Divided by } \Delta x$$

i.e., $$\frac{\sin\Delta y}{\cos(y+\Delta y)\cos y.\Delta x} = 1$$

i.e., $$\frac{\sin\Delta y}{\Delta y\cos(y+\Delta y)\cos y} \times \frac{\Delta y}{\Delta x} = 1$$

i.e., $$\lim_{\Delta x \to 0}\left[\frac{\sin\Delta y}{\Delta y\cos(y+\Delta y)\cos y} \times \frac{\Delta y}{\Delta x}\right] = 1$$

$$\lim_{\Delta x \to 0}\left[\frac{\sin\Delta y}{\Delta y\cos(y+\Delta y)\cos y} \times \lim_{\Delta x \to 0}\left(\frac{\Delta y}{\Delta x}\right)\right] = 1$$

$$\frac{1}{\cos(y+0)\cos y}.\frac{dy}{dx} = 1$$

i.e., $$\frac{1}{\cos^2 y}.\frac{dy}{dx} = 1$$

$$\sec^2 y\frac{dy}{dx} = 1, \frac{dy}{dx} = \frac{1}{\sec^2 y} = \frac{1}{1+\tan^2 y} = \frac{1}{1+x^2}$$

$$\therefore \quad \frac{d}{dx}(\tan^{-1}x) = \frac{1}{1+x^2}$$

Note:

(a) In finding the derivatives of inverse trigonometric functions from first principles, it is assumed that $\Delta y \to 0$ when $\Delta x \to 0$.

(b) You can apply similar method to find the derivatives of other inverse trigonometric functions from first principles.

(c) You have to memorize the following formulae:

1. $\frac{d}{dx}(\sin^{-1}x) = \frac{1}{\sqrt{1-x^2}}$
2. $\frac{d}{dx}(\cos^{-1}x) = \frac{-1}{\sqrt{1-x^2}}$
3. $\frac{d}{dx}(\tan^{-1}x) = \frac{1}{1+x^2}$
4. $\frac{d}{dx}(\cot^{-1}x) = \frac{-1}{1+x^2}$
5. $\frac{d}{dx}(\sec^{-1}x) = \frac{1}{x\sqrt{x^2-1}}$
6. $\frac{d}{dx}(\mathrm{cosec}^{-1}x) = \frac{-1}{x\sqrt{x^2-1}}$

Worked Examples

Differentiate w.r.t. x

1. $x^2\sin^{-1}x$

Take $y = x^2\sin^{-1}x;\ \frac{dy}{dx} = \frac{d}{dx}(x^2\sin^{-1}x)$

$$= x^2.\frac{d}{dx}(\sin^{-1}x) + \sin^{-1}x.\frac{d}{dx}(x^2)$$

$$= x^2.\frac{1}{\sqrt{1-x^2}} + \sin^{-1}x.\,2x$$

$$= \frac{x^2}{\sqrt{1-x^2}} + 2x\sin^{-1}x$$

2. $y = \sqrt{x^2-1}\,\sec^{-1}x$

$$\frac{dy}{dx} = \frac{d}{dx}\left[\sqrt{x^2-1}\right]\sec^{-1}x$$

$$= \sqrt{x^2-1}\frac{d}{dx}\left(\sec^{-1}x\right) + \sec^{-1}x\frac{d}{dx}\sqrt{x^2-1}$$

$$= \sqrt{x^2-1}\frac{1}{x\sqrt{x^2-1}} + \sec^{-1}x\frac{1}{2\sqrt{x^2-1}}2x$$

$$= \frac{1}{x} + \frac{x\sec^{-1}x}{\sqrt{x^2-1}}$$

3. $y = \dfrac{x\cos^{-1}x}{\sqrt{1+x^2}}$

$$\frac{dy}{dx} = \frac{d}{dx}\left(\frac{x\cos^{-1}x}{\sqrt{1-x^2}}\right)$$

$$= \frac{\sqrt{1-x^2}\frac{d}{dx}(x\cos^{-1}x) - x\cos^{-1}x\frac{d}{dx}(\sqrt{1-x^2})}{\left(\sqrt{1-x^2}\right)^2}$$

$$= \frac{\sqrt{1-x^2}\left[x.\frac{-1}{\sqrt{1-x^2}} + \cos^{-1}x.1\right] - x\cos^{-1}x\frac{1}{2\sqrt{1-x^2}}(-2x)}{1-x^2}$$

$$= \frac{-x + \sqrt{1+x^2}\cos^{-1}x + \frac{x^2\cos^{-1}x}{\sqrt{1-x^2}}}{1+x^2}$$

$$= \frac{-x + \sqrt{1-x^2} + (1-x^2)\cos^{-1}x + x^2\cos^{-1}x}{(1-x^2)\sqrt{1-x^2}}$$

$$= \frac{\cos^{-1}x - x\sqrt{1-x^2}}{(1-x^2)\sqrt{1-x^2}}$$

6.6 FUNCTION OF A FUNCTION OR A COMPOSITE FUNCTION

Consider $(x^2 + 6x + 8)^7$. Writing $(x^2 + 6x + 8) = u$, $y = u^7$, $u = x^2 + 6x + 8$. Here y is a function of u and u is a function of x. So y is a composite function of x.

$y = \sin^3(x)$, $y = \sqrt{a^2 + x^2}$, $y = \log_e(\sin x)$, $y = e^{\cos x}$, $y = \cos(\sqrt{x})$ etc., are examples of a function of a function of x.

Next consider, $y = \sin^3(x^2 + 1)$. Take $x^2 + 1 = u$ then $y = \sin^3 u$.

Take $\sin u = v$ then $y = v^3$ i.e., $y = v^3$, $v = \sin u$ and $u = x^2 + 1$.

Here y is a function of v, v is a function of u and u is a function of x. So y is a function of a function of a function x, or y is a composite function of x.

Differentiation of a function of x. (Chain rule) If y is a function of u, u is a function of x then.

$$\frac{dy}{dx} = \frac{dy}{du}.\frac{du}{dx}$$

Change x to x + Δx; then let u change to u + Δu; and y to y + Δy

Now $\frac{\Delta y}{\Delta x} = \frac{\Delta y}{\Delta u}.\frac{\Delta u}{\Delta x}$

Taking limits as $\Delta x \to 0$

$$\lim_{\Delta x \to 0}\left(\frac{\Delta y}{\Delta x}\right) = \lim_{\Delta x \to 0}\left(\frac{\Delta y}{\Delta u}\frac{\Delta v}{\Delta x}\right)$$

$$\frac{dy}{dx} = \lim_{\Delta x \to 0}\left(\frac{\Delta y}{\Delta u}\right)\lim_{\Delta x \to 0}\left(\frac{\Delta u}{\Delta x}\right) \quad \text{when } \Delta x \to 0, \Delta u \to 0$$

$$= \frac{dy}{du}.\frac{du}{dx}$$

$$\therefore \quad \frac{dy}{dx} = \frac{dy}{du}.\frac{du}{dx} \qquad \text{(Chain rule)}$$

Similarly, if y is a function of u, u is a function of v, and v is a function of x then

$$\frac{dy}{dx} = \frac{dy}{du}.\frac{du}{dv}.\frac{dv}{dx} \qquad \text{(Chain rule)}$$

Worked Examples

1. $(x^2 + 6x + 8)^7$

I Method: Take $y = (x^2 + 6x + 8)^7$

Put $x^2 + 6x + 8 = u$, then $y = u^7$

$$\frac{dy}{du} = \frac{d}{du}(u^7) = 7u^6; \quad \frac{du}{dx} = \frac{d}{dx}(x^2 + 6x + 8) = 2x + 6$$

Using the chain rule,

$$\therefore \quad \frac{dy}{dx} = \frac{dy}{du}.\frac{du}{dx}$$

$$= 7\,u^6\,(2x + 6)$$

$$= 7\,(x^2 + 6x + 8)^6.\,(2x + 6)$$

II Method: $y = (x^2 + 6x + 8)^7$

$$\frac{dy}{dx} = \frac{d}{dx}(x^2 + 6x + 8)^7$$

$$= 7(x^2 + 6x + 8)^6 . \frac{d}{dx}(x^2 + 6x + 8)$$

$$= 7(x^2 + 6x + 8)^6 (2x + 6)$$

Note: It is better to follow the second method. After practice you can write the answer in one step. If we differentiate x^7, we get $7x^6$ and so if we differentiate $(x^2 + 6x + 8)^7$, we get $7(x^2 + 6x + 8)^6$ which should be multiplied by the derivative of $x^2 + 6x + 8$.

In general, if $y = f(x)^n$ $\left[\text{then } \frac{dy}{dx} = \frac{d}{dx}\{f(x)\}^n = [nf(x)^{n-1}\frac{d}{dx}[f(x)]\right]$

2. $y = (2 - x^4)^{10}$

$$\frac{dy}{dx} = \frac{d}{dx}(2 - x^4)^{10}$$

$$= 10(2 - x^4)^9(-4x^3) = -40x^3(2 - x^4)^9$$

3. $y = \sin^2 x$

$$\frac{dy}{dx} = \frac{d}{dx}\sin^2 x$$

$$= 2\sin x \frac{d}{dx}(\sin x) = 2\sin x \cos x$$

4. $y = \cos^2 x$

$$\frac{dy}{dx} = \frac{d}{dx}\cos^2 x$$

$$= 2\cos x \frac{d}{dx}(\cos x) = 2\cos x(-\sin x)$$

$$= -2\sin x \cos x$$

5. $y = \tan^3 x$

$$\frac{dy}{dx} = \frac{d}{dx}\tan^3 x$$

$$= 3\tan^2 x \frac{d}{dx}(\tan x) = 3\tan^2 x \sec^2 x$$

6. $y = \text{cosec}^2 x$

$$\frac{dy}{dx} = \frac{d}{dx}(\text{cosec}^2 x)$$

$$= 2\text{coscex}(-\text{cosce}\,x \cot x) = -2\text{cosce}^2 x \cot x$$

7. $y = (1 + \log x)^5$

$$\frac{dy}{dx} = \frac{d}{dx}(1 + \log x)^5 = 5(1 + \log x)^4 . \frac{1}{x}$$

8. $y = \sqrt{a^2 + x^2}$

$$\frac{dy}{dx} = \frac{d}{dx}\sqrt{a^2 + x^2}$$

$$= \frac{1}{(2\sqrt{a^2 + x^2})} \frac{d}{dx}(a^2 + x^2)$$

$$= \frac{1}{2\sqrt{a^2 + x^2}} 2x = \frac{x}{a^2 + x^2} \qquad \text{since} \frac{d}{dx}(\sqrt{x}) = \frac{1}{2\sqrt{x}}$$

9. $y = \frac{1}{\text{sinx} + \text{cosx}}$

$$\frac{dy}{dx} = \frac{d}{dx}\left(\frac{1}{\sin x + \cos x}\right)$$

$$= \frac{-1}{(\sin x + \cos x)^2 dx} \frac{d}{dx}(\sin x + \cos x) \qquad \text{since} \frac{d}{dx}\left(\frac{1}{x}\right) = \frac{-1}{x^2}$$

$$= \frac{-1(\cos x - \sin x)}{(\sin x + \cos x)^2} = \frac{\sin x - \cos x}{(\sin x + \cos x)^2}$$

10. $y = \sin^3(\sqrt{x})$

I Method: $y = \sin^3(\sqrt{x})$ put $\sqrt{x} = u.$ then $y = \sin^3 u$

Put sin u = v then y = v^3

$\therefore\ y = v^3,\ c = \sin u,\ u = \sqrt{x}$

$$\frac{dy}{dx} = 3v^2,\ \frac{dv}{du} = \cos u,\ \frac{du}{dx} = \frac{1}{2\sqrt{x}}$$

$$\frac{dy}{dx} = \frac{dy}{dv}.\frac{dv}{du}.\frac{du}{dx} \qquad \text{(Chain rule)}$$

$$= 3v^2.\cos u.\frac{1}{2\sqrt{x}} = 3\sin^2 u \cos(\sqrt{x}).\frac{1}{2\sqrt{x}}$$

$$= \sin^2(\sqrt{x}).\cos(\sqrt{x}).\frac{1}{2\sqrt{x}}$$

II Method: $y = \sin^3(\sqrt{x})$

$$\frac{dy}{dx} = \frac{d}{dx}\left[\sin(\sqrt{x})\right]^3$$

6.7 LOGARITHMIC DIFFERENTIATION

Consider the derivative of x^x w.r.t. x

Let $y = x^x$ .....(1)

Note that $\frac{dy}{dx}(x^n) = nx^{n-1}$ only when n is a constant $\frac{d}{dx}(x^x) \neq x.x^{x-1}$ as index x is not a constant. So whenever there is a function of x in the index, we take logarithms and then differentiate both sides w.r.t. x. This is known as "logarithmic differentiation".

Taking logarithms on both sides of eq.(1)

$$\log_e y = \log_e x^x = x \log_e x$$

Differentiate w.r.t. x $\quad \frac{d}{dx}(\log_e y) = \frac{d}{dx}(x \log_e x)$

$$\frac{1}{y}\frac{dy}{dx} = x\frac{1}{x} + \log_e x.1$$

$$\frac{dy}{dx} = y(1 + \log_e x) = x^x(1 + \log_e x)$$

Worked Examples

1. Find the derivatives of a^x w.r.t. x

   Let $y = a^x$. Take logarithms

   $$\log_e y = \log_e a^x = x \log_e a$$

   $$\frac{d}{dx}(\log_e y) = \frac{d}{dx}(x \log_e a)$$

$$\frac{1}{y}\frac{dy}{dx} = 1.\log_e a$$

$$\therefore \quad \frac{dy}{dx} = y\log_e a = a^x \log_e a$$

$$\therefore \quad \frac{d}{dx}(a^x) = a^x \log_e a$$

2. Differentiate w.r.t x, $\cos\left(x\log_e^x\right)$

Let $y = \cos\left(x\log_e^x\right)$ take $(x\log_e^x) = u$

Then $y = \cos u$; $\frac{dy}{dx} = -\sin u.\frac{du}{dx}$ .....(1)

$$u = \left(x\log_e^x\right); \log_e u = \log_e\left(x\log_e^x\right)$$

$$= \log_e x\,(\log_e x) = (\log_e x)^2$$

$$\frac{d}{dx}(\log_e u) = \frac{d}{dx}(\log_e x)^2$$

$$\frac{1}{u}\frac{du}{dx} = 2(\log_e x)\frac{1}{x}$$

$$\frac{du}{dx} = \frac{2u(\log_e x)}{x} = \frac{2.x^{(\log_e^x)}.\log_e x}{x}$$

Using this in eq.(1), $\frac{dy}{dx} = \frac{-\sin(x^{(\log_e x)}).2.x^{(\log_e x)}.\log_e x}{x}$

3. Find $\frac{dy}{dx}$, if $y = (\tan x)^{\log x} + x^x$

Let $u = (\tan x)^{\log x}$, $v = x^x$

$$\log u = \log x \ \log(\tan x)$$

Differentiating w.r.t. 'x', we get

$$\frac{1}{u}\frac{du}{dx} = \log x\frac{1}{\tan x}\sec^2 x + \frac{1}{x}\log(\tan x)$$

$$\therefore \quad \frac{du}{dx} = \tan x^{\log x}\left[\frac{\log x}{\sin x\cos x} + \frac{\log(\tan x)}{x}\right]$$

$$\log v = x\log x$$

Differentiating w.r.t. 'x', we get

$$\frac{1}{v}\frac{dv}{dx} = 1 + \log x$$

$$\therefore \quad \frac{dv}{dx} = x^x(1 + \log x)$$

$$\therefore \quad \frac{dy}{dx} = \frac{du}{dx} + \frac{dv}{dx}$$

$$\frac{dy}{dx} = (\tan x)^{\log x}\left[\frac{\log x}{\sin x \cos x} + \frac{\log(\tan x)}{x}\right] + x^x(1 + \log x)$$

4. Differentiate $(\sin x)^x + x^{\sin x}$ w.r.t. 'x'

Let $y = (\sin x)^x + x^{\sin x}$

Let $u = (\sin x)^x$, $\quad v = x^{\sin x}$

$\text{Log}(u) = \log(\sin x)^x = x\log(\sin x)$

Differentiating w.r.t 'x', we get

$$\frac{1}{u}\frac{du}{dx} = x \cot x + \log \sin x$$

$\log v = \sin x \log x$

Differentiating w.r.t 'x', we get

$$\frac{1}{v}\frac{dv}{dx} = \frac{\sin x}{s} + \cos x \log x$$

$$\frac{dv}{dx} = x^{\sin x}\left[\frac{\sin x}{x} + \cos x \log x\right]$$

Now, $\quad \dfrac{dy}{dx} = \dfrac{du}{dx} + \dfrac{dv}{du}$

$$= (\sin x)^x[x \cot x + \log \sin x] + x^{\sin x}\left[\frac{\sin x}{x} + \cos x \log x\right]$$

5. If $y = x^{\sin^{-1}x} + (\sin^{-1}x)^x$, Find $\dfrac{dy}{dx}$

let $u = x^{\sin^{-1}x}$, $v = (\sin^{-1}x)^x$

$\log u = \sin^{-1}x \log x$

Differentiating w.r.t 'x', we get

$$\frac{1}{u}.\frac{du}{dx}=\frac{\sin^{-1}x}{x}+\frac{\log x}{\sqrt{1-x^2}}$$

$$\therefore \quad \frac{dy}{dx}=x^{\sin^{-1}x}\left[\frac{\sin^{-1}x}{x}+\frac{\log x}{\sqrt{1-x^2}}\right]$$

$\log v = x \log (\sin^{-1}x)$

Differentiating w.r.t. 'x', we get

$$\frac{1}{v}.\frac{dv}{dx}=\frac{x}{\sin^{-1}x\sqrt{1-x^2}}+\log(\sin^{-1}x)$$

$$\therefore \quad \frac{dv}{dx}=(\sin^{-1}x)^x\left[\frac{x}{\sin^{-1}x\sqrt{1-x^2})}+\log(\sin^{-1}x)\right]$$

$$\therefore \quad \frac{dy}{dx}=\frac{du}{dx}+\frac{dv}{dx}$$

$$=x^{\sin^{-1}x}\left[\frac{\sin^{-1}x}{x}+\frac{\log x}{\sqrt{1-x^2}}\right]+(\sin^{-1}x)^x\left[\frac{x}{\sin^{-1}x\sqrt{1-x^2}}+\log\sin^{-1}x\right]$$

6.8 DIFFERENTIATION OF IMPLICIT FUNCTIONS

In functions like $y = x^2 + a^2$, $y = \sin^{-1}(x^3)$, $y=\sqrt{x^2+x+1}$ etc., y is directly expressed as a function of x. **Such functions are known as explicit functions.**

Consider $x^2+y^2=a^2$, $x^3+y^3=3axy$, $x+y=\sqrt{xy}$ etc. here y is not directly expressed as a function of x. Such functions are known as implicit functions. $y = f(x)$ is an example of an explicit function. $f(x, y) = c$ where c is a constant is an example of an implicit function.

Worked Examples

1. Find $\frac{dy}{dx}$ if $2x^2-3xy+4y^2=1$

$2x^2-3xy+4y^2=1$

Differentiate both sides w.r.t x

$$2\frac{d}{dx}(x^2) - 3\frac{d}{dx}(xy) + 4\frac{d}{dx}(y^2) = \frac{d}{dx}(1)$$

$$2(2x) - 3\left[x\frac{dy}{dx} + y.1\right] + 4.\left(2y\frac{dy}{dx}\right) = 0$$

$$4x - 3x\frac{dy}{dx} - 3y + 8y\frac{dy}{dx} = 0$$

i.e.,
$$8y\frac{dy}{dx} - 3x\frac{dy}{dx} = 3y - 4x$$

or
$$\frac{dy}{dx}(8y - 3x) = 3y - 4x$$

$$\therefore \quad \frac{dy}{dx} = \frac{3y-4x}{8y-3x}$$

Note: The given equation is differentiated both sides w.r.t. x

You should not take $y = 2x^2 - 3xy + 4y^2$

2. If $x^2 + 2xy + 3y^2 + x + y - 1 = 0$ find $\frac{dy}{dx}$ when x = 1, y = 2

$$x^2 + 2xy + 3y^2 + x + y - 1 = 0$$

$$\frac{d}{dx}(x^2) + 2\frac{d}{dx}(xy) + 3\frac{d}{dx}(y^2) + \frac{d}{dx}(x) + \frac{d}{dx}(y) - \frac{d}{dx}(1) = 0$$

$$2x + 2x\frac{dy}{dx} + 2y + 6y\frac{dy}{dx} + 1 + \frac{dy}{dx} = 0$$

6.9 MAXIMA AND MINIMA

Thus a function y = f(x), which is continuous is said to be maximum at $x = a$ if $f(a) > f(a + h)$ and $f(a) > f(a - h)$. Where h is a small positive number. f(a) is the maximum if f(x) at x = a.

Similarly, y = f(x), is said to be minimum if

$f(a) < f(a + h)$ and $f(a) < f(a - h)$. Where h is a small positive number. f(a) is the minimum of f(x) at x = a.

6.9.1 Conditions for a Function to be a Maximum or a Minimum at a Point

Consider a curve y = f(x), which is continuous. Let A be a point on the curve at which y is a maximum. Let the x-coordinate of A be a.

Then $f(a) > f(a + h)$ and $f(a) > f(a - h)$. Let B and C be points on the curve to the left and right of the point A respectively. At the point B, the tangent to the curve makes an angle ψ_1 with the positive direction of axis.

Since ψ_1 is acute, $\frac{dy}{dx} = \tan\psi_1$ is positive. At point A, the tangent to the curve is parallel at x-axis and so $\frac{dy}{dx} = 0$

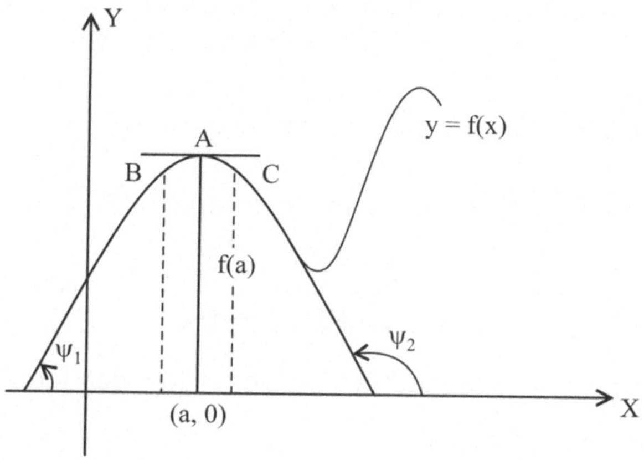

At the point C, the tangent to the curve makes an angle ψ_2 is obtuse, $\frac{dy}{dx} = \tan\psi_2$ is negative.

Now as x takes the value to through a (from left to right,) $\frac{dy}{dx}$ changes from positive value to negative value. This means that $\frac{dy}{dx}$ decreases and so its derivative namely $\frac{d^2y}{dx^2}$ is negative at A.

So for y = f(x), be maximum at A (x = a) the conditions are:

(i) $\frac{dy}{dx} = 0$ and

(ii) $\frac{d^2y}{dx^2}$ must be negative at A i.e., at the point x = a. The maximum value of the function is f(a).

Similarly, it can be shown that for y = f(x), to be minimum at x = a, the conditions are:

(i) $\frac{dy}{dx} = 0$ and

(ii) $\frac{d^2y}{dx^2}$ must be positive at x = a.

Note:

1. A maximum value is not necessarily the greatest value, the function can have, not the minimum the least. A function may have many maxima and minima.
2. The maxima and minima values occur alternately.
3. The function is neither maximum nor minimum if $\frac{dy}{dx} = 0$ and $\frac{d^2y}{dx^2} = 0$

Worked Examples

1. Find the maximum and minimum values of the function

$$2x^3 - 3x^2 - 36x + 10$$

Let $y = 2x^3 - 3x^2 - 36x + 10$ .....(1)

$$\frac{dy}{dx} = 6x^2 - 6x - 36 \quad .....(2)$$

$$\frac{d^2y}{dx^2} = 12x - 6 \quad .....(3)$$

For the function to be maximum or minimum $\frac{dy}{dx} = 0$

$\therefore$ $6x^2 - 6x - 36 = 0$

i.e., $x^2 - x - 6 = 0$

i.e., $(x - 3)(x + 2) = 0$

$x = 3$ or $x = -2$

When x = 3, $\frac{dy}{dx}=0$, $\frac{d^2y}{dx^2}=36-6=30$ (positive)

Therefore the function is minimum at x = 3. The minimum value is got by putting x = 3 in (1)

$$y\ min = 2.3^3 - 3.3^2 - 36.3 + 10 = 54 - 27 - 108 + 10 = -71$$

When x = – 2, $\frac{dy}{dx}=0$, $\frac{d^2y}{dx^2}=-24-6=-30$ (negative)

Therefore the function is maximum at x = –2

The maximum value is got by putting x = –2 in (1)

$$y\ max = 2(-2)^3 - 3(-2)^2 - 36(2) + 10 = -16 - 12 + 72 + 10 = 54$$

2. Show that sin x(1+cos x) is maximum when $x = \frac{\pi}{3}$

Let y = sin x(1 + cos x) .....(1)

$$\frac{dy}{dx} = \sin x(-\sin x) + (1+\cos x)\cos x = -\sin^2 x + \cos x + \cos^2 x$$

i.e., $\frac{dy}{dx} = \cos^2 x - \sin^2 x + \cos x$ .....(2)

$$\frac{d^2y}{dx^2} = -2\cos x \sin x - 2\sin x \cos x - \sin x \quad .....(3)$$

For y to be maximum or minimum $\frac{dy}{dx}=0$

i.e., $\cos^2(x) - \sin^2(x) + 1 = 0$

$\cos(2x) + \cos(x) = 0$

$2\cos^2(x) - 1 + \cos(x) = 0$

$2\cos^2(x) + 2\cos(x) - \cos(x) - 1 = 0$

$2\cos(x)(\cos(x) + 1) - 1(\cos(x) + 1) = 0$

$(\cos(x) + 1)(2\cos(x) - 1)$

$(\cos(x) + 1) = 0$ or $2\cos(x) - 1 = 0$

$\cos x = -1$ or $\cos x = \frac{1}{2}$

i.e., $x = \pi$ or $x = \frac{\pi}{3}$

when $x = \frac{\pi}{3}\ \frac{dy}{dx} = 0,\ \frac{d^2(y)}{dx^2} = -ve$

The function is maximum at $x = \frac{\pi}{3}$

$$\text{Max Value} = \sin\frac{\pi}{3}\left(1+\cos\frac{\pi}{3}\right) = \frac{\sqrt{3}}{2}\left(1+\frac{1}{2}\right) = \frac{3\sqrt{3}}{4}$$

Exercise 6.1

1. Find the derivative of $\frac{1}{x^3}$
2. Find dy/dx when $y = \frac{1}{x} + \frac{2}{x^2} + \frac{3}{x^3} + \frac{4}{x^4}$
3. If $f(x) = 2x^3 + 3x^2 + 5x - 3$ find $f^1(0)$
4. If $y = \sin x + \cos x + e^x$ find dy/ dx
5. If $y = x \tan x$ find $\frac{dy}{dx}$ when $x = \frac{\pi}{4}$
6. If $y = x^3 e^x$ find $\frac{dy}{dx}$
7. If $y = 4e^x + 4\tan x + \sin x + \log(x)$ find $\frac{dy}{dx}$
8. If $y = x \sin x$, find $\frac{dy}{dx}$
9. If $y = x^4 \tan x$, find $\frac{dy}{dx}$
10. If $y = \sqrt{x} \sin x$, find $\frac{dy}{dx}$
11. Differentiate each w.r.t.x
    (a) $(3x^4 - 7x^3 + 10x^2 + 1)(x^2 + x - 1)$
    (b) $(3x^2 - 1)(4x^4 + 2x^2 - 1)$
    (c) $X^n(\sqrt{x} - 1)$

12. $\frac{1-x^2}{1+x^2}$ 13. $\frac{x}{x^3+1}$ 14. $\frac{e^x}{1+e^x}$

15. $x\sin^{-1}x$

16. $\sqrt{1-x^2}\cos^{-1}x$

17. $x^2\sec^{-1}x$

18. $x^2e^{a\sin^{-1}x}$

19. $\sin(m\sin^{-1}x)$

20. $x^2\sec^{-1}(x^2)$

21. $\dfrac{e^{3x}}{\log x}$

Answers

1. $\dfrac{-3}{x^4}$

2. $-\dfrac{1}{x^2}-\dfrac{4}{x^3}-\dfrac{9}{x^4}-\dfrac{16}{x^5}$

3. 5

4. $\cos x-\sin x+e^x$

5. $\dfrac{\pi}{2}+1$

6. $e^x(x^3+3x^2)$

7. $4e^x+4\sec^2(x)+\cos(x)+\dfrac{1}{x}$

8. $x\cos(x)+\sin(x)$

9. $x^4\sec^2x+\tan x\,(4x^3)$

10. $\sqrt{x}\cos x+\sin x\dfrac{1}{2\sqrt{x}}$

11. (a) $(x^2+x-1)(12x^3-21x^2+20x)+(3x^4-7x^3+10x^2+1)(2x+1)$

(b) $(3x^2-1)(16x^3+4x)+(4x^4+2x^2-1)(6x)$

(c) $X^n\dfrac{1}{2\sqrt{x}}+(\sqrt{x}-1)(nX^{n-1})$

12. $\dfrac{(-4x)}{(1+x^2)^2}$

13. $\dfrac{1-2x^3}{(x^3+1)^2}$

14. $\dfrac{e^x}{(1+e^x)^2}$

15. $\dfrac{x}{\sqrt{1-x^2}}+\sin^{-1}x$

16. $-1+\dfrac{x\cos^{-1}(x)}{\sqrt{1-x^2}}$

17. $x^2\dfrac{1}{x\sqrt{x^2-1}}+2x\sec^{-1}x$

18. $a\,x^2e^{a\sin^{-1}(x)}\dfrac{1}{\sqrt{1-x^2}}$

19. $m\cos(m\sin^{-1}x)\dfrac{1}{\sqrt{1-x^2}}$

20. $2x\left[\dfrac{1}{\sqrt{x^4-1}}+\sec^{-1}(x^2)\right]$

21. $\dfrac{3\log(x)e^{3x}-\dfrac{e^{3x}}{x}}{(\log x)^2}$

Problems

1. The amount of drug that distributes in the body is given by the function $X = X_0 e^{-kt}$ where X_0 is the amount drug injected (i.e., dose) when time is 0 and k is first elimination rate constant for a drug. Find X_0 and also obtain the value of $\frac{dx}{dt}$ when $t = 0$.
2. The Cumulative amount of unchanged drug excreted from body at time t is given by the function $X_u = \frac{k_e X_0}{K}(1 - e^{-kt})$ where k_e is apparent first-order rate constant for renal excretion and k is elimination rate constant. Obtain $\frac{dx_u}{dt}$ and also find $\frac{dx_u}{dt}$ when time is 0
3. The metabolite Concentration in the Plasma (c_m) is given by the function $C_m = k_f X_0/V_m\ (k - k_m)\ (e^{-kmt} - e^{-kt})$, find $\frac{dc_m}{dt}$, where k_f and k_m are apparent first order constants for metabolite formation and elimination.
4. The concentration of drug when it is administered intravenously at a constant rate is given by the function $c = \frac{k_0}{VK}(1 - e^{-kt})$. Find $\frac{dc}{dt}$ where k_0 is rate of drug infusion, expressed in terms of amount per unit time, k is first order elimination constant and v is volume distribution.
5. A drug that decomposes with regard to the time is given by a linear equation $c_d = kt$. Find dc/dt
6. The Plasma concentration versus time profile can be obtained by the concentration function $c_p = c_1 e_1^{-\lambda t} + c_2 e_2^{-\lambda t}$. Find $\frac{d_{cp}}{dt}$ when $t = 0$ (Journal of Pharmaceutical Sciences Vol – 77–2, Feb – 1988)
7. The function which is used for the calculation rate of diffusion of through a layer is given by the function $x = 1 - (1 - \sqrt{kt})^3$ find $\frac{dx}{dt}$ (Journal of Pharmaceutical Sciences Vol – 77-4, 1988).
8. The concentration of drug in the plasma when it is administered intravenously at a constant rate is given by the function $c = \frac{kaFX_0}{V(Ka - k)} e^{-kt}$. Find $\frac{dc}{dt}$ where k_a is apparent first order rate constant, k is first order elimination constant, F is fraction of administered dose, X_0 that is absorbed and v is volume distribution.

9. If $\log(y) = -BX + \log A$, find $\frac{dy}{dt}$

10. If the simple first order kinetic relationship is given by the equation $Y = Ae^{-kt}$, Prove $\frac{dy}{dt} = -kAe^{-kt}$

11. If a solution initially containing 2 moles/liter of Y and 1 mole/liter of Z is allowed to react at time t is given by the function of $x(t) = \frac{-2+2e^{ki}}{-1+2e^{kt}}$.

    Find $\frac{dx}{dt}$ and show that $\frac{dx}{dt} = 0$ when $t = 0$

12. The concentration of drug in the plasma when it is administered intravenously at a constant rate is obtained by function $F(t) = \frac{Q_0}{k}(1-e^{-kt})$ where Q_0 and k are constants. Prove that $\frac{d(F(t))}{dt} = \frac{Q_0}{k}e^{-kt}$.

13. The amount of drug that has been absorbed into systemic circulation, X_A, at any time after administration will be equal to the sum of the amount of drug in the body, X and the cumulative amount of drug eliminated, X_E by urinary excretion, by metabolism and by all other routes at that time is given by the function $X_A = X + X_E$. Prove that $\frac{dX_A}{dt} = \frac{dX}{dt} + \frac{dX_E}{dt}$

14. The observed plasma concentration and the plasma concentration at the time of first order input into the body is given by the equation

$$C = \frac{k_a FX_0}{V(k_a - K)}e^{-kt} - \frac{k_a FX_0}{V(k_a - K)}e^{-k_a t}.$$

Prove that

$$\frac{dc}{dt} = \frac{k^2 aFX_0}{V(k_a - K)}e^{-k_a t} - \frac{k_a FX_0}{V(k_a - K)}e^{-kt}.$$

CHAPTER **7**

INTEGRATION

7.1 INTRODUCTION

This branch of calculus arose initially in connection with the summation of infinitely large numbers to infinitely small quantities. For example the area under a given curve can be expressed as summation of infinitely small known areas. Such situations lead to the development of the concept known as integration. In this chapter we define integration of a function and study the techniques of integration. The technique of integration and its application in solving/deriving the pharmacokinetic equation.

Definition

So far we have considered the problem of differentiation. That is, given y = f(x) or f(x, y) = c, we have found $\frac{dy}{dx}$. Now, we consider the converse problem, finding of a function whose derivative is known, which is called integration.

Integration is the Inverse Process of Differentiation

Consider $\frac{d}{dx}(x^4) = 4x^3$. i.e., the derivative of x^4 w.r.t.x is $4x^3$. Now it is said that the integral of $4x^3$ w.r.t. x is x^4. x^4 is also called the antidervative of $4x^3$. In symbols this is written as $\int 4x^3\,dx = x^4$ (Read it as the integral of $4x^3$ dx is equal to x^4. It is to be noted that the integral of a function ($4x^3$) is that function (x^4) whose derivatives is the function ($4x^3$)

$$\frac{d}{dx}(x^4) = 4x^3 \qquad \therefore \qquad \int 4x^3\,dx = x^4$$

$$\frac{d}{dx}(x^4 + 3) = 4x^3 \qquad \therefore \qquad \int 4x^3\,dx = x^4 + 3$$

($\because$ the derivative of a constant is 0)

$$\frac{d}{dx}(x^4 + c) = 4x^3 \quad \therefore \quad \int 4x^3\,dx = x^4 + c$$

C is called the Constant of Integration

Thus, if $\frac{d}{dx}[\phi(x)] = f(x)$ then $\int f(x)\,dx = \phi(x) + c$

$\int f(x)\,dx$ is called as indefinite integration of f(x) w.r.t. x.

f(x) is called the integrand and x is the variable of integration.

Example:

1. $\frac{d}{dx}(\sin^2 x) = 2\sin x \cos x \quad \therefore \quad \int 2\sin x \cos x dx = \sin^2 x + c$

2. $\frac{d}{dx}(\log_e \sin x) = \frac{1}{\sin x}.\cos x = \cot x \quad \therefore \quad \int \cot x dx = \log_e \sin x + c$

3. $\frac{d}{dx}(\tan x) = \sec^2 x \quad \therefore \quad \int \sec^2 x dx = \tan x + c$

Standard Formulae

1. $\int x^n dx = \frac{x^{n+1}}{n+1} + c\ (n \neq -1) \qquad \left[\because \frac{d}{dx}\left(\frac{x^{n+1}}{n+1}\right) = \frac{(n+1)x^n}{(n+1)} = x^n\right]$

2. $\int \frac{1}{x} dx = \log_e x + c \qquad \left[\because \frac{d}{dx}(\log_e x) = \frac{1}{x}\right]$

3. $\int \sin x\,dx = -\cos x + c$

4. $\int \cos x\,dx = \sin x + c$

5. $\int \tan x\,dx = \log_e \sec x + c \qquad \left[\because \frac{d}{dx}(\log_e \sec x) = \frac{1}{\sec x} \sec x \tan x = \text{tax}\right]$

6. $\int \cot(x) x\,dx = \log_e \sin x + c$

7. $\int \sec x\,dx = \log_e(\sec x + \tan x) + c$

$$\left[\because \frac{d}{dx}\left(\log_e(\sec x + \tan x)\right) = \frac{1}{(\sec x + \tan x)}(\sec x \tan x + \sec x^2 x\right]$$

$$= \left[\frac{\sec x(\sec x + \tan x)}{\sec x + \tan x} = \sec x\right]$$

8. $\int \text{cosec}x\, dx = -\log_e(\text{cosec}x + \cot x) + c$

9. $\int \sec^2 x\, dx = \tan x + c$

10. $\int \text{cosec}^2 x\, dx = -\cot x + c$

11. $\int \sec x \tan x\, dx = \sec x + c$

12. $\int \text{cosec}x \cot x\, dx = -\text{cosec}x + c$

13. $\int \sinh x\, dx = \cosh x + c$

14. $\int \cosh x\, dx = \sinh x + c$

15. $\int k\, dx = kx + c$ where k is a constant

16. $\int e^x\, dx = e^x + c \qquad \left(\because \frac{d}{dx}(e^x) = e^x\right)$

From Formula (1)

$$\int x dx = \frac{x^{1+1}}{1+1} = \frac{x^2}{2}; \int x^2 dx = \frac{x^{2+1}}{2+1} = \frac{x^3}{3}; \int x^3 dx = \frac{x^4}{4};$$

$$\int \frac{1}{x^2} dx = \int x^{-2} dx = \frac{x^{-2+1}}{-2+1} = -\frac{1}{x}$$

$$\int \sqrt{x} dx = \int x^{\frac{1}{2}} dx = \frac{x^{\frac{1}{2}+1}}{\frac{1}{2}+1} = \frac{x^{\frac{3}{2}}}{\frac{3}{2}} = \frac{2}{3} x^{\frac{3}{2}}$$

$$\int \frac{1}{\sqrt{x}} dx = \int x^{-\frac{1}{2}} dx = \frac{x^{-\frac{1}{2}+1}}{-\frac{1}{2}+1} = \frac{x^{\frac{1}{2}}}{\frac{1}{2}} = 2\sqrt{x}$$

$$\int \frac{1}{\sqrt[3]{x^2}} dx = \int x^{-\frac{2}{3}} dx = \frac{x^{-\frac{2}{3}+1}}{-\frac{2}{3}+1} = \frac{x^{\frac{1}{3}}}{\frac{1}{3}} = 3.x^{\frac{1}{3}}$$

(The constant c is considered to be understood)

7.2 RULES OF INTEGRATION

Rule 1: $\int kf(x)dx = k\int f(x)dx$ where k is a constant

Examples

1. $\int 3x^4 dx = 3\int x^4 dx = 3\frac{x^5}{5}$
2. $\int \frac{2}{3x^6} dx = \frac{2}{3}\int x^{-6} dx = \frac{2}{3}\frac{x^{-5}}{-5} = -\frac{2}{15x^5}$
3. $\int 3\sin x dx = 3(-\cos x) = -3\cos x$

Rule 2: $\int [f(x) \pm g(x) \pm h(x) \pm ...]dx$

$$= \int f(x)dx \pm \int g(x)dx \pm \int h(x)dx \pm ...$$

Examples

1. $\int (x^3 + 3x^2 + 7x - 13)dx$

$$= \int x^3 dx + \int 3x^2 dx + \int 7x dx - \int 13 dx$$

$$= \frac{x^4}{4} + 3\frac{x^3}{3} + 7\frac{x^2}{2} - 13x + c$$

2. $\int \left(\sqrt{x} + \frac{1}{\sqrt{x}}\right) dx = \int \left(x^{\frac{1}{2}} + x^{-\frac{1}{2}}\right) dx$

$$= \frac{x^{\frac{3}{2}}}{\frac{3}{2}} + \frac{x^{\frac{1}{2}}}{\frac{1}{2}} + c = \frac{2}{3}x^{\frac{3}{2}} + 2x^{\frac{1}{2}} + c$$

3. $\int \left(2x^3 - \frac{1}{3x^2}\right) dx$

$$= \int \left(2x^3 - \frac{x^{-2}}{3}\right) dx = 2\frac{x^4}{4} - \frac{x^{-1}}{3(-1)} + c = \frac{x^4}{2} + \frac{1}{3x} + c$$

4. $\int (a \sin x + b \cos x + c)dx$

$$= a(-\cos x) + b \sin x + cx + c^1 = -a \cos x + b \sin x + cx + c^1$$

5. $\int \left(e^x + x^e + e^e\right) dx = e^x + \frac{x^{e+1}}{e+1} + e^e x + c$

Worked Examples

Integrate each of the following with respect to x

1. $3x^4 - 4x^2 + \frac{1}{x} + \frac{1}{x^2}$

$$\int \left(3x^4 - 4x^2 + \frac{1}{x} + \frac{1}{x^2}\right)dx = 3\frac{x^5}{5} - 4\frac{x^3}{3} + \log_e x + \frac{x^{-1}}{-1} + c$$

$$= \frac{3x^5}{5} - \frac{4x^3}{3} + \log_e x - \frac{1}{x} + c$$

2. $(x^2 + 1)(2x^3 - 3)$

$$\int (x^2 + 1)(2x^3 - 3)dx = \int (2x^5 + 2x^3 - 3x^2 - 3)dx$$

$$= 2\frac{x^6}{6} + 2\frac{x^4}{4} - 3\frac{x^3}{3} - 3x + c = \frac{x^6}{3} + \frac{x^4}{2} - x^3 - 3x + c$$

3. $\left(x^3 - \frac{2}{x^3}\right)^2$

$$\int \left(x^3 - \frac{2}{x^3}\right)^2 dx = \int \left(x^6 + \frac{4}{x^6} - 4\right)dx = \frac{x^7}{7} + \frac{4x^{-5}}{-5} - 4x + c$$

$$= \frac{x^7}{7} - \frac{4}{5x^5} - 4x + c$$

4. $\left(x + \frac{1}{x}\right)^3$

$$\int \left(x + \frac{1}{x}\right)^3 dx = \int x^3 + \frac{1}{x^3} + 3x.\frac{1}{x}\left(x + \frac{1}{x}\right)dx$$

$$= \int \left(x^3 + x^{-3} + 3x + \frac{3}{x}\right)dx$$

$$= \frac{x^4}{4} - \frac{1}{2x^2} + \frac{3x^2}{2} + 3\log_e x + c$$

5. $\frac{x^3+3x^2+4}{\sqrt{x}}$

$$\int\frac{x^3+3x^2+4}{\sqrt{x}}dx=\int\left(\frac{x^3}{\sqrt{x}}+\frac{3x^2}{\sqrt{x}}+\frac{4}{\sqrt{x}}\right)dx$$

$$=\int\left(x^{3-\frac{1}{2}}+3x^{2-\frac{1}{2}}+4x^{-\frac{1}{2}}\right)dx$$

$$=\int\left(x^{\frac{5}{2}}+3x^{\frac{3}{2}}+4x^{-\frac{1}{2}}\right)dx$$

$$=\frac{x^{\frac{5}{2}+1}}{\frac{5}{2}+1}+3.\frac{x^{\frac{3}{2}+1}}{\frac{3}{2}+1}+4.\frac{x^{-\frac{1}{2}+1}}{-\frac{1}{2}+1}+c$$

$$=\frac{x^{\frac{7}{2}}}{\frac{7}{2}}+3.\frac{x^{\frac{5}{2}}}{\frac{5}{2}}+4.\frac{x^{\frac{1}{2}}}{\frac{1}{2}}+c=\frac{2}{7}x^{\frac{7}{2}}+\frac{6x^{\frac{5}{2}}}{5}+8x^{\frac{1}{2}}+c$$

6. $\frac{1}{1-\sin x}$

$\int\frac{1}{1-\sin x}dx$ multiply both N and D by 1 + sin x

$$=\int\frac{(1+\sin x)}{(1-\sin x)(1+\sin x)}dx=\int\frac{1+\sin x}{1-\sin^2 x}dx=\int\frac{1+\sin x}{\cos^2 x}dx$$

$$=\int\left(\frac{1}{\cos^2 x}+\frac{\sin x}{\cos^2 x}\right)dx=\int\left(\sec^2 x+\frac{\sin x}{\cos x}.\frac{1}{\cos x}\right)dx$$

$$=\int(\sec^2 x+\tan x\sec x)dx=\sec x+\tan x+c$$

7. $\sqrt{1+\sin^2 x}$

$$\int\sqrt{1+\sin^2 x}dx=\int\sqrt{\sin^2 x+\cos^2 x+2\sin x\cos x}dx \qquad (\because 1=\sin^2 x+\cos^2 x)$$

$$\int\sqrt{(\sin x+\cos x)^2}dx=\int(\sin x+\cos x)dx$$

$$=-\cos x\ x+\sin x+c$$

8. $\int \frac{\cos x}{\sin^2 x} dx = \int \frac{\cos x}{\sin x} \cdot \frac{1}{\sin x} dx = \int \cot x \ \text{cosec} x \ dx$

$= -\text{cosec} x + c$

9. $2 \cos x + 3 \sin x$

$\int (2\cos x + 3 \sin x) dx = 2 \sin x + 3 \cos x + c$

10. $\cos x + 4 \sin x$

$\int (\cos x + 4 \sin x) dx = \sin x - 4 \cos x + c$

11. $\frac{1}{\sin^2 x \cos^2 x}$

$$\int \frac{1}{\sin^2 x \cos^2 x} dx = \int \frac{\sin^2 x + \cos^2 x}{\sin^2 x \cos^2 x} dx$$

$$= \int \left(\frac{1}{\cos^2 x} + \frac{1}{\sin^2 x} \right) dx$$

$$= \int \left(\sec^2 x + \text{cosec}^2 x \right) dx$$

$$= \tan x - \cot x + c$$

12. $\tan^2 x$

$$\int \tan^2 x \ dx = \int (\sec^2 x - 1) dx$$

$$= \tan x - x + c$$

7.3 METHOD OF SUBSTITUTION

Integrals of the form: $\int (ax + b)^n dx, \int \sin(ax + b) dx$ etc.

1. $\int (ax + b)^n dx \quad (n \neq -1)$

put $ax + b = t$

differentiate w.r.s.t x

$ax + b = t$

$$a = \frac{dt}{dx}$$

$a dx = dt$

$$dx = \frac{dt}{a}$$

$$\int t^n \frac{dt}{a} = \frac{1}{a}\frac{t^{n+1}}{n+1} + c$$

$$= \frac{(ax+b)^{n+1}}{a(n+1)} + c$$

$$\therefore \quad \int (ax+b)^n dx = \frac{(ax+b)^{n+1}}{a(n+1)} + c$$

2. $\int \frac{1}{ax+b} dx$

put ax + b = t

differentiate w.r.s.t x

$$ax + b = t$$

$$a = \frac{dt}{dx}$$

$$adx = dt$$

$$dx = \frac{dt}{a}$$

$$\int \frac{1}{ax+b} dx = \int \frac{1}{t}\frac{dt}{a} = \frac{1}{a}\log_e t + c = \frac{1}{a}\log_e (ax+b) + c$$

$$\therefore \quad \int \frac{1}{ax+b} dx = \frac{1}{a}\log_e (ax+b) + c$$

3. $\int \sin(ax+b)dx$

put ax + b = t

differentiate w.r.s.t x

$$ax + b = t$$

$$a = \frac{dt}{dx}$$

$$adx = dt$$

$$dx = \frac{dt}{a}$$

$$\int \sin(ax+b)dx = \int \sin t \frac{dt}{a} = \frac{1}{a}(-\cos t) + c = -\frac{\cos(ax+b)}{a} + c$$

In particular, when b = 0, $\int \sin axdx = \frac{\cos ax}{a} + c$

Similarly, $\int \cos ac\ dx = \frac{\sin ax}{a} + c$; $\int e^{ax} dx = \frac{e^{ax}}{a} + c$

$$\int \sec^2 axdx = \frac{\tan ax}{a} + c \text{ etc.}$$

Examples

1. $\int (2x+3)^6 dx = \frac{(2x+3)^7}{2(7)} + c = \frac{(2x+3)^7}{14} + c$
2. $\int \frac{1}{3x+5} dx = \frac{1}{3}\log_e(3x+5) + c$
3. $\int \sin 3x\ dx = -\frac{\cos 3x}{3} + c$
4. $\int \cos 4x\ dx = \frac{\sin 4x}{4} + c$
5. $\int e^{2x} dx = \frac{e^{2x}}{2} + c$

Worked Examples

Integrate each of the following w.r.t. x:

1. $\frac{1}{(2x+1)^3}$

$$\int \frac{1}{(2x+1)^3} dx = \int (2x+1)^{-3} dx = \frac{(2x+1)^{-3+1}}{2(-3+1)} + c$$

$$= \frac{(2x+1)^{-2}}{-4} + c = -\frac{1}{4(2x+1)^2} + c$$

2. $\dfrac{1}{\sqrt{4-3x}}$

$$\int\frac{1}{\sqrt{4-3x}}dx=\int(4-3x)^{-\frac{1}{2}}dx=\frac{(4-3x)^{-\frac{1}{2}+1}}{-3\left(-\frac{1}{2}+1\right)}+c$$

$$=-\frac{2}{3}(4-3x)^{\frac{1}{2}}+c=-\frac{2}{3}\sqrt{4-3x}+c$$

3. $\dfrac{1}{1-8x}$

$$\int\frac{1}{1-8x}dx=\frac{1}{-8}\log_e(1-8x)+c=-\frac{1}{8}\log_e(1-8x)+c$$

4. $\dfrac{1}{\cos^2 4x}$

$$\int\frac{1}{\cos^2 4x}dx=\int\sec^2 4x\,dx=\frac{\tan 4x}{4}+c$$

5. $\dfrac{\sin 3x}{\cos^2 4x}$

$$\int\frac{\sin 3x}{\cos^2 3x}dx=\int\frac{\sin 3x}{\cos 3x}.\frac{1}{\cos 3x}dx$$

$$=\int\tan 3x\sec 3x\,dx=\frac{\sec 3x}{3}+c$$

6. $\sqrt{1+\cos x}$

$$\int\sqrt{1+\cos x}\,dx=\int\sqrt{2\cos^2\frac{x}{2}dx}$$

Use the formula $1+\cos x=2\cos^2\left(\frac{x}{2}\right)$

$$=\sqrt{2}\int\cos\left(\frac{x}{2}\right)dx$$

$$=\sqrt{2}.\frac{\sin\left(\frac{x}{2}\right)}{\frac{1}{2}}+c=2\sqrt{2}\sin\left(\frac{x}{2}\right)+c$$

7. $\int \sec x \, dx$

$\int \sec x \, dx = \int \frac{\sec x(\sec x + \tan x)}{(\sec x + \tan x)} dx$ Multiply both Nr and Dr

by sec x + tan x

$$= \int \frac{\left(\sec^2 x + \sec x \tan x\right) dx}{(\sec x + \tan)}$$

by sec x + tan x

Put sec x + tan x = t

Differentiating

$$= \int \frac{dt}{t} \qquad \sec x \tan x + \sec^2 x = \frac{dt}{dx}$$

$$= \log_e t + c \qquad \therefore \ (\sec x \tan x + \sec^2 x) dx = dt$$

$$= \log_e (\sec x + \tan x) + c$$

8. $\int \frac{\sin x - \cos x}{\sin x + \cos x} dx$

$$= -\int \frac{1}{t} dt \qquad \text{Put } \sin x + \cos x = t$$

$$= -\log t \qquad (\cos x - \sin x) dx = dt$$

$$= -\log(\sin x + \cos x) + c \qquad (\sin x - \cos x)\, dx = -dt$$

9. $\sin^2 x$

$$\int \sin^2 x dx = \int \frac{1}{2}(1 - \cos 2x) dx \qquad \text{Use the formula } \sin^2 x = \frac{1}{2}(1 - \cos 2x)$$

$$= \frac{1}{2}\left[x - \frac{\sin 2x}{2}\right] + c$$

10. $\cos^2 x$ $\qquad \cos^2 x = \frac{1}{2}(1 + \cos 2x)$

$$\int \cos^2 x dx = \int \frac{1}{2} + (1 + \cos 2x) dx = \frac{1}{2}\left[x + \frac{\sin 2x}{2}\right] + c$$

Exercise 7.1

1. Integrate each of the following with respect to x

1. $(2x+3)^3$
2. $\sqrt{1-x}$
3. $\frac{1}{\sqrt{1-x}}$
4. $\frac{1}{5x-3}$
5. $\frac{1}{1-x}$
6. $\tan^2 2x$
7. $\sin^2 3x$
8. $\sin x \cos x$
9. $\frac{1}{\sin^2 3x}$
10. $\frac{\cos 2x}{\sin^2 2x}$
11. $\frac{\sin 3x}{\cos^2 3x}$
12. $e^{\frac{x}{3}}$
13. $(\sin x + \cos x)^2$

II Integrate w.r.t. x

1. $\sin 4x \,.\, \cos x$
2. $\sin 2x \cos 4x$
3. $\cos 2x \cos x$
4. $\sin 4x \sin 2x$
5. $\sin^2 x \cos 3x$
6. $\cos^2 x \sin 4x$
7. $\sec^2 x \tan^3 x$
8. $\sqrt{\cos x \sin x}$
9. $\sqrt{\tan x}\,.\sec^2 x$

III. Integrate w.r.t. x

1. $\sin^4 x$
2. $\sin^3 x$
3. $\cos^3 x$
4. $\cos^4 x$
5. $\tan^3 x$
6. $\cot^3 x$
7. $\tan^4 x$
8. $\cot^4 x$
9. $\sec^4 x$
10. $\operatorname{cosec}^4 x$

Answers

I. 1. $\frac{1}{8}(2x+3)^4$
2. $\frac{-2}{3}(1-x)^{3/2}+c$
3. $-2\sqrt{1-x}+c$
4. $\frac{1}{5}\log(5x-3)$
5. $-\log(1-x)+c$
6. $\frac{\tan 2x}{2}+c$
7. $\frac{x}{2}-\frac{\sin 6x}{12}+c$
8. $-\frac{\cos 2x}{4}+c$
9. $-\frac{\cot 3x}{3}+c$
10. $-\frac{\cos 2x}{2}+c$
11. $\frac{\sec 3x}{3}+c$
12. $3\ 3e^{\frac{x}{3}}+c$
13. $x-\frac{\cos 2x}{2}$

II. 1. $\frac{-\cos 5x}{10} - \frac{\cos 3x}{6} + c$

2. $\frac{-\cos 6x}{12} + \frac{\cos 2x}{4} + c$

3. $\frac{\sin 3x}{6} - \frac{\sin x}{2} + c$

4. $\frac{\sin 2x}{4} - \frac{\sin 6x}{12} + c$

5. $\frac{-\sin 5x}{20} - \frac{\sin x}{4} + \frac{\sin 3x}{6} + c$

6. $\frac{-\cos 6x}{24} + \frac{\cos 4x}{8} - \frac{\cos 2x}{8} + c$

7. $\frac{\tan^4 x}{4} + c$

8. $2/3\ (\cos x)^{3/2}$

9. $2/3\ (\tan)^{3/2}$

III 1. $\frac{3}{8}x + \frac{\sin 4x}{32} - \frac{\sin 2x}{4} + C$

2. $-\cos x + \cos^3 x + C$

3. $\sin x - \frac{\sin^2 x}{3} + c$

4. $\frac{3}{8}x + \frac{\sin 4x}{32} + \frac{\sin 2x}{4} + C$

5. $\frac{\tan^2 x}{2} - \log(\sec x) + c$

6. $-\frac{\cot^2 x}{2} - \log(\sin x) + c$

7. $\frac{\tan^2 x}{3} - \tan x + x + c$

8. $-\frac{\cos^2 x}{3} + \cot x + x + c$

9. $\tan x + \frac{\tan^2 x}{3} + c$

10. $-\cot x - \frac{\cot^2 x}{3} + c$

7.4 METHOD OF PARTIAL FRACTIONS

Integrate with respect to x

1. $\frac{1}{(x-1)(x+2)(x-3)}$

$$\int \frac{(2x+5)dx}{(x-1)(x+2)(x-3)}$$

Resolve $\frac{2x+5}{(x-1)(x+2)(x-3)}$ into partial fractions

Let $\frac{2x+5}{(x-1)(x+2)(x+3)} = \frac{A}{x-1} + \frac{B}{x+2} + \frac{C}{x-3}$

$\therefore \quad A(x+2)(x-3)+B(x-1)(x-3)+C(x+2)(x-1)=2x+5$

Put $x=1$, $A(3)(-2)=7$ $\therefore \ A=-\dfrac{7}{6}$

Put $x=-2$, $B(-3)(-5)=1$ $\therefore \ B=\dfrac{1}{15}$

Put $x=3$, $C(5)(2)=11$ $\therefore \ C=\dfrac{11}{10}$

$$\therefore \quad \frac{2x+5}{(x-1)(x+2)(x+3)}=\frac{-\frac{7}{6}}{x-1}+\frac{\frac{1}{15}}{x+2}+\frac{\frac{11}{10}}{x-3}$$

$$\therefore \quad \int\frac{(2x+5)dx}{(x-1)(x+2)(x-3)}=-\frac{7}{6}\int\frac{dx}{x-1}+\frac{1}{15}\int\frac{dx}{x-1}+\frac{11}{10}\int\frac{dx}{x-3}$$

$$=-\frac{7}{6}\log(x-1)+\frac{1}{15}\log(x+2)+\frac{11}{10}\log(x-3)+c$$

2. $\dfrac{x^2}{(x+1)(2x-1)^2}$

$$\int\frac{x^2dx}{(x+1)(2x-1)^2}$$

Resolve $\dfrac{x^2}{(x+1)(2x-1)^2}$ into partial fractions.

Let $\dfrac{x^2}{(x+1)(2x-1)^2}=\dfrac{A}{x+1}+\dfrac{B}{2x-1}+\dfrac{C}{(2x-1)}$

$\therefore \quad A(2x-1)^2+B(x+1)(2x-1)+C(x+1)=x^2$ .....(1)

Put $x=-1$, $A(-3)^2=1$ $\therefore \ A=\dfrac{1}{9}$

$x=\dfrac{1}{2}, C\left(\dfrac{3}{2}\right)=\dfrac{1}{4}$ $\therefore \ C=\dfrac{1}{6}$

Compare the coefficients of x^2 in (1)

$4A+2B=1 \ \dfrac{4}{9}+2B=1$ $\therefore \ B=\dfrac{5}{18}$

$$\therefore \quad \frac{x^2}{(x+1)(2x-1)^2} = \frac{\frac{1}{9}}{x+1} + \frac{\frac{5}{18}}{2x-1} + \frac{\frac{1}{6}}{(2x-1)^2}$$

$$\therefore \quad \int \frac{x^2 dx}{(x+1)(2x-1)^2} = \frac{1}{9}\int \frac{dx}{x+1} + \frac{5}{18}\int \frac{dx}{2x-1} + \frac{1}{6}\int \frac{dx}{(2x-1)^2}$$

$$= \frac{1}{9}\log(x+1) + \frac{5}{36}\log(2x-1) - \frac{1}{12(2x-1)} + c$$

3. $\dfrac{(x+1)}{x(x^2+1)}$

$$\int \frac{(x+1)dx}{x(x^2+1)}$$

Let $\dfrac{(x+1)}{x(x^2+1)} = \dfrac{A}{x} + \dfrac{Bx+C}{x^2+1}$

$\therefore \quad A(x^2+1) + x(Bx+C) = x+1$

i.e., $(A + B)x^2 + Cx + A = x + 1$

$\therefore \quad A + B = 0, C = 1, A = 1$

$\therefore \quad B = -A = -1$

$$\frac{(x+1)}{x(x^2+1)} = \frac{1}{x} + \frac{-x+1}{x^2+1}$$

$$\int \frac{(x+1)\,dx}{x(x^2+1)} = \int \frac{1}{x}dx - \int \frac{x}{x^2+1}dx + \int \frac{1}{x^2+1}dx$$

$$= \log x - \frac{1}{2}\log(x^2+1) + \tan^{-1}x + c$$

4. $\dfrac{\sin x}{\cos x(4+\cos x)}$

$$\int \frac{\sin x\, dx}{\cos x(4+\cos x)}$$

Put $\cos x = t$

$$\int \frac{-dt}{t(4+t)} = -\int \frac{dt}{t^2+4t}$$

$\because \quad -\sin x = \dfrac{dt}{dx}$

$\sin x\, dx = -dt$

$$= -\int \frac{dt}{(t+2)^2 - 2^2} \qquad \because \; t^2 + 4t = (t+2)^2 - 4$$

$$= -\frac{1}{2.2}\log\left[\frac{t+2-2}{t+2+2}\right] + c$$

$$= -\frac{1}{4}\log\left[\frac{\cos x}{\cos x + 4}\right] + c$$

5. $\int \frac{2x+1}{x^2 - 3x + 2} dx$

Let $\frac{2x+1}{x^2-3x+2} = \frac{2x+1}{(x-1)(x-2)} = \frac{A}{x-1} + \frac{B}{x-2}$

i.e., $2x + 1 = A(x-2) + B(x-1)$

Put, $x = 1, 3 = -A$ $\quad \therefore A = -3$

$x = 2, 5 = B$ $\quad \therefore B = 5$

$$\therefore \int \frac{2x+1}{x^2-3x+2} dx$$

$$= \int \left(\frac{-3}{x-1} + \frac{5}{x-2}\right) dx$$

$$= -3\log(x-1) + 5\log(x-2) + c$$

$$= \log\frac{(x-2)^5}{(x-1)^3} + c$$

6. $\int \frac{x+2}{(x+3)(x+1)} dx$

Let $\frac{x+2}{(x+3)(x+1)} = \frac{A}{x+3} + \frac{B}{x+1}$

$x + 2 = A(x+1) + B(x+3)$

$\Rightarrow$ Put $x = -3 \Rightarrow -1 = -2A$ $\quad \therefore A = \frac{1}{2}$

$\Rightarrow \frac{X}{lc} = -1 \Rightarrow 1 = 2B$ $\quad \therefore B = \frac{1}{2}$

$$\therefore \quad \int \frac{x+2}{(x+3)(x+1)} dx$$

$$= \frac{1}{2} \int \left(\frac{1}{x+3} + \frac{1}{x+1} \right) dx$$

$$= \frac{1}{2} [\log(x+3) + \log(x+1)] + c$$

7. $\int \frac{2x+3}{(x-1)(x-2)} dx$

Let $\frac{2x+3}{(x-1)(x-2)} = \frac{A}{x-1} + \frac{B}{x-2}$

$$2x + 3 = A(x-2) + B(x-1)$$

Put $x = 1$, $5 = -A$ $\therefore A = -5$

$x = 2$, $7 = B$ $\therefore B = 7$

$\therefore$ Given integral $= \int \left(\frac{-5}{x-1} + \frac{7}{x-2} \right) dx$

$$= -5\log(x-1) + 7\log(x-2) + c$$

8. $\int \frac{dx}{x^2 + 3x + 2}$

Let $\frac{1}{x^2+3x+2} = \frac{1}{(x+1)(x+2)} = \frac{A}{x+1} + \frac{B}{x+2}$

$\therefore 1 = A(x+2) + B(x+1)$

Put, $x = -1$, $1 = A$ $\therefore A = 1$

$x = -2$ $1 = -B$ $B = -1$

Given integral $= \int \left(\frac{1}{x+1} - \frac{1}{x+2} \right) dx = \log \frac{x+1}{x+2} + c$

9. $\int \frac{dx}{1+e^x}$

Put $1 + e^x = t$ so that $e^x = t - 1$

$e^x \, dx = dt$

$$\therefore \quad dx = \frac{1}{t-1} dt$$

$$\therefore \quad G.I = \int \frac{1}{t(t-1)} dt = \int \left(\frac{1}{t-1} - \frac{1}{t} \right) dt$$

(By resolving fraction into partial fractions)

$= \log(t - 1) - \log t + c$

$= \log e^x - \log(1 + e^x) + c$

$= x - \log(1 + e^x) + c$

Exercise 7.2

I Integrate w.r.t. x

1. $\frac{1}{x^2 + 4x - 5}$
2. $\frac{1}{(x-1)(x+2)}$
3. $\frac{1}{x^2(x-1)}$
4. $\frac{1}{x(x^2+1)}$
5. $\frac{1}{x^3(x^4+1)}$
6. $\frac{\sec^2 x}{\tan x(1+\tan x)}$
7. $\frac{1}{1+2e^x}$

II Integrate w.r.t x

1. $\frac{x^2+1}{(x-1)^2(x+1)}$
2. $\frac{3x+1}{(x+1)^2(x-2)}$
3. $\frac{x^2+1}{x(x^2-4)}$
4. $\frac{x}{(x^2+1)(x-1)}$
5. $\frac{\sin x}{(\cos^2 x+1)(2+\cos x)}$
6. $\frac{e^x}{(e^x+1)(e^{2x}+3)}$
7. $\frac{1}{x(\log x+1)(\log x-2)}$

Answers

I. 1. $\frac{1}{6}\log\left(\frac{x-1}{x+5}\right) + c$

2. $\frac{1}{3}\log\frac{x-1}{x+2} + c$

3. $-\log x + \frac{1}{x} + \log(x-1) + c$

4. $\log x - \frac{1}{2} + \log(x^2+2) + c$

5. $\frac{1}{2}\left[-\frac{1}{x^2}-\tan^{-1}x^2\right]+c$

6. $\log\frac{\tan x}{1+\tan x}+c$

7. $\log\left(\frac{e^x}{1+2e^x}\right)$

II 1. $\frac{1}{2}\log\left(x^2-1\right)-\frac{1}{x-1}+c$

2. $-\frac{7}{9}\log(x+1)-\frac{2}{3(x+1)}+\frac{7}{9}\log(x-2)+c$

3. $-\frac{1}{4}\log(x)-\frac{5}{8}\log(x-2)+\frac{5}{8}\log(x+2)+c$

4. $-\log(x^2+1)+\frac{1}{2}\tan^{-1}x+\frac{1}{2}\log(x-1)+c$

5. $-\frac{1}{10}\log\left(\cos^2 x+1\right)+\frac{2}{5}\tan^{-1}(\cos x)-\frac{1}{5}\log(\cos x+2)+c$

6. $-\frac{1}{4}\log(ex+1)+\frac{1}{8}\log(e2x+3)+\frac{1}{4\sqrt{3}}\tan^{-1}\left(\frac{e^x}{\sqrt{3}}\right)+c$

7. $\frac{1}{3}\log\left(\frac{\log x-2}{\log x+1}\right)+c$

7.5 INTEGRATION BY PARTS

If u and v are functions of x, then $\int u\,dv = uv - \int v\,du$

From the product rule, $\frac{d}{dx}(uv) = u\frac{dv}{dx} + v\frac{dv}{dx}$

where u and v are functions of x.

Integrate both sides w.r.t. x.

$$\int \frac{d}{dx}(uv)dx = \int u\frac{dv}{dx}dx + \int v\frac{dv}{dx}dx$$

i.e., $$uv = \int u\,dv + \int v\,du$$

$\therefore$ $$uv - \int v\,du = \int u\,dv \text{ or } \int u\,dv = uv - \int v\,du$$

This is the formula for integration by parts. It can also be written as,

$$\int u\,v' = u\,v - \int v\,u'$$

Note:

Take u = first function, dv = second function.

Then du = differential of first function, v = integral of second function

$$\int u\,dv = u\,v - \int v\,du$$

= (integral of first function) (Differentiation of second function)

$$-\int(\text{integral of second function}) \times (\text{Differential of first function})$$

Examples

1. $\int x \sin x\,dx$

   $u = x,\ dv = \sin x\,dx$

   $= x(-\cos x) - \int(-\cos x)dx$

   $du = dx,\ v = -\cos x$

   $= -x\cos x + \int \cos x\,dx$

   $= -x\cos x + \sin x + c$

2. $\int x\cos x\,dx = x\sin x - \int \sin x\,dx = x\sin x + \cos x + c$

Worked Examples

---

1. x sin3x

   $$\int x \sin 3x\,dx = x\left(-\frac{\cos 3x}{3}\right) - \int -\left(\frac{\cos 3x}{3}\right)dx$$

   $$= -\frac{x\cos 3x}{3} + \frac{1}{3}\frac{\sin 3x}{3} + c = -\frac{x\cos 3x}{3} + \frac{\sin 3x}{9} + c$$

2. $x^2 \sin x$

   $$\int x^2 \sin x dx = x^2(-\cos x) - \int(-\cos x)2x dx$$

$$= -x^2\cos x + 2\int x\cos\, dx$$

$$= -x^2\cos x + 2[x\sin x] - \int \sin x\, dx + c$$

$$= -x^2\cos x + 2[x\sin x + \cos x] + c$$

$$= -x^2\cos x + 2x\sin x + 2\cos x + c$$

3. $\int x^2\sin^2 x dx$

$$= \int x^2 \frac{1}{2}(1-\cos 2x)dx = \frac{1}{2}\int (x^2 - x^2\cos 2x)dx$$

$$\left(\because \sin^2 x = \frac{1}{2}(1-\cos 2x)\right)$$

$$= \frac{1}{2}\int x^2 dx - \frac{1}{2}\int x^2\cos 2dx$$

$$= \frac{1}{2}\frac{x^3}{3} - \frac{1}{2}\left[x^2\frac{\sin 2x}{2} - \int \frac{\sin 2x}{2}2xdx\right]$$

$$= \frac{x^3}{6} - \frac{1}{2}\left[\frac{x^2\sin 2x}{2} - \int x\sin\, xexdx\right]$$

$$= \frac{x^3}{6} - \frac{1}{2}\left[\frac{x^2\sin 2x}{2} - \left\{x\left(-\frac{\cos 2x}{2}\right) - \int -\frac{\cos 2x}{2}dx\right\}\right]$$

$$= \frac{x^3}{6} - \frac{x^2\sin 2x}{4} - \frac{x\cos 2x}{4} + \frac{\sin 2x}{8} + c$$

4. $\int x\sin 3x\cos x\, dx$

$$= \int x\frac{1}{2}[\sin 4x + \sin 2x]dx$$

$$\sin 3x\cos x = \frac{1}{2}[\sin 4x + \sin 2x]$$

$$\frac{1}{2}\int x\sin 4xdx + \frac{1}{2}\int x\sin 2x\, dx$$

$$\frac{1}{2}\left[x\left(-\frac{\cos 4x}{4}\right) - \int -\frac{\cos 4x}{4}dx\right] + \frac{1}{2}\left[x\left(-\frac{\cos 2x}{2}\right) - \int -\frac{\cos 2x}{2}dx\right]$$

$$= -\frac{x\cos4x}{8} + \frac{1}{8}\frac{\sin4x}{32} - \frac{x\cos2x}{4} + \frac{1}{4}\frac{\sin2x}{2}$$

$$= -\frac{x\cos4x}{8} + \frac{\sin4x}{32} - \frac{x\cos2x}{4} + \frac{\sin2x}{8} + c$$

5. $x^3e^{ax}dx$

$$= x^3\frac{e^{ax}}{a} - \int\frac{e^{ax}}{a}3x^2dx = \frac{x^3e^{ax}}{a} - \frac{3}{a}\int x^2e^{ax}dx$$

$$= \frac{x^3e^{ax}}{a} - \frac{3}{a}\left[x^2\frac{e^{ax}}{a} - \int\frac{e^{ax}}{a}2xda\right]$$

$$= \frac{x^3e^{ax}}{a} - \frac{3}{a^2}x^2e^{ax} + \frac{6}{a^2}\left[x\frac{e^{ax}}{a} - \int\frac{e^{ax}}{a}dx\right]$$

$$= \frac{x^3e^{ax}}{a} - \frac{3}{a^2}x^2e^{ax} + \frac{6xe^{ax}}{a^3} - \frac{6e^{ax}}{a^4} + c$$

$$= e^{ax}\left[\frac{x^3}{a} - \frac{3x^2}{a^2} + \frac{6x}{a^3} - \frac{6}{a^4}\right] + c$$

6. $\int \log_e x\, dx$

$$\int \log_e x.1dx = \log_e x(x) - \int (x)\frac{1}{x}dx$$

$$= x\log_e x - \int 1dx = x\log_e x - x + c$$

7. $\int x\sin^{-1} xdx$

$$= \int \sin^{-1} x.x.dx = \sin^{-1}x\frac{x^2}{2} - \int\frac{x^2}{2}\frac{1}{\sqrt{1-x^2}}dx$$

$$= \frac{x^2\sin^{-1}x}{2} - \frac{1}{2}\int\frac{x^2}{\sqrt{1-x^2}}dx$$

Put $x = \sin\theta$

$$= \frac{x^2\sin^{-1}x}{2} - \frac{1}{2}\int\frac{\sin^2\theta\cos\theta}{\sqrt{1-\sin^2\theta}}d\theta$$

$\therefore\ dx = \cos\theta d\theta$

$$= \frac{x^2 \sin^{-1}x}{2} 2 - \frac{1}{2}\int \sin^2\theta d\theta \qquad \sin\theta = x$$

$$= \frac{x^2 \sin^{-1}x}{2} - \frac{1}{2}\int \frac{1}{2}(1-\cos 2\theta) d\theta \ \theta = \sin^{-1} x$$

$\cos\theta = \sqrt{1-x^2}$

$$= \frac{x^2 \sin^{-1}x}{2} - \frac{1}{4}\left[\theta - \frac{\sin 2\theta}{2}\right] + c$$

$$= \frac{x^2 \sin^{-1}x}{2} - \frac{1}{4}\left[\sin^{-1}x - x.\sqrt{1-x^2}\right] + c$$

7.6 DEFINITE INTEGRALS AND THEIR APPLICATIONS

Definite Integrals

If $\int f(x)\,dx = \phi(x) + c$, then

$$\int_a^b f(x)\,dx = [\phi(x)+c]_a^b = [\phi(b)+c] = \phi(b) - j(a)$$

$$\int_a^b f(x)\,dx$$

[Read it as "integral a to b f(x) dx"] is called a definite integral, a and b are called limits of integration, a is called the lower limit and b is called the upper limit.

To evaluate a definite integral, integrate the function as usual. Then take the difference between the values you get by substituting the upper and lower limits for x respectively. Note that the constant of integration gets cancelled. So the constant of integration need not be written when you evaluate definite integrals. A definite integral can also be defined as the limit of a sum.

Examples:

1. $\int_2^3 x^2 dx = \left[\frac{x^3}{3}\right]_2^3 = \frac{3^3}{3} - \frac{2^3}{3} = \frac{19}{3}$

2. $\int_0^{\frac{\pi}{2}} \sin x dx = [-\cos x]_0^{\frac{\pi}{2}} = -\cos\frac{\pi}{2} - (-\cos 0) = 0 - (-1) = 1$

Worked Examples

1. $\int_0^{\frac{\pi}{2}} \sec^2 3x dx$

$$= \left[\frac{\tan 3x}{3}\right]_0^{\frac{\pi}{2}} = \frac{\tan\frac{3\pi}{4}}{3} - \frac{\tan 0}{3} = \frac{1}{3}[-1-0] = -\frac{1}{3}$$

2. $\int_0^{\frac{\pi}{4}} \tan^2 x dx$

$$= \int_0^{\frac{\pi}{4}} (\sec^2 x - 1)dx = [\tan x - x]_0^{\frac{\pi}{4}} = \tan\frac{\pi}{4} - \frac{\pi}{4} - 0 = 1 - \frac{\pi}{4}$$

3. $\int_0^{\frac{\pi}{2}} \sin^2 x dx$

$$= \int_0^{\frac{\pi}{2}} \frac{1}{2}(1-\cos 2x)dx = \frac{1}{2}\left[x - \frac{\sin 2x}{2}\right]_0^{\frac{\pi}{2}}$$

$$= \frac{1}{2}\left[\left(\frac{\pi}{2} - \frac{\sin\pi}{2}\right) - \left(0 - \frac{\sin 0}{2}\right)\right] = \frac{1}{2}\left(\frac{\pi}{2} - 0\right) = \frac{\pi}{4}$$

4. $\int_0^{\frac{\pi}{2}} \sin^3 x dx$

Put $\cos x = t$; $\sin x = \frac{dt}{dx}$

$$= \int_0^{\frac{\pi}{2}} \sin^2 x \sin x\, dx \qquad \therefore \quad \sin x\, dx = -dt$$

When $x = 0$, $t = \cos 0 = 1$

$$\int_0^{\frac{\pi}{2}} (1-\cos^2 x)\sin x dx$$

When $x = \frac{\pi}{2}$, $t = \cos\frac{\pi}{2} = 0$

$$= \int_1^0 (1-t^2)(-dt)$$

$$= -\left[t - \frac{t^3}{3}\right]_1^0$$

$$= -\left[(0-0) - \left(1 - \frac{1}{3}\right)\right] = \frac{2}{3}$$

5. $\int_0^{\frac{\pi}{2}} \sin 3x \cos x dx$

$$= \int_0^{\frac{\pi}{2}} \frac{1}{2}[\sin(3x+x) + \sin(3x-x)]dx$$

$$= \frac{1}{2}\int_0^{\frac{\pi}{2}} (\sin 4x + \sin 2x)dx$$

$$= \frac{1}{2}\left[\frac{-\cos 4x}{4} - \frac{\cos 2x}{2}\right]_0^{\frac{\pi}{2}}$$

$$= \frac{1}{2}\left[\left(\frac{-\cos 2\pi}{4} - \frac{\cos \pi}{2}\right) - \left(-\frac{\cos 0}{4} - \frac{\cos 0}{2}\right)\right]$$

$$= \frac{1}{2}\left[\left(-\frac{1}{4} + \frac{1}{2}\right) - \left(-\frac{1}{4} - \frac{1}{2}\right)\right] = \frac{1}{2}$$

6. $\int_0^{\frac{\pi}{2}} (1 + 2\cos x)^3 \sin x dx$

$$= \int_3^1 t^3 \left(-\frac{dt}{2}\right)$$

Put $1 + 2 \cos x = t$

$$-2\sin x = \frac{dt}{dx}$$

$$= \frac{1}{2}\int_{3}^{1} t^{3}dt = -\frac{1}{2}\left[\frac{t^{4}}{4}\right]_{3}^{1} \qquad \therefore \quad \sin x dx = -\frac{dt}{2}$$

when x = 0, $\quad t = 1 + 2 = 3$

$$= -\frac{1}{2}\left[\frac{1^{4}}{4} - \frac{3^{4}}{4}\right] = 10 \qquad \text{when } x = \frac{\pi}{2},\ t = 1 + 0 = 1$$

7.6.1 Application

1. Calculate Area under the Plasma Concentration time curve, AUC between 0 to ∞ when $C_p(t) = c_p 0_e^{-kelt}$

***Solution*:**

Given that $\quad C_p(t) = c_p 0_e^{-kelt}$

But $\quad C_p 0 = \frac{DOSE}{V} e^{-kelt}$

$$AUC = \frac{DOSE}{V}\int_{0}^{\infty} e^{-kelt}dt$$

$$= \frac{DOSE}{V}\left[e^{-kelt}\right]_{t=0}^{t=\infty}$$

Apply limit t = 0 and t = ∞

$$AUC = \frac{DOSE}{V}\left[0 - \frac{1}{-kelt}\right]$$

$$AUC = \frac{DOSE}{V}\frac{1}{kelt}$$

2. The rapid intravenous injection of a drug that distribute in the body according to two compartment model system with elimination occurring from the central compartment is as shown in model and the amount of drug in the central compartment a_{sc} is given by equation (function)

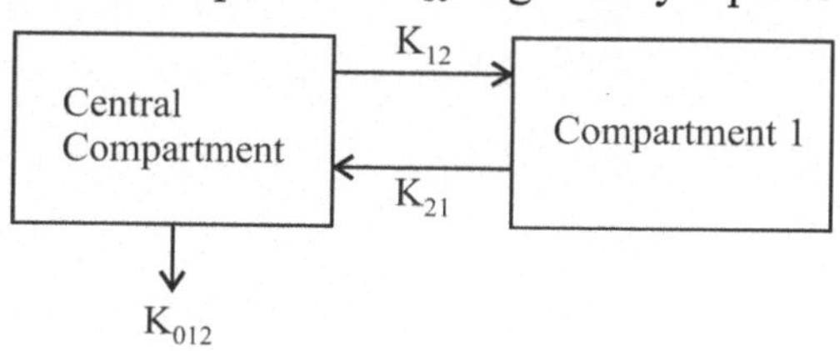

$$a_{sc} = X_0 \frac{(S+E_2)}{(S+\lambda_1)(S+\lambda_2)}$$

Calculate the total amount of drug in the central compartment (X_c) after time t hours (Concentration in the central compartment)

***Solution*:**

To calculate concentration of drug in the central compartment, we have to resolve the $\frac{(S+E_2)}{(S+\lambda_1)(S+\lambda_2)}$ into partial fraction.

After resolution into partial fraction, will arrive into the equation

$$\frac{(S+E_2)}{(S+\lambda_1)(S+\lambda_2)} = \frac{A}{S+\lambda_1} + \frac{B}{S+\lambda_2}$$

$$= \frac{E_2 - \lambda_1}{(\lambda_2 - \lambda_1)(S+\lambda_1)} - \frac{E_2 - \lambda_2}{(\lambda_2 - \lambda_1)(S+\lambda_2)}$$

Integrating w. r. t. t

$$Xc = \int a_{sc} dt = x_0 \int \frac{E_2 - \lambda_1}{(\lambda_2 - \lambda_1)(S+\lambda_1)} dt - \int \frac{E_2 - \lambda_2}{(\lambda_2 - \lambda_1)(S+\lambda_2)} dt$$

$$= \frac{x_0}{(\lambda_2 - \lambda_1)} \int \frac{E_2 - \lambda_1}{(S+\lambda_1)} dt - \int \frac{E_2 - \lambda_2}{(S+\lambda_2)} dt$$

$$X_c = \frac{x_0}{(\lambda_2 - \lambda_1)} \left[(E_2 - \lambda_1) e^{-\lambda 1t} - (E_2 - \lambda_1) e^{-\lambda 2t} \right]$$

3. If amount drug that dissolve in the body is given by the equation $c(t) = e^{2t}$. Calculate the total amount of drug that dissolve between 0 to 2 hours, where 2 is elimination rate constant.

***Solution*:**

$$\oint_0^2 e^{2t} dt = \left[\frac{e^{2t}}{2} \right]_{t=0}^{t=\infty}$$

$$= \frac{1}{2}\left[e^4 - e^0 \right]$$

$$= \frac{1}{2}\left[e^4 - 1 \right]$$

CHAPTER 8

DIFFERENTIAL EQUATIONS

In this chapter we consider the topic of ordinary differential equations which plays a basic role in Pharmacokinetics. Some standard methods of solving ordinary differential equations of first–order and first degree are presented. Some examples illustrating applications of differential equations in solving the Pharmacokinetics equations are presented.

8.1 SOME BASIC DEFINITIONS

An equation involving a function of one or more independent variables and/or its derivatives is called a differential equation.

If the derivatives present in a differential equation are all ordinary derivatives, then the differential equation is called an ordinary differential equation.

On the other hand, if the derivatives present in a differential equation are partial derivatives, then the differential equation is called a partial differential equation.

Evidently, ordinary differential equations are associated with functions of one independent variable and partial differential equations are associated with functions of two or more independent variables.

For Example:

(a) If y is a function of an independent variable x, then

$$\frac{dy}{dx} = xy \qquad .....(1)$$

$$\left(\frac{dy}{dx}\right)^4 = x^2y^3 \qquad \text{.....(2)}$$

$$\frac{d^2y}{dx^2} + 2x\left(\frac{dy}{dx}\right)^3 = \cos x \qquad \text{.....(3)}$$

$$\left(\frac{d^2y}{dx^2}\right)^4 + 4y\left(\frac{d^3y}{dx^3}\right)^2 + x = 0 \qquad \text{.....(4)}$$

are all ordinary differential equations, and

(b) If z is a function of two independent variables x and y, then

$$x\frac{\partial z}{\partial x} + y\frac{\partial z}{\partial y} = 0 \qquad \text{.....(5)}$$

$$\frac{\partial^2 z}{\partial x^2} + y\frac{\partial^2 z}{\partial y^2} = 0 \qquad \text{.....(6)}$$

are partial differential equations.

In this chapter, we discuss more about ordinary differential equations with their applications in solving Pharmacokinetics equations.

8.1.1 Order and Degree

The differential equation in which the highest derivative appearing in an ordinary differential equation is called the order of the differential equation.

For example, in the differential equation $\left(\frac{d^2y}{dx^2}\right)^4 + 4y\left(\frac{d^3y}{dx^3}\right)^2 + x = 0$ the highest – order derivative present is d^3y/dx^3 and its order is 3. Hence the differential equation is of third order. Evidently, the differential equations (1) and (2) are of first-order and the differential equation (3) is of second – order.

On the other hand, the degree of a differential equation is the positive integral power to which the highest – order derivative present in the equation is raised.

As another example, consider the differential equation.

$$\left(\frac{d^2y}{dx^2}\right)^2 = \left[1 + \left(\frac{dy}{dx}\right)^2\right]^{3/2} \qquad \text{.....(1)}$$

In this equation a term with fractional power appears. This fractional power can be cleared by squaring both sides. Thus we get.

$$\left(\frac{d^2y}{dx^2}\right)^4 = \left[1+\left(\frac{dy}{dx}\right)^2\right]^3$$

From this, we note that the differential equation (1) is of second–order and fourth degree.

Equations of First–Order and First-Degree

In this section we consider ordinary differential equations of first-order and first – degree. If x is an independent variable and y is the dependent variable, such equations are of the form

$$\varphi\left(x, y, \frac{dy}{dx}\right) = 0 \qquad .....(1)$$

in which dy/dx appears with first-degree. The general solution of this equation is a relation of the form.

$$F(x, y, c) = 0 \qquad .....(2)$$

Where c is an arbitrary constant, which satisfies the equation.

When a particular value is assigned to c, the general solution becomes a particular solution.

The general solution (2) is to be obtained by solving equation (1). The actual procedure of solving equation (1) depends upon the nature of the function φ. In the following sub-section, we consider some standard forms of equation (1), which can be solved by some standards techniques.

Equations in Separable Form

Suppose the differential equation to be solved is in the form

$$\frac{dy}{dx} = \frac{f(x)}{g(y)} \qquad .....(1)$$

where f(x) is a function of x only and g(y) is a non-zero function of y only.

Equation (1) may be rewritten as

$$f(x)\, dx - g(y)\, dy = 0$$

or

$$f(x)\, dx = g(x)\, dy$$

in which the variables x and y are separated. Integrating this, we obtain

$$\int f(x)\,dx = \int g(y)\,dy + c \qquad \ldots..(2)$$

where c is an arbitrary constant. This is the general solution of equation (1). For a particular value of c. this becomes a particular solution.

Example 1: Solve $\frac{dy}{dx} = 1 + x^2 + y^2 + x^2y^2$

The given equation may be rewritten as

$$\frac{dy}{dx} = (1+x^2)(1+y^2), \text{ or } \frac{dy}{1+y^2} = (1+x^2)\,dx$$

in which the variables x and y are separated, Integrating this,

we get

$$\tan^{-1}y = x + \frac{x^3}{3} + \text{constant.}$$

This is the general solution of the given equation.

Example 2: Solve $(e^y+1)\cos x\,dx + e^y \sin x\,dy = 0.$

He given equation may be written as

$$(e^y+1)\cos x\,dx = -e^y \sin x\,dy$$

or

$$\frac{\cos x}{\sin x}dx = -\frac{e^y}{e^y+1}dy$$

in which the variables x and y are separated. Integrating this,

we get

$$\frac{\cos x}{\sin x}dx = -\frac{e^y}{e^y+1}dy$$

$$\log(\sin x) = -\log(e^y+1) + c$$

or $$\log\{(\sin x)(e^y+1)\} = c$$

or $$\{(\sin x)(e^y+1)\} = c$$

This is the general solution of the given equation.

Example 3: Solve $3e^x \tan y\, dx + (1 - e^x)\sec^2 y\, dy = 0$

The given equation may be rewritten as

$$3e^x \tan y\, dx = (e^x - 1)\sec^2 y\, dy$$

or
$$\frac{3e^x}{e^x - 1} dx = \frac{\sec^2 y}{\tan y} dy$$

in which the variables *x* and *y* are separated. Integrating this, we get

$$3\log(e^x - 1) = \log \tan y + c$$

or
$$\log(e^x - 1)^3 - \log \tan y = c$$

or
$$\log\left\{\frac{\left(e^x - 1\right)^3}{\tan y}\right\} = c$$

or
$$\frac{\left(e^x - 1\right)^3}{\tan y} = c$$

This is the general solution of the given equation

Example 4: Solve $(xy - x)\, dx + (xy + y)\, dy = 0$

The given equation may be rewritten as

$$x(y - 1)dx = -y(x + 1)dy$$

or
$$\frac{x}{x+1} dx = -\frac{y}{y-1} dy,$$

or
$$\frac{(x+1)-1}{x+1} dx = -\frac{(y-1)+1}{y-1} dy,$$

or
$$\left(1 - \frac{1}{x+1}\right) dx = -\left(1 + \frac{1}{y-1}\right) dy$$

Integrating this, we get

$$x - \log(x + 1) = -\{y + \log(y - 1)\} + c$$

or
$$x + y - \log(x + 1) + \log(y - 1) = \text{constant},$$

or
$$(x + y) + \log\left(\frac{y-1}{x+1}\right) = c$$

This is the general solution of the given equation

Example 5: Solve $\left(x^2+y^2\right)^2\left(x\frac{dy}{dx}+y\right)=xy\left(1+\frac{dy}{dx}\right)$

To solve the given equation, we set

$$u=x+y, \quad v=xy,$$

so that

$$\frac{du}{dx}=1+\frac{dy}{dx}, \text{ and } \frac{dv}{dx}=x+\frac{dy}{dx}+y$$

using these, the given equation becomes

$$u^2\frac{dv}{dx}=v\frac{du}{dx}, \text{ or } \frac{1}{v}\frac{dv}{dx}=\frac{1}{u^2}\frac{du}{dx}, \text{ or } \frac{d}{dx}(\log v)=\frac{d}{dx}\left(-\frac{1}{u}\right)$$

integration of this yields

$$\log v=-\frac{1}{u}+c, \text{ or } \log xy=-\frac{1}{x+y}+c$$

This is the general solution of the given equation

8.2 HOMOGENEOUS EQUATIONS

Suppose the differential equation to be solved of the form

$$\frac{dy}{dx}=f(x, y) \qquad \text{.....(1)}$$

where f(x, y) is a function of *x* and *y*, which can be rewritten as a function of y/x or as a function of x/y. (Such functions are called homogeneous functions of x and *y* of degree zero*). The (1) is called a homogeneous differential equation.

If f(x, y) is rewritten as a function of y/x, then we put y = vx, where v = v(x), so that

$$\frac{dy}{dx}=v+x\frac{dv}{dx} \qquad \text{.....(2)}$$

Substituting for y and $\frac{dy}{dx}$ into (1), we get an equation involving v and x, which may be solved by separating the variables. See example 1 to 14 below.

One the other hand, if f(x, y) can be rewritten as a function of x/y, then we put x = vy, where v = v(y), so that

$$\frac{dx}{dy} = v + y\frac{dv}{dy} \qquad .....(3)$$

Then (1) becomes an equation involving *v* and *y*, which may be solved by separating the variables. See examples 15 to 18 below.

Example 6: Solve $\frac{dy}{dx} = \frac{y}{x} + \sin\frac{y}{x}$

Since the right hand side is a function of *(y/x)*, the given equation is homogeneous. Setting y = vx, the equation becomes

$$v + x\frac{dv}{dx} = v + \sin v,$$

or $$\text{cosec } v \, dv = \frac{dx}{x}$$

Integrating this, we get

$$\log(\text{cosec } v - \cot v) = \log x + \text{constant},$$

or $$\log(\text{cosec } v - \cot v) - \log x = \text{constant}$$

or $$\log\left\{\frac{\text{cosec } v - \cot v}{x}\right\} = \text{constant},$$

or $$\frac{1}{x}(\text{cosec } v - \cot v) = c, \text{ a constant},$$

Substituting for v, this becomes

$$\text{cosec } (y/x) - \cot(y/x) = cx$$

This is the general solution of the given equation.

Example 7: Solve $x\frac{dy}{dx} + \frac{y^2}{x} = y$

The given equation may be rewritten as

$$x\frac{dy}{dx} = y - \frac{y^2}{x}, \text{ or } \frac{dy}{dx} = \frac{y}{x} - \frac{y^2}{x^2}$$

which is in homogeneous form. Setting y = vx, this equation becomes

$$v + x\frac{dv}{dx} = v - v^2, \text{ or } x\frac{dv}{dx} = -v^2 \text{ or } -\frac{dv}{v^2} = \frac{dx}{x}$$

Integrating this, we get

$$\frac{1}{v} = \log x + c(\text{constant})$$

Substituting for v, this becomes

$$\frac{x}{y} = \log x + c$$

This is the general solution of the given equation.

Example 8: Solve $x\frac{dy}{dx} = y(\log y - \log x + 1)$

The given equation may be rewritten as

$$\frac{dy}{dx} = \frac{y}{x}\left(\log\frac{y}{x} + 1\right)$$

which is in homogeneous form, setting $y = vx$, this equation becomes

$$v + x\frac{dv}{dx} = v(\log v + 1), \quad \text{or } x\frac{dv}{dx} = v\log v, \quad \text{or } \frac{(1/v)dv}{\log v} = \frac{dx}{x}$$

Integrating this, we get

$$\log(\log v) = \log x + \text{constant, or } \log\left(\frac{\log v}{x}\right) = \text{constant,}$$

or $$\frac{\log v}{x} = c, \text{ a constant}$$

Substituting for *v*, this becomes

$$\log\left(\frac{y}{x}\right) = cx$$

This the general solution of the given equation

Example 9: Solve $\left(x^2 - y^2\right)dx - xy\,dy = 0$

The given equation may be rewritten as

$$\frac{dy}{dx} = \frac{x^2 - y^2}{xy} = \frac{1-(y/x)^2}{(y/x)}$$

which is in homogeneous form, setting $y = vx$, this equation becomes

$$v + x\frac{dv}{dx} = \frac{1-v^2}{v}, \text{ or } x\frac{dv}{dx} = \frac{1-v^2}{v} - v = \frac{1-2v^2}{v}$$

or $$\frac{v}{1-2v^2}dv = \frac{dx}{x}, \text{ or } \frac{4v}{2v^2-1}dv = -4\frac{dx}{x}$$

Integrating this, we get

$$\log(2v^2-1) = -4\log x + \text{constant}$$

or $$\log(2v^2-1) + 4\log x = \text{constant}, \text{ or } \log(2v^2-1)x4 = \text{constant}$$

or $$(2\left(\frac{y}{x}\right)^2 - 1)x^4 = c, \text{ a constant}$$

or $$\left(\frac{2y^2}{x^2-1}\right)x^4 = c, \text{ or } x^2\left(2y^2 - x^2\right) = c$$

This is the general solution of the given equation

Example 10: Solve $(x^2 - xy + y^2)\,dx - xy\,dy = 0$

The given equation may be rewritten as

$$\frac{dy}{dx} = \frac{x^2-xy+y^2}{xy} = \frac{x^2\{1-(y/x)+(y^2/x^2)\}}{xy} = \frac{1-(y/x)+(y/x)^2}{\left(\frac{y}{x}\right)}$$

which is in homogeneous form, setting $y = vx$, this equation becomes

$$v + x\frac{dv}{dx} = \frac{1-v-v^2}{v},$$

or $$x\frac{dv}{dx} = \frac{1-v+v^2}{v} - v = \frac{1-v}{v},$$

or $$\frac{dx}{x} = \frac{v}{1-v}dv = \frac{(v-1)+1}{1-v}dv = -\left[1 + \frac{1}{v-1}\right]dv$$

Integrating this, we get

$$\log x = -[v + \log(v-1)] + c, \text{ or } \log x + \log(v-1) = c - v$$

or $$\log x(v-1) = c - v, \text{ or} \log x\left(\frac{y}{x} - 1\right) = c - \frac{y}{x},$$

or $$\log(y-x) = c - \left(\frac{y}{x}\right)$$

This is general solution of the given equation

8.3 LINEAR EQUATIONS

Suppose the equation to be solved is of the form

$$\frac{dy}{dx} + P(x)y = Q(x) \qquad .....(1)$$

where P and Q are known functions of *x*. such an equation is called a linear differential equation*.

Let us take

$$R = R(x) = e^{\int Pdx} \qquad .....(2)$$

Then we find that

$$\frac{dR}{dx} = e^{\int Pdx} \frac{d}{dx} \int Pdx = RP \qquad .....(3)$$

and $$\frac{d}{dx}(Ry) = R\frac{dy}{dx} + y\frac{dR}{dx} = R\frac{dy}{dx} + y(RP) \qquad .....(4)$$

on using (3). Hence, on multiplying by R, equation (1) takes the form

$$\frac{d}{dx}(Ry) = RQ$$

Integrating this, we get

$$Ry = \int RQ\,dx + c,$$

where *c* is a constant. Using (2), this reads

$$Pe^{\int Pdx} = \int Q(x)\,e^{\int Pdx}\,dx + c \qquad .....(5)$$

$$P(IF) = \int Q(x)\,(IF)\,dx + c$$

Here $IF = e^{\int Pdx}$ is called as integrating factor

This is the general solution of equation (1)

Example 11: Solve: $\frac{dy}{dx} - \left(\frac{2}{x}\right)y = x + x^2$

We observe that the given equation is a linear differential equation of the form (1), with $P = -\frac{2}{x}$ and $Q = x + x^2$ we note that

$$\int Pdx = \int\left(-\frac{2}{x}\right)dx = -2\log x^{-2} = \log\frac{1}{x^2}$$

Hence

$$I.F = \int_e Pdx = e^{\log(1/x^2)} = \frac{1}{x^2}$$

Accordingly, the general solution of the given equation is [by formula (5)]

$$y\frac{1}{x^2} = \int (x+x^2)\frac{1}{x^2}dx + c = \int\left(\frac{1}{x}+1\right)dx + c = (\log x + x) + c$$

$$y\frac{1}{x^2} = (\log x + x) + c$$

Example 12: Solve: $\frac{dy}{dx} + y\cot x = \cos x$

The given equation is a linear equation with $P = \cot x$, $Q = \cos x$. Therefore,

$$\int Pdx = \int \cot x\, dx = \log \sin x,$$

so that $$I.F = \int_e Pdx = e^{\log \sin x} = \sin x$$

Hence, the general solution of the given equation is [by formula (5)]

$$y \sin x = \int \cos x \sin x\, dx + c = \frac{1}{2}\sin^2 x\, dx + c$$

or $$y = \frac{1}{2}\sin x + c\,\mathrm{cosec}x$$

Example 13: Solve: $(x+1)\frac{dy}{dx} - y = e^{3x}(x+1)^2$

Dividing throughout by (x + 1), the given equation becomes

$$\frac{dy}{dx} - \frac{1}{x+1}y = (x+1)e^{3x}$$

which is a linear differential equation with $P = -\frac{1}{x+1}$ and $Q = (x+1)e^{3x}$

We note that

$$\int Pdx = -\int \frac{dx}{x+1} = -\log(x+1) = \log\frac{1}{x+1}$$

so that

$$\text{IF} = e^{\log\left(\frac{1}{1+x}\right)} = \frac{1}{1+x}$$

Therefore, the general solution of the given equation is

$$y\frac{1}{x+1} = \int (x+1)e^{3x}\frac{1}{x+1}dx + c = \int e^{3x}dx + c = \frac{1}{3}e^{3x} + c$$

$$\text{or } y = (x+1)\left(\frac{1}{3}e^{3x} + c\right)$$

Example 14: Solve: $(1+x^2)\frac{dy}{dx} + x = \sinh^{-1}x$

The given equation may be rewritten as

$$\frac{dy}{dx} + \frac{x}{1+x^2} = \frac{\sinh^{-1}x}{1+x^2}$$

which is a linear differential equation with $P = \frac{x}{1+x^2}$ and $Q = \frac{\sinh^{-1}x}{1+x^2}$

we note that

$$\int Pdx = \int \frac{x}{1+x^2}dx = \frac{1}{2}\int \frac{2x}{1+x^2} = \frac{1}{2}\log(1+x^2) = \log\sqrt{1+x^2}$$

so that

$$\text{I.F} = e^{\int Pdx} = \sqrt{1+x^2}$$

Therefore, the general solution of the given equation is

$$y\sqrt{1+x^2} = \int \frac{\sinh^{-1}x}{1+x^2}\sqrt{1+x^2}dx + c = \int \frac{\sinh^{-1}x}{\sqrt{1+x^2}}dx + c$$

$$= \int t\,dt + c, \text{ on putting } \sinh^{-1}x = t, \text{ so that } \frac{1}{\sqrt{1+x^2}}dx = dt$$

$$= \frac{1}{2}t^2 + c = \frac{1}{2}\left(\sinh^{-1}x\right)^2 + c$$

Example 15: Solve $(1+x^2)(dy - dx) = 2xydx$

The given equation may be rewritten as

$$dy - dx = \frac{2xy}{1+x^2}dx, \text{ or } \frac{dy}{dx} - 1 = \frac{2xy}{1+x^2}, \text{ or } \frac{dy}{dx} - \frac{2x}{1+x^2}y = 1,$$

which is a linear differential equation with $P = \frac{2x}{1+x^2}$ and $Q = 1$

We note that

$$\int P dx = -\int \frac{2x}{1+x^2} dx = -\log(1+x^2) = \log\left(\frac{1}{1+x^2}\right)$$

so that

$$I.F = e^{\int P dx} = \frac{1}{1+x^2}$$

Therefore, the general solution of the given equation is

$$y\frac{1}{1+x^2} = \int 1.\frac{1}{1+x^2} + c = \tan^{-1}x + c$$

or

$$y = (1+x^2)(\tan^{-1}x + c)$$

Example 16: Solve $(1+xy)dx - (1+x^2)dy = 0,$ given that $y(1) = 0$

The given equation may be rewritten as

$$\frac{dy}{dx} = \frac{1+xy}{1+x^2}, \text{ or } \frac{dy}{dx} - \frac{x}{1+x^2}y = \frac{1}{1+x^2} \qquad (1)$$

which is a linear differential equation with $P = -\frac{x}{1+x^2}$ and $Q = \frac{1}{1+x^2}$

Therefore,

$$\int P dx = -\int \frac{x}{1+x^2} dx = -\frac{1}{2}\int \frac{2x}{1+x^2} dx = -\frac{1}{2}\log(1+x^2) = \log\frac{1}{\sqrt{1+x^2}}$$

so that

$$I.F\, e^{\int P dx} = e^{\log\left(\frac{1}{\sqrt{1+x^2}}\right)} = \frac{1}{\sqrt{1+x^2}}$$

Accordingly the general solution of the given equation is

$$y\frac{1}{\sqrt{1+x^2}} = \int \frac{1}{1+x^2}.\frac{1}{\sqrt{1+x^2}} dx + c = \int \frac{dx}{(1+x^2)^{3/2}} + c$$

$$= \int \frac{\sec^2 \theta \, d\theta}{\sec^3 \theta} + c \quad \text{on setting } x = \tan \theta$$

$$= \int \cos\theta \, d\theta + c = \sin \theta + c = \sin(\tan^{-1} x) + c \qquad .....(2)$$

It is given that y(1) = 0; that is, y = o when x = 1. Using this in (ii), we get

$$0.\frac{1}{\sqrt{1+1}} = \sin(\tan^{-1} 1) + c = \sin\frac{\pi}{4} + c = \frac{1}{\sqrt{2}} + c$$

so that $c = -1\sqrt{2}$ using this in (ii), we get

$$\frac{y}{\sqrt{1+x^2}} = \sin(\tan^{-1} x) - \frac{1}{\sqrt{2}}$$

This is the required solution

8.4 EXACT EQUATIONS

Suppose the equation to be solved is of the form

$$M(x, y)\, dx + N(x, y)\, dy = 0 \qquad .....(1)$$

where *M* and *N* are functions of *x* and *y* such that

$$\frac{\partial M}{\partial y} = \frac{\partial N}{\partial x} \qquad .....(2)$$

Let us put

$$F = F(x, y) = \int M(x, y)\, dx, \qquad .....(3)$$

with *y* kept constant while integrating M, then

$$\frac{\partial F}{\partial x} = M \text{ and } \frac{\partial}{\partial y}\left(\frac{\partial F}{\partial x}\right) = \frac{\partial M}{\partial y} = \frac{\partial N}{\partial x}, \text{ using (2)} \qquad .....(4)$$

thus,

$$\frac{\partial}{\partial x}\left(\frac{\partial F}{\partial y} - N\right) = 0,$$

or

$$\frac{\partial F}{\partial x} - N = \varphi'(y)(\text{say}) \qquad .....(5)$$

where $\varphi'(y)$ is a function of y

Since F = F (x, y), we have

$$dF = \frac{\partial F}{\partial x}dx + \frac{\partial F}{\partial y}dy$$

on using expressions (4) and (5), this becomes

$$dF = M\,dx + \{N + \varphi'(y)\}\,dy$$

or

$$M\,dx + N\,dy = dF - \varphi'(y)\,dy = dF - d\varphi$$

$$d(F - \varphi) \qquad .....(6)$$

This shows that the left-hand side of the given equation is an exact differential of the function (F - φ). For this reason, when the condition (2) holds, equation (1) is called an exact differential. Then the equation can be rewritten as

$$d(F - \varphi) = 0$$

Integrating this, we get

$$F - \varphi = c, \text{ a constant}$$

This is the general solution of the equation (1)

In view of the definitions of F(x, y) and φ(y) the following working rule is used to write down the general solution of exact differential equation.

Working Rule

1. Integrate M(x, y) w.r.t. *x* treating y as constant. Let I_1 be this integral.
2. Integrate w.r.t *y* only those terms in *N*(*x, y*) that do not contain x. Let I_2 be this integral.
3. Then the sum of the above integrals equated to a constant c; that is $I_1 + I_2 = c$, is the general solution of the given equation.

Example 17: Solve $3x(xy - 2)\,dx + (x^3 + 2y)\,dy = 0$

The given equation is of the form M dx + N dx = 0 with M = 3x(xy – 2), $N = x^3 + 2y$ we find that

$$\frac{\partial M}{\partial y} = 3x^2 \text{ and } \frac{\partial N}{\partial x} = 3x^2. \text{ Thus, } \frac{\partial M}{\partial y} = \frac{\partial N}{\partial x}$$

therefore, the given equation is exact.

Integrating M w.r.t. x, treating y as constant, we get the integral

$$I_1 = x^3y - 3x^2$$

Integrating w.r.t. y only those terms in N which do not contain x, we get the integral

$$I_2 = y^2$$

hence, the general solution of the given equation is

$$I_1 + I_2 = x^3y - 3x^2 + y^2 = c, \text{ a constant}$$

Example 18: Solve $(x^2 + y^2 - a^2)xdx + (x^2 - y^2 - b^2)y\,dy = 0$

The given equation is of the form M dx + N dy = 0, with

$$M = x(x^2 + y^2 - a^2), N = y(x^2 - y^2 - b^2)$$

we find that

$$\frac{\partial M}{\partial y} = 2xy = \frac{\partial N}{\partial x}$$

Therefore, the given equation is exact

Integrating M w.r.t x., treating *y* as constant, we get the integral

$$I_1 = \frac{x^4}{4} + (y^2 - a^2)\frac{x^2}{2}$$

Integrating w.r.t. *y* only those terms in N which do not contain x, we get the integral

$$I_2 = -\frac{y^4}{4} - b^2\frac{y^2}{2}$$

Hence, the general solution of the given equation is

$$I_1 + I_2 = \frac{x^4}{4} + (y^2 - a^2)\frac{x^2}{2} - \frac{y^4}{4} - b^2\frac{y^2}{2} = c$$

or

$$x^4 + 2x^2(y^2 - a^2) - y^4 - 2b^2y^2 = 2c$$

Example 19: Solve $(3x^2y^2 + x^2)dx + (2x^3y + y^2)dy = 0$

The given equation is of the form M dx + N dy = 0, with

$$M = (3x^2y^2 + x^2)\ N = (2x^3y + y^2)$$

we find that

$$\frac{\partial M}{\partial y} = 6x^2y = \frac{\partial N}{\partial x}$$

Therefore, the given equation is exact

Integrating M w.r.t *x*., treating y as constant, we get the integral

$$I_1 = x^3y^2 + \frac{x^3}{3}$$

Integrating w.r.t. y only those terms in N which do not contain x, we get the integral

$$I_2 = \frac{y^3}{3}$$

Hence, the general solution of the given equation is

$$I_1 + I_2 = x^3y^2 + \frac{x^3}{3} + \frac{y^3}{3} = c$$

or

$$x^3 + y^3 + 3x^3y^2 = 3c$$

Example 20: Solve $(y^3 - 3x^2y)\,dx - (x^3 - 3xy^2)\,dy = 0$

The given equation is of the form M dx + N dy = 0, with

$$M = y^3 - 3x^2y, \quad N = -(x^3 - 3xy^2)$$

We find that

$$\frac{\partial M}{\partial y} = 3y^2 - 3x^2 = \frac{\partial N}{\partial x}$$

therefore, the given equation is exact

Integrating M w.r.t x., treating y as constant, we get the integral

$$I_1 = y^3x - x^3y$$

We observe that every term in N contains x. Therefore, we do not integrate N, and take

$$I_2 = 0$$

Hence, the general solution of the given equation is

$$I_1 = y^3x - x^3y \times c, \text{ a constant}$$

Example 21: Solve $(5x^4 + 3x^2y^2 - 2xy^3)dx + (2x^3y - 3x^2y^2 - 5y^4)dy = 0$

The given equation is of the form M dx + N dy = 0 with

$$M = 5x^4 + 3x^2y^2 - 2xy^3,\ N = 2x^3y - 3x^2y^2 - 5y^4$$

Application

1. In a certain culture of bacteria, the rate at which bacteria increase is proportional to the instantaneous number present. If the original number doubles in one hour, in how many hour will it triple?

***Solution*:**

Let N be the number at time t

$$\frac{dN}{dt} \propto N$$

$$\frac{dN}{dt} = KN \qquad \text{.....(1)}$$

K is Positive Constant

Solving this equation 1 by the method of variable

$$\frac{dN}{N} = Kdt$$

Integrate both side

$$\int_0^N \frac{dN}{N} = \int_0^N Kdt$$

$$\log N = Kt + \log C$$

$$\log N - \log C = Kt$$

$$\log(N / C) = Kt$$

Take exponential both side

$$\frac{N}{C} = e^{Kt}$$

$$N = Ce^{Kt}$$

For $t = 0$ then $N = N_0$

Put $\quad C = N_0$

$$N = N_0 e^{kt} \qquad .....(2)$$

This gives the number of bacteria at time $t \geq 0$, if K is known

It is given that $N = 2\ N_0$ When $t = 1$

Substitute in equation 2

$$2N_0 = N_0 e^{Kt}$$

$$e^{K.1} = 2$$

Therefore $N = N_0 e^{kt}$ can be written as $N = N_0 2^t$

Suppose the original triples in T (hours). Then $N = 3N_0$ when $t = T$

Then $\quad 3N_0 = N_0 2^T$

$$3 = 2^T$$

Take log both side

$$\log^3 = T \log^2$$

$$T = \frac{\log 3}{\log 2} = \frac{0.4771}{0.3010} = 1.6 \text{ (1 hour and 36 minutes)}$$

2. Suppose that a solution initially containing 2 moles/liter of Y and 1 mole/liter of Z is allowed to react. Find an expression for the amount of X at time t.

***Solution*:**

We have to solve the initial value problem

$$\frac{dx}{dt} = k(2 - x)(1 - x), \ x(0) = 0$$

(The constants 2 and 1 come from the initial concentrations.) Separating variable we get

$$\frac{dx}{(2 - x)(1 - x)} = kdt$$

we integrate both sides with respect to t

$$\int \frac{dx}{(2 - x)(1 - x)} = \int kdt$$

The left hand value is obtained by partial fraction method and solution is

$$\frac{1}{(2-x)(1-x)} = \frac{A}{2-x} + \frac{B}{1-x}$$

$$\frac{1}{(2-x)(1-x)} = \frac{A(1-x)+B(2-x)}{(2-x)(1-x)} \qquad .....(1)$$

Cancel Denominator term of LHS and RHS

$$1 = A(1-x) + B(2-x)$$

Put $1 - x = 0$ then $x = 1$

Substitute x = 1 in the equation 2

$$1 = A \times 0 + B(2-1)$$

$$1 = B \text{ or } B = 1$$

Put $2 - x = 0$ then $x = 2$

Substitute x = 2 in the equation 2

$$1 = A(1-2) + B \times 0$$

$$1 = -A \text{ or } A = -1$$

Substitute A and B in equation 2 $\dfrac{1}{(2-x)(1-x)} = \dfrac{A}{2-x} + \dfrac{B}{1-x}$

$$\frac{1}{(2-x)(1-x)} = \frac{-1}{2-x} + \frac{1}{1-x}$$

$$\int \frac{dx}{(2-x)(1-x)} = \int kdt$$

$$\int \frac{-1dx}{2-x} + \int \frac{dx}{1-x} = \int kdt$$

$$\int \frac{1dx}{x-2} - \int \frac{dx}{x-1} = \int kdt$$

$$ln(x-2) - ln(x-1) = kt + c$$

$$ln\left(\frac{x-2}{x-1}\right) = kt$$

Take e both side

$$\frac{x-2}{x-1} = e^{kt+c}$$

$$(x-2) = e^{kt+c}(x-1)$$

$$x - xe^{kt+c} = -2 - e^{kt+c}$$

$$x(1-e^{kt+c}) = -2 - e^{kt+c}$$

$$x(t) = -2 - e^{kt+c} / 1 - e^{kt+c}$$

We now obtain an explicit solution for x(t) and use the initial condition to determine c.

subs(t = 0);

$$0 = -2 + e^{c} / 1 - e^{c}$$

$$e^{c} = 2$$

So the explicit solution to the initial value problem is

$$X(t) = \frac{-2 + 2e^{ki}}{-1 + 2e^{kt}}$$

3. The time course for which the drug is administered intravenously (Infusion) at a constant rate is set into the system of linear differential equation $\frac{dF(t)}{dt} = -kF(t) + Q_0$ where F(t) - Amount of drug present at time t and Q_0 is drug flow rate into the compartment in units of amount / time. Prove that $F(t) = \frac{Q_0}{k}(1-e^{-kt})$

Solution:

$$\frac{dF(t)}{dt} = -kF(t) + Q_0$$

$$\frac{dF(t)}{dt} + k\,F(t) = +Q_0$$

{The above mentioned differential can be solved Linear differential equation or Leibnitz's theorem $\frac{dy}{dx} + Py = Q$ (Leibnitz's theorem)

P – Function of X

Q – Function of X

We know that $\frac{d(uv)}{dx} = u\frac{dv}{dx} + v\frac{du}{dx}$

$$\frac{dy}{dx} + Py = Q$$

Multiply both side by $e\int Pdx$

$$\left(\frac{dy}{dx} + Py = Q\right)e^{\int Pdx}$$

$$\frac{dy}{dx}e^{\int Pdx} + y\,e^{\int Pdx}\,P = Q\,e^{\int Pdx}$$

This can be reduced into the form of

We know that

$$\frac{d(uv)}{dx} = u\frac{dv}{dx} + v\frac{du}{dx}$$

$$\frac{d}{dx}(y\,e^{\int Pdx}) = Q\,e^{\int Pdx}$$

Integrate both side

$$ye^{\int Pdx} = \int Q\,e^{\int Pdx}dx + c \Big\}$$

The above equation should be used for solving

$$\frac{dF(t)}{dt} + k\,F(t) = Q_0 \text{ (K and } Q_0 \text{ are functions of t)}$$

$$F(t)e^{\int Kdt} = \int Q_0 e^{\int kdt}dt + c$$

$$F(t)e^{kt} = Q_0\int e^{kt}dt + c$$

$$t = Q_0\left[\frac{e^{kt}}{k}\right]_0^t \quad 0$$

Apply upper limit and lower limit

$$= Q_0\left(\frac{e^{kt}}{k} - \frac{e^0}{k}\right)$$

$$F(t)\,e^{kt} = \frac{Q_0}{k}(e^{kt} - 1)$$

Divide both side by e^{kt}

$$F(t) = \frac{Q_0}{k}(1 - e^{-kt})$$

4. The amount of drug dissolved in the body is proportional to the amount present in the capsule. If 30% of 500 mg dissolved in 1 hour, calculate the time taken to dissolve 500 mg

Solution:

$$\frac{dc}{dt} = -kc$$

$$\int \frac{dc}{c} = \int -k\,dt$$

$$\log c = -kt + \log c_0$$

$$\log(c/c_0) = -kt$$

Take exp both side

$$c = c_0 e^{-kt}$$

When $c = 500$ and $t = 0$

Since 30% is dissolved in 60 mints then

$$c = 500 - (30/100) \times 500$$

$$c = 500 - 150$$

$c = 350$ after 1 hour

$$c = c_0 e^{-kt}$$

$$350 / e^{-kt} = c_0$$

$c = c_0$ when $t = 0$

$$350 / e^{-kt} = c_0$$

$$e^{60k} = \frac{500}{350} = \frac{10}{7}$$

Take log both side

$$60\,k = \log(10/7)$$

If 90% is dissolved in T hours

$C = 50$ mg $t = T$

$$e^{kt} = \frac{c_0}{50} = \frac{500}{50}$$

$$e^{kT} = 10$$

$$kT = \log(10)$$

$$T = \frac{\log(10)}{K}$$

$$T = \frac{\log(10)}{\log\left(\frac{10}{7}\right)} = 6.45 \text{ hours} = 7 \text{ hours}$$

5. When two molecules of the same reactant are involved in the chemical reaction, then the rate of second order reaction with respect to time would be expressed as

$$r = \frac{dx}{dt} = k(a-x)^2$$

$$r = \frac{dx}{dt} = K(a-x)^2$$

$$\frac{dx}{dt} = K(a-x)^2 \Rightarrow \frac{dx}{(a-x)^2} = Kt$$

To calculate K – value, we have to find the partial fraction of $\frac{1}{(a-x)^2}$.

since the factor (a – x) is repeated, then the equation $\frac{1}{(a-x)^2}$ should be expressed as

$$\frac{1}{(a-x)^2} = \frac{A}{a-x} + \frac{B}{(a-x)^2}$$

$$\frac{1}{(a-x)^2} = \frac{A(a-x)+B}{(a-x)^2}$$

$1 = A(a-x) + B \quad .....(1)$

put $a - x = 0 \rightarrow x = a$

substitute $x = a$ in (1)

$1 = 0 + B$

$B = 1$

Compare coefficient of constants both side of the equation.

$1 = A(a-x) + B$

$1 = Aa + B$

$1 = Aa + 1$ because B = 1

$1 - 1 = Aa$

$0 = Aa$

$A = 0$

$$\therefore \quad \frac{1}{(a-x)^2} = \frac{A}{a-x} + \frac{B}{(a-x)^2}$$

$$\frac{1}{(a-x)^2} = \frac{0}{a-x} + \frac{1}{(a-x)^2}$$

$$\frac{dx}{dt} = K(a-x)^2 \Rightarrow \frac{dx}{(a-x)^2} = Kdt$$

$$\frac{dx}{(a-x)^2} = Kdt$$

$$(a-x)^{-2}\,dx = K\,dt$$

Integrating both side

$$\int_0^x (a-x)^{-2}dx = \int_0^t kdt$$

$$(a-x)^{-2+1}/-2+1 = kt$$

$$\frac{1}{-1}\left(\frac{(a-x)^{-2+1}}{-2+1}\right) = kt$$

$$\frac{1}{-1}\left(\frac{(a-x)^{-1}}{-1}\right) = kt$$

$$\left(\frac{1}{(a-x)}\right) = kt$$

Applying limit x from 0 to x and t from 0 to t we get

$$\left(\frac{1}{(a-x)} - \frac{1}{a}\right) = kt - k0$$

$$\left(\frac{1}{(a-x)} - \frac{1}{a}\right) = kt$$

$$\left(\frac{1}{(a-x)t} - \frac{1}{at}\right) = k$$

6. If the third order $2X + Y \rightarrow Z$, the differential rate is given by the equation $\frac{dy}{dx} = k(a-2x)^2(b-x)$ a and b initial molar concentration of X and Y respectively and x is concentration of the product formed at time t. Prove that.

$$Kt = \frac{1}{(2b-a)^2}\left\{\ln\left[\frac{(a-2x)/(b-x)}{a/b}\right] + (2b-a)\left[\frac{a-(a-2x)}{a(a-x)}\right]\right\}$$

$$Kt = \frac{1}{(2b-a)^2}\left\{\ln\left[\frac{b(a-2x)}{a(b-x)}\right] + \left[\frac{(2b-a)(2x)}{a(a-x)}\right]\right\}$$

Solution:

$$\frac{dy}{dx} = k(a-2x)^2(b-x)$$

Given equation is in the form of differential equation

To solve this apply variable separable method

$$\frac{dx}{(a-2x)^2(b-x)} = kdt$$

Integrate both side

$$\frac{dx}{(a-2x)^2(b-x)} = kdt$$

Find the partial fraction of $\frac{dx}{(a-2x)^2(b-x)}$

$$\frac{1}{(a-2x)^2(b-x)} = \frac{A}{(a-2x)^2} + \frac{B}{(a-2x)} + \frac{C}{(b-x)}$$

Take LCM for RHS side rational functions

$$\frac{1}{(a-2x)^2(b-x)} = \frac{A(b-x) + B(a-2x)(b-x) + C(a-2x)^2}{(b-x)(a-2x)^2}$$

Cancel denominators of LHS and RHS

$1 = A(b-x) + B(a-2x)(b-x) + C(a-2x)^2$ .....(1)

Put $b - x = 0$ then $x = b$

Substitute $x = b$ in equation (1)

$$1 = 0 + 0 + C(a - 2b)^2 \rightarrow C = \frac{1}{(a - 2b)^2}$$

Put a –2x = 0 then x = a/2

Substitute x = b in equation (1)

$$1 = A(b - a/2) + 0 + 0$$

$$1 = A\left(\frac{(2b - a)}{2}\right)$$

$$A = \frac{2}{(2b - a)}$$

To find B compare the coefficient of x both side of the equation (1)

$$0 = -A + B(-2b - a) + C(-4a)$$

$$A + 4Ca = B(-2b - a) \qquad \text{.....(2)}$$

Substitute the value of A and C in equation 2 and simplify

$$B = \frac{-2}{(a - 2b)^2}$$

$$\frac{1}{(a - 2x)^2(b - x)} = \frac{2}{(2a - b)(a - 2x)^2} - \frac{2}{(a - 2b)^2(a - 2x)} + \frac{C_1}{(a - 2b)^2(b - x)}$$

7. Problems about restricted Growth

No organism and No population grow indefinitely

Let Y-be the individual value

Let B- be the upper bound

If y = y(t) approaches B

Then the growth rate dy/dt tends to (B-y)

$$\frac{dy}{dt} \propto (B - y)$$

$$\frac{dy}{dt} = k(B - y)$$

Apply Variable separable form

$$\frac{dy}{(B - y)} = kdt$$

Integrate both side

$$\int \frac{dy}{(B-y)} = \int kdt$$

$$-1(B-y) = ce^{-kt}$$

$$Y = Ce^{-kt} + B$$

Assume When $t = 0 \quad y = 0$

$$B = -C$$

$$Y = B(1-e^{-kt})$$

8. Diffusion Problem

Let the Cell contains constant volume of solute of concentration C_0

Let $C = C(t)$ be the concentration when time is t

By diffusion the molecules of the solute will enter the cell from the surrounding liquid

Let $m = m(t)$ be mass of solute in the cell

Let A = Area of the cell Membrane

Let V = Volume of the cell

But $m(t) = V.C(t)$

According to Fick's Law

$$\frac{dm}{dt} = K\,A(c_0 - c)$$

If $c < c_0$ then $\frac{dm}{dt}$ is directly proportional to the area of the membrane and to the difference in concentration on both side of the membrane

But $$\frac{dm}{dt} = V\frac{dc}{dt}$$

$$\frac{dc}{dt} = \frac{1}{V}\frac{dm}{dt}$$

$$\frac{dc}{dt} = \frac{KA(c_0 - c)}{V}$$

$$\frac{dc}{(c_0 - c)} = \frac{KA}{V} dt$$

$$\int \frac{dc}{(c_0 - c)} = \int \frac{KA}{V} dt$$

$$\log(c - c_0) = \frac{KA}{V} t$$

Apply If t = 0 and t = t

$$\log(c - c_0) = \frac{KA}{V} t + K$$

Take Exp both side

$$c - c_0 = e^{(KA/V)t+K}$$

$$c - c_0 = e^{(KA/V)t} + e^{k}$$

$$c - c_0 = Ke^{(KA/V)t}$$

$$c = Ke^{(KA/V)t} + c_0$$

Exercise 8.1

I. Solve the following differential equations by separating the variables

1. $\left(e^{y}+1\right) \cos x \, dx + e^{y} \sin y \, dy = 0$
2. $xy\frac{dy}{dx} = y + 2$
3. $X\sqrt{1+y^2}dx + y\sqrt{1+x^2}dy = 0$
4. $\frac{e^x}{e^y} = \frac{dy}{dx}$
5. $\frac{dy}{dx} = e^{2x-3y} + 4x^2e^{-3y}$
6. $\frac{dy}{dx} = \frac{y^2(x+1)}{x^2(y-1)}$

II. Solve the following differential equations by reducing into variable separable form

7. $\frac{dy}{dx} + 1 = e(x + y)$
8. $\frac{dy}{dx} = (4x + y + 1)^2$

9. $\frac{dy}{dx} = \frac{(x+y-1)}{(x+y+1)}$

10. $\frac{dy}{dx} = \cos(x+y)$

11. $\frac{dy}{dx} = 1 + e^{(x-y)}$

Answers

1. $\sin x \left(e^{y}\right) = c$

2. $y - 2\log(y+2) = \log x + c$

3. $\sqrt{1+x^2}\,dx + \sqrt{1+y^2}\,dy = c$

4. $e^{x} = e^{y} + c$

5. $3e^{2x} - 2e^{3y} + 8x^3 = c$

6. $\log(y/x) = \frac{1}{x} - \frac{1}{y} + c$

7. $x + e^{-(x+y)} + c = 0$

8. $4x + y + 1 = 2(\tan(2x + 2c))$

9. $x - y + c = \log(x+y)$

10. 10. $x + c = \tan\left(\frac{x+y}{2}\right)$

11. $x - e^{-(x-y)} = c$

CHAPTER 9

LAPLACE TRANSFORMS

Introduction

The Laplace transforms is a powerful tool for solving linear differential equations with given boundary values. Normally, to find the solution of an equation with given boundary conditions, we first find the general solution of the equation, then evaluate the value of the arbitrary constants involved in the solution by using the boundary values. But the method of solving linear equations using Laplace transform has the advantage of getting the solution directly with said boundary values. Further, by applying the method of Laplace transform the problem of solving differential equation can be reduced to mere algebraic manipulations. Just as simplifying the tedious arithmetic calculation by the use of logarithms, the differential operations on a function *f(t)* can be replaced by simple algebraic operations such as multiplication or division.

In this chapter we shall introduce the Laplace transformation, develop its fundamental properties and illustrate its use to solve linear differential equations with boundary values.

9.1 LAPLACE TRANSFORM

***Definition*:** Let f(t) be a function of real variable '*t*' defined for $t \geq 0$. Laplace transform of f(t) is denoted by L[f(t)] and is defined by.

$$L[f(t)] = \int_0^\infty e^{-st} f(t)dt$$

Provided the integral on right hand side exists, where *s* is a parameter real or complex number.

The operator L is called the Laplace transform operator.

Clearly, the L[*f(t)*] is a function of the parameter *s*. we shall denote this function by F(s).

Thus

$$L[f(t)] = \int_0^\infty e^{-st} f(t)dt = F(s)$$

If F(s) is the Laplace transform of *f(t)*, then *f(t)* is called the inverse Laplace transform of F(s) and is denoted by $L^{-1}[F(s)]$.

Thus if $L[f(t)] = F(s)$

Then $f(t) = L^{-1}[F(s)]$

9.1.1 Properties of Laplace Transform

Theorem 1: (Linearity property). If f(t) and g(t) are two functions whose Laplace transform exist and if *a* and *b* are any constants, then

$$L[a\,f(t) + b\,g(f(t))] = a\,L[f(t)] + b\,L[g(t)]$$

Proof: By definition

$$L[a\,f(t) + b\,g(f(t))] = \int_0^\infty e^{-st}[a\,f(t) + bg(t)dt]$$

$$= a\int_0^\infty e^{-st} f(t)dt + b\int_0^\infty e^{-st} g(t)dt$$

$$= a\,L[f(t)] + b\,L[g(t)]$$

Hence

$$L[a\,f(t) + b\,g(f(t))] = a\,L[f(t)] + b\,L[g(t)]$$

Theorem 2 (First shifting property). If the Laplace transform of f(t) is F(s) then the Laplace transform of

$$L\{e^{st}[f(t)]\} = F(s-a)$$

i.e., if $L[f(t)] = F(s)$, then $L\left[e^{st} f(t)\right] = F(s-a)$

Proof: By definition of Laplace transform

$$L\{e^{st}[f(t)]\} = \int_0^\infty e^{-st} e^{st} f(t)dt$$

$$L\{e^{st}[f(t)]\} = \int_0^\infty e^{-rt} f(t)dt \qquad \text{[where } s - a = r\text{]}$$

$$L\left[e^{st} f(t)\right] = F(r) = F(s-a)$$

9.1.2 Laplace Transforms of Elementary Functions

We shall consider the Laplace transforms of some standard elementary functions – like exponential, trigonometric and f lynomial. Here we assume the convergence of integral involved – i.e., F(s) exists in the definition of Laplace transform.

1. Laplace transform of e^{kt}

By definition

$$L\left[e^{kt}\right]=\int_0^\infty e^{-st}e^{kt}dt$$

$$=\int_0^\infty e^{-(s-k)t}dt$$

$$=\left[\frac{-e^{-(s-k)}}{s-k}\right]_0^\infty$$

$$=0+\frac{1}{s-k} \qquad [\text{if } s-k>0]$$

$$\therefore \quad L\left[e^{kt}\right]=\frac{1}{s-k} \qquad \text{provided } s-k>0$$

If $s-k\le 0$, the power of e is positive or zero and the integral diverges.

Similarly

$$\therefore \quad L\left[e^{-kt}\right]=\frac{1}{s+k} \qquad \text{provided } s+k>0$$

In particular if $k = 0$, we have

$$L[1]=\frac{1}{s} \qquad \text{for } s>0$$

2. Laplace transform of cos m t and sin m t

We know that

$$e^{imt}=\cos mt+i\sin mt$$

$$\therefore \quad L\left[e^{imt}\right]=L[\cos mt]+iL[\sin mt]$$

[using linearity property]

Now $$L\left[e^{imt}\right]=\int_0^\infty e^{-st}.e^{imt}\,dt$$

$$=\frac{1}{s-im}=\frac{s}{s^2+m^2}+i\frac{m}{s^2+m^2}$$

L [cos m t] = real part of L [e ^{imt}]

L [sin m t] = Imaginary part of l [e ^{imt}]

$\therefore$ $$L[\cos mt]=\frac{s}{s^2+m^2}$$

and $$L[\sin mt]=\frac{m}{s^2+m^2}$$

3. Laplace transform of t^n, when *n* is a positive integer

By definition $L[t^n]=\int_0^\infty e^{-st}.t^n\,dt$

Integrating by parts

$$L[t^n]=-\left[\frac{t^n e^{-st}}{s}\right]_0^\infty+\int_0^\infty e^{-st}.t^{n-1}\,dt$$

$$L[t^n]=0+\frac{n}{s}L[t^{n-1}]$$

[Because for s > 0, and n > 0, then first term is zero]

$\therefore$ $$L[t^n]=\frac{n}{s}L[t^{n-1}] \qquad .....(1)$$

Again $$L\left[t^{n-1}\right]=\frac{n-1}{s}L\left[t^{n-2}\right] \qquad .....(2)$$

$\therefore$ $$L\left[t^n\right]=\frac{n}{s}\cdot\frac{n-1}{s}L\left[t^{n-2}\right] \qquad \text{[from (1) and (2)]}$$

Repeating the process, we get

$$L\left[t^n\right]=\frac{n(n-1)(n-2)...2.1}{s^n}L\left[t^0\right]$$

But we know that

$$L\left[t^0\right]=L[1]=\frac{1}{s}$$

If n is a positive integer

$$L\left[t^n\right]=\frac{n!}{s^{n+1}},\ s>0$$

In particular

$$L[t]=\frac{1}{s^2},\ L\left[t^2\right]=\frac{2}{s^3},\ \text{etc}$$

By applying the theorem 2 (First shifting property) we obtain the following results.

4. $L\left[e^{at.t^n}\right]=\frac{n!}{(s-a)^{n+1}}$

5. $L\left[e^{at}\cos mt\right]=\frac{s-a}{(s-a)^2+m^2}$

6. $L\left[e^{at}\sin mt\right]=\frac{m}{(s-a^2)+m^2}$

9.1.3 Existence of Laplace Transform

We shall state a condition for the existence of Laplace transform for a given condition.

If f(t) is continuous and $\lim_{n\to\infty} L\left[e^{-at}f(t)\right]$ is finite, the Laplace transform of f(t)

i.e., $\int_0^\infty e^{-at}f(t)dt$ exists for $s>a$

The above condition is only sufficient condition but not necessary. For example consider the function; $f(t)=\frac{1}{\sqrt{t}}$ the function is $\frac{1}{\sqrt{t}}$ is not a continuous function at $t=0$. But $L=\left[\frac{1}{\sqrt{t}}\right]$ exists and $L\left[\frac{1}{\sqrt{t}}\right]=\frac{\sqrt{\pi}}{s}$.

Example 1: Obtain L $[t^2+3t+5]$

Solution: By linearity property, we have

$$L[t^2+3t+5]=L[t^2]-3L[t]+5L[1]$$

$$= \frac{2}{s^3} - 3.\frac{1}{s^2} + 5.\frac{1}{s}, \qquad s > 0$$

$$= \frac{2 - 3s + 5s^2}{s^3}$$

Example 2: Evaluate $L[e^{-4t} + 3e^{-2t}]$

Solution: We have

$$L[e^{-4t} + 3e^{-2t}] = L[e^{-4t}] + 3L[e^{-2t}]$$

$$= \frac{1}{s+4} + 3.\frac{1}{s+2}$$

$$= \frac{2(2s+7)}{(s+4)(s+2)}$$

Example 3: Find the laplace transform of cos 3t sin2t

Solution: $\cos 5t \sin 2t = \frac{1}{2}[\sin 5t - \sin t]$

$$\therefore \quad L[\cos 3t \sin 2t] = \frac{1}{2}\{L[\sin 5t] - L[\sin t]\}$$

$$= \frac{1}{2}\left[\frac{5}{s^2+25} - \frac{1}{s^2+1}\right]$$

$$= \frac{3(s^2-5)}{(s^2+25)(s^2+1)}$$

Example 4: Show that $L[\sin 2t] = \frac{2}{s(s^2+4)}$

Solution: We have

$$\sin^2 t = \frac{1}{2}(1 - \cos 2t)$$

$$L[\sin^2 t] = \frac{1}{2}L[1 - \cos 2t]$$

$$= \frac{1}{2}\{[1] - L[\cos 2t]\}$$

$$= \frac{1}{2}\left\{\frac{1}{s} - \frac{s}{s^2+4}\right\}$$

$$= \frac{2}{s(s^2+4)}$$

Example 5: Find the laplace transform of cos3t sin2t

Solution: $\cos 3t \sin 2t = \frac{1}{2}[\sin 5t - \sin t]$

$$\therefore \quad L[\cos 3t \sin 2t] = \frac{1}{2}\{L[\sin 5t] - L[\sin t]\}$$

$$= \frac{1}{2}\left[\frac{5}{s^2+25} - \frac{1}{s^2+1}\right]$$

$$= \frac{2(s^2-5)}{(s^2+25)(s^2+1)}$$

Example 6: Show that $L[\sin^2 t] = \frac{2}{s(s^2+4)}$

Solution: We have

$$\sin^2 t = \frac{1}{2}(1 - \cos 2t)$$

$$L[\sin^2 t] = \frac{1}{2}L[1 - \cos 2t]$$

$$= \frac{1}{2}\left\{\frac{1}{s} - \frac{s}{s^2+4}\right\}$$

$$= \frac{2}{s(s^2+4)}$$

Example 7: Evaluate L[t sin at] and L[t cos at]

Solution: We have $L(t) = \frac{1}{s^2}$

$$\therefore \quad L[t.e^{iat}] = \frac{1}{(s-ia)^2} \qquad \text{[Using first shifting property]}$$

$$= \frac{(s+ia)^2}{(s^2+a^2)^2}$$

$$= \frac{(s^2 - a^2) + 2ias}{(s^2 + a^2)^2}$$

$$\therefore \quad L[t\cos at + i\, t\sin at] = \frac{s^2 - a^2}{(s^2 + a^2)^2} + i\frac{2as}{(s^2 + a^2)^2}$$

Applying linearity property to the left side and equating the real and imaginary parts on both sides we have,

$$L[t\cos at] = \frac{s^2 - a^2}{(s^2 + a^2)^2}$$

$$L[t\sin at] = \frac{2as}{(s^2 + a^2)^2}$$

Example 8: Find the Laplace transform of

(i) $e^{at}(2t^2 - 3t + 4)$

(ii) $e^{-3t}(2\cos 5t - 3\sin 5t)$

Solution: By applying linearity property we have

(i) $L[e^{at}(2t^2 - 3t + 4)] = 2L[e^{at}.t^2] - 3L[e^{at}.t] + 4L[e^{at}]$

$$= 2\frac{2}{(s-2)^3} - 3\frac{1}{(s-2)^2} + 4\frac{1}{(s-2)}$$

(Applying the first shifting property)

$$= \frac{4s^2 - 11s + 26}{(s-2)^3}$$

(ii) $L[e^{-3t}(2\cos 5t - 3\sin 5t)]$

$$= 2L[e^{-3t}\cos 5t] - 3L[e^{-3t}\sin 5t]$$

$$= 2.\frac{s+3}{(s+3)^2 + 25} - 3.\frac{5}{(s+3)^2 + 25}$$

$$= \frac{2s - 9}{(s+3)^2 + 25}$$

Example 9: Find the Laplace transform of

(i) a^t (ii) 6^t

Solution: we know that $A^B = e^{B\log A}$

(i) $L[a^t] = L[e^t \log a] = \dfrac{1}{s - \log a}$

(ii) $L[6^t] = L[e^{t\log 6}) = \dfrac{1}{s - \log 6}$

9.2 INVERSE LAPLACE TRANSFORMS

We have seen that if,

$$L[f(t)] = F(s), \quad \text{then} \quad L^{-1}[F(s)] = f(t)$$

The L^{-1} denotes the inverse Laplace transform.

We have observed that L[f(t)] is a simple rational function of s. This suggests that the most obvious way of finding f(t) for which the given function may have its Laplace transform, is by resolving the given function into partial fractions and to look out the table of Laplace transform and get the functions whose transform is the different partial fraction.

Following is the table of transforms and inverse transforms of some standard elementary functions.

	F(t)	L[f(t)] = F(s)	F(s)	L^{-1}[F(s)] = f(t)
1.	1	$\frac{1}{s}$	$\frac{1}{s}$	1
2.	t	$\frac{1}{s^2}$	$\frac{1}{s^2}$	t
3.	t^2	$\frac{1}{s^2}$	$\frac{2}{s^3}$	$\frac{1}{2}t^2$
4.	t^n	$\frac{n!}{s^{n+1}}$	$\frac{1}{s^n}$	$\frac{t^{n-1}}{(n-1)!}$
5.	e^{kt}	$\frac{1}{s-k}$	$\frac{1}{s-k}$	e^{kt}
6.	cos at	$\frac{s}{s^2+a^2}$	$\frac{s}{s^2+a^2}$	cos at
7.	sin at	$\frac{a}{s^2+a^2}$	$\frac{a}{s^2+a^2}$	sin at

Contd...

	F(t)	L[f(t)] = F(s)	F(s)	$L^{-1}[F(s)] = f(t)$
8.	$e^{kt}.t^n$	$\frac{n!}{(s-k)^{n+1}}$	$\frac{1}{(s-k)^n}$	$e^{kt}\frac{t^{n-1}}{(n-1)}$
9.	$e^{kt}\sin at$	$\frac{a}{(s-k)^2+a^2}$	$\frac{a}{(s-k)^2+a^2}$	$\frac{1}{a}.e^{kt}\sin at$
10.	$e^{kt}\cos at$	$\frac{s-k}{(s-k)^2+a^2}$	$\frac{s-k}{(s-k)^2+a^2}$	$e^{kt}\cos at$
11.	$t\sin at$	$\frac{2as}{(s^2+a^2)^2}$	$\frac{s}{(s^2+a^2)^2}$	$\frac{1}{2a}t\sin at$
12.	$t\cos at$	$\frac{a^2+s^2}{(s^2+a^2)^2}$	$\frac{a^2-s^2}{(s^2+a^2)^2}$	$t\cos at$

Example 10: Find the inverse Laplace transform of the following

(i) $\frac{s}{(s+4)^2}$ (ii) $\frac{1}{(s-4)^3}$

(iii) $\frac{s+2}{(s^2-4s+13)}$ (iv) $\frac{s+1}{(s^2+2s-8)}$

Solution:

(i) $$L^{-1}\left[\frac{s}{(s+4)^2}\right] = L^{-1}\left[\frac{(s+4)-4}{(s+4)^2}\right]$$

$$= L^{-1}\left[\frac{1}{(s+4)} - \frac{4}{(s+4)^2}\right]$$

$$= L^{-1}\left[\frac{1}{(s+4)}\right] - 4L^{-1}\left[\frac{1}{(s+4)^2}\right]$$

$$= e^{-4t} - 4t.e^{-4t}$$

$$= e^{-4t}[1-4t]$$

(ii) $$L^{-1}\left[\frac{1}{(s-4)^3}\right] = \frac{1}{2}.L^{-1}\left[\frac{2!}{(s-4)^3}\right]$$

$$= \frac{1}{2}.e^{4t}\,t^2 \qquad \left(\text{Because } L^{-1}\left[\frac{1}{s^3}\right] = \frac{t^2}{2!}\right)$$

(iii) $L^{-1}\left[\dfrac{s+2}{(s^2-4s+13}\right]$

Consider $s^2 - 4s + 13 = s^2 - 4s + 4 + 9$

$= (s-2)^2 + 3^2$ (completing the square)

$$\therefore \quad L^{-1}\left[\frac{s+2}{(s^2-4+13}\right] = L^{-1}\left[\frac{s+2}{(s-2)^2+3^2}\right]$$

$$= L^{-1}\left[\frac{(s-2)+4}{(s-2)^2+3^2}\right]$$

$$= L^{-1}\left[\frac{(s-2)}{(s-2)^2+3^2}\right] + L^{-1}\left[\frac{4}{(s-2)^2+3^2}\right]$$

$$= L^{-1}\left[\frac{(s-2)}{(s-2)^2+3^2}\right] + \frac{4}{3}L^{-1}\left[\frac{3}{(s-2)^2+3^2}\right]$$

$$= e^{2t}\cos 3t + \frac{4}{3}e^{2t}\sin 3t$$

Example 11: Find the Inverse Laplace transform of the following functions

(i) $\dfrac{3s+2}{(2s^2-4s+3)}$ (ii) $\dfrac{3+4s}{(9s^2-16)}$ (iii) $\dfrac{2s-1}{(s^2-2s+10)}$

Solution:

(i) $L^{-1}\left[\dfrac{3s+2}{(2s^2-4s+3)}\right]$

Consider, $2s^2 - 4s + 3 = 2\left(s^2 - 2s + 1 + \dfrac{1}{2}\right)$

$$= 2\left[(s-1)^2 + \frac{1}{2}\right]$$

$$\therefore \quad L^{-1}\left[\frac{3s+2}{(2s^2-4s+3)}\right] = L^{-1}\left[\frac{3s+2}{\left\{2(s-1)^2+\frac{1}{2}\right\}}\right]$$

$$= \frac{1}{2} L^{-1}\left[\frac{3s+2}{(s-1)^2 + \frac{1}{2}}\right]$$

$$= \frac{1}{2} L^{-1}\left[\frac{3(s-1)+5}{(s-1)^2 + \frac{1}{2}}\right]$$

$$= \frac{1}{2} 3L^{-1}\left[\frac{s-1}{(s-1)^2 + \left(\frac{1}{\sqrt{2}}\right)^2}\right] + 5\sqrt{2}L^{-1}\left[\frac{\frac{1}{\sqrt{2}}}{(s-1)^2 + \left(\frac{1}{\sqrt{2}}\right)^2}\right]$$

$$= \frac{3}{2} e^t \cos\left(\frac{t}{\sqrt{2}}\right) + \frac{5}{\sqrt{2}} e^t \sin\left(\frac{t}{\sqrt{2}}\right)$$

$$= \frac{e^t}{2}\left[3\cos\left(\frac{t}{\sqrt{2}}\right) + 5\sqrt{2}\sin\left(\frac{t}{\sqrt{2}}\right)\right]$$

(ii) $L^{-1}\left[\frac{3+4s}{(9s^2-16)}\right]$

Consider, $9s^2 - 16 = 9\left(s^2 - \frac{16}{9}\right) = 9\left[s^2 - \left(\frac{4}{3}\right)^2\right]$

$$\therefore \quad L^{-1}\left[\frac{3+4s}{(9s^2-16)}\right] = \frac{1}{9} L^{-1}\left[\frac{3+4s}{s^2 - \left(\frac{4}{3}\right)^2}\right]$$

$$= \frac{1}{9}\left\{L^{-1}\left[\frac{3}{s^2 - \left(\frac{4}{3}\right)^2}\right] + L^{-1}\left[\frac{4s}{s^2 - \left(\frac{4}{3}\right)^2}\right]\right\}$$

$$= \frac{1}{9}\left\{\frac{9}{4}L^{-1}\left[\frac{\frac{4}{3}}{s^2-\left(\frac{4}{3}\right)^2}\right]+4L^{-1}\left[\frac{s}{s^2-\left(\frac{4}{3}\right)^2}\right]\right\}$$

$$= \frac{1}{4}\sinh\left(\frac{4t}{3}\right)+\frac{4}{9}\cosh\left(\frac{4t}{3}\right)$$

(iii) $L^{-1}\left[\frac{2s-1}{(s^2-2s+10)}\right]$

Consider $s^2-2s+10 = s^2-2s+1+9 = (s-1)^2+3^2$

$$\therefore \quad L^{-1}\left[\frac{2s-1}{(s^2-2s+10)}\right] = L^{-1}\left[\frac{2s-1}{(s-1)^2+3^2}\right]$$

$$= L^{-1}\left[\frac{2(s-1)+1}{(s-1)^2+3^2}\right]$$

$$= 2L^{-1}\left[\frac{s-1}{(s-1)^2+3^2}\right]+\frac{1}{3}L^{-1}\left[\frac{3}{(s-1)^2+3^2}\right]$$

$$= 2s^t\cos 3t + \frac{1}{3}e^t\sin 3t$$

$$= \frac{e^t}{3}\left[6\cos 3t + e^t\sin 3t\right]$$

9.3 LAPLACE TRANSFORM OF DERIVATIVES

We shall express the Laplace transform of the derivative of a function in terms of the function itself. This property of Laplace transform is very useful, as the operation of differentiation may be replaced by simple algebraic operation of the Laplace transforms.

Definition: A continuous functions f(t) for $t > 0$ is said to be of exponential order if

$$\lim_{t\to\infty} e^{-st}f(t) = 0$$

Theorem 1: Let f (t) be of exponential order and have $f'(t)$ which is continuous.

If

$$L[f(t)] = F(s)$$

Then $$L[f'(t)] = sF(s) - f(0)$$

Proof: By definition, we have

$$L[f'(t)] = \int_0^{\infty} e^{-st} f'(t)\, dt$$

$$L[f'(t)] = \left[e^{-st} f(t)\right]_0^{\infty} + s\int_0^{\infty} e^{-st} f(t)\, dt$$

[Integration by parts]

$$= 0 - f(0) + s\, L[f(t)]$$

[Because f(t) is of exponential order]

$\therefore$ $$L[f'(t)] = s\, L[f(t)] - f(0)$$

or $$L[f'(t)] = s\, F(s) - f(0)$$

The above result can be extended to 2nd order derivatives.

Corollary: $L[f''(t)] = s^2F(s) - f(0) - f'(0)$

Proof: Consider

$$F[f''(t)] = L\{[f'(t)]'\}$$

$$= sL[f'(t)] - f'(0) \qquad \text{[By theorem 1]}$$

$$= s\{sL[f(t)] - f(0)\} - f'(0)$$

$$= s^2 L[f(t) - sf(0) - f'(0)$$

$$= s^2 F(s) - sf(0) - f'(0)$$

or $$L[f''(t)] = s^2F(s) - s^2F(s) - sf(0) - f'(0)$$

In general, we have

$$L[f^n(t)] = s^n F(s) - s^{n-1} f(0) - s^{n-2} f'(0) \ldots - f^{n-1}(0),$$

provided f(t) and all its derivatives up to order (n – 1) are of exponential order and that $f'(t)$ is continuous.

Theorem 2: If $L[f(t)] = F(s)$ than $L\left[t\, f'(t)\right] = -F'(s)$

Proof: By definition, we have

$$F(s) = L[f(t)] = \int_0^\infty e^{-st} f(t)dt$$

$$\therefore \quad F'(s) = \frac{d}{ds}\int_0^\infty e^{-st} f(t)dt$$

$$= \int_0^\infty \frac{d}{ds}[e^{-st} f(t)]\, dt$$

$$= \int_0^\infty -t\, e^{-st} f(t)\, dt$$

$$= -\int_0^\infty e^{-st}[t\, f(t)]dt = -L[t\, f(t)]dt$$

$$\therefore \quad L[t\, f(t)] = -F'(s)$$

The above result can be extended.

Corollary: $L[t^2\, f(t)] = (-1)^2 F''(s)$

Proof: By theorem 2, we have

$$F'(s) = -\int_0^\infty e^{-st} t[t\, f(t)]dt$$

$$\therefore \quad F''(s) = -\int_0^\infty -t\, e^{-st}[t\, f(t)]dt$$

or

$$F''(s) = -\int_0^\infty e^{-st}[t^2\, f(t)]dt$$

$$F''(s) = (-1)^2\, L[t^2 f(t)]$$

$$\therefore \quad L[t^2 f(t)] = (-1)^2 F''(s)$$

In general we have

$$L[t^n f(t)] = (-1)^n F^n(s)$$

where n is a positive integer

Example 12: Find the Laplace transform of

(i) t cos at (ii) t^2 sin at (iii) $t\, e^{-t} \cosh t$

Solution:

(i) $$L[\cos at] = \frac{s}{s^2 + a^2}$$

Now $$L[t \cos at] = \frac{d}{ds}[L(\cos at)]$$

$$= \frac{d}{ds}\left[\frac{s}{s^2 + a^2}\right]$$

$$= \frac{s^2 - a^2}{(s^2 + a^2)^2}$$

(ii) $$L[\sin at] = \frac{a}{s^2 + a^2} = F(a)$$

$\therefore$ $$L[t^2 \sin at] = (-1)^2 F''(s)$$

$$= \frac{d^2}{ds^2}\left[\frac{a}{s^2 + a^2}\right]$$

$$= \frac{d}{ds}\left[\frac{-2as}{(s^2 + a^2)}\right]$$

(iii) Now $$L[t\, e^{-t} \cosh t] = \frac{s + a}{(s + 1)^2 - 1} = \frac{s + 1}{s^2 + 2s}$$

$\therefore$ $$L[t\, e^{-t} \cosh t] = \frac{d}{ds}\left[\frac{s + 1}{s^2 + 2s}\right] = \frac{s^2 + 2s + 2}{(s^2 + 2s)^2}$$

Example 13: Show that

$$L^{-1}\left[\frac{1}{\left(s^2 + a^2\right)^2}\right] = \frac{1}{2a^3}[\sin at - at \cos at]$$

$$L[\sin at - at \cos at] = 2a^3\left[\frac{1}{\left(s^2 + a^2\right)^2}\right]$$

$$L[\sin at] = \frac{a}{(s^2 + a^2)}$$

By example 1. (i), we have

$$L[t \cos at] = \frac{s^2 - a^2}{(s^2 + a^2)^2}$$

$$\therefore \quad L[\sin at - at \cos at] = L[\sin at] - a\, L[t \cos at]$$

$$= \frac{a}{(s^2 + a^2)} - a \frac{s^2 - a^2}{(s^2 + a^2)^2}$$

$$= \frac{as^2 + a^3 - as^2 + a^3}{(s^2 + a^2)^2}$$

$$\therefore \quad L^{-1}\left[\frac{1}{(s^2 + a^2)^2}\right] = \frac{1}{2a^3}[\sin at - at \cos at]$$

9.4 APPLICATION TO SOLVE LINEAR DIFFERENTIAL EQUATIONS

9.4.1 Transformation of Ordinary Differential Equations

One of the very important applications of Laplace transformation lies in solving linear differential equations with constant coefficients. By applying the method of Laplace transform, the problem of solving differential equation can be reduced to mere algebraic manipulations such as multiplication or division. Moreover, this method gives us directly the particular solutions of the equation.

Consider the linear differential equation,

$$a_0 y''(t) + a_1 y'(t) + a_2 y(t) = Q$$

where Q is a function of t and a_0, a_1, a_2 are constants, with the conditions $y = C_1$ and $y' = C_2$ when $t = 0$, i.e., $y(0) = C_1$ and $y'(0) = C_2$.

Applying the Laplace transform both sides we get.

$$L[a_0 y''(t) + a_1 y'(t) + a_2 y(t)] = L[Q]$$

$$L[a_0 y''(t)] + L[a_1 y'(t)] + L[a_2 y(t)] = L[Q]$$

or

$$a_0[s^2y(s) - s\,y(0) - y'(0)] + a_1[s\,\gamma(s) - y(0)] + a_2\gamma(s) = L[Q]$$

[using theorem 1]

where y(s) is the function L [y (t)]

but by data y (0) = C_1 and y' (0) = C_2

$$\therefore \qquad a_0[s^2\gamma(s) - C_1\,s - C_2] + a_1[s\,\gamma(s) - C_1] + a_2\gamma(s) = L[Q]$$

or $$(a_0s^2 + a_1s + a_2)\gamma(s) - a_0C_1s - a_0C_2 - a_1C_1 = L[Q]$$

or $$\gamma(s) = \frac{L[Q] + a_0C_1s - a_0C_2 - a_1C_1}{a_0s^2 + a_1s + a_2} = F(s) \qquad \text{(say)}$$

Taking inverse transform of both sides, we get

$$L^{-1}[\gamma(s)] = L^{-1}[F(s)]$$

or y = f (t), which is the required solution.

9.4.2 Working Rule to Solve Differential Equations

Step 1: Take the Laplace transformation on both sides of the equation and use the initial conditions given in the problem. This reduces the differential equation to an algebraic equation.

Step 2: Solve the algebraic Laplace transform equation obtained in step 1., for Υ (s), where L [y (t)] = Υ (s). Let Υ(s), = F (s)

Step 3: Take inverse Laplace transform on both sides of $\Upsilon(s)$, = F (s). This gives $L^{-1}[\gamma(s)] = L^{-1}[F(s)]$, that is y = f(t), is the required solution. Here f (t) = L^{-1} [F (s)] which has to be evaluated.

Example 14: Solve $y' - 5y = e^{5x}$ given $y(0) = 2$

Solution: Taking Laplace transform on both sides of the equation, we get

$$L[y' - 5y] = L\left[e^{5x}\right]$$

$$s\,F(s) - y(0) - 5F(s) = \frac{1}{s-5}$$

$$F(s)=\frac{2s-9}{(s-5)^2}$$

$$F(s)=\frac{2}{s-5}+\frac{1}{(s-5)^2}$$

$$y=L^{-1}[F(s)]=2L^{-1}\left[\frac{1}{s-5}\right]+L^{-1}\left[\frac{1}{(s-5)^2}\right]$$

$$y=2e^{5x}+xe^{5x}$$

Therefore the solution is $y=2e^{5x}+xe^{5x}$

Exercise 9.1

I Solve the following differential equations by Laplace transform method:

1. $y'-5y=0$ given $(0)=2$
2. $y'+y=\sin x$ given $y(0)=2$
3. $y'-5y=0$ given $y(\pi)=2$
4. $y'+y=\sin x$ given $y(0)=1$
5. $\frac{dQ}{dt}+2Q=1$ given $Q(0)=0$
6. $\frac{dN}{dt}=kN$ given $N(0)=250$, k constant

Answers

1. $Y=2\,e^{5t}$
2. Y = ½ e-x – 1/2cosx + ½ sinx
3. $y=2\,e^{5(x-\pi)}$
4. $Y=3/2e^{-x}\ -1/2\cos x\ +1/2\ \sin x$
5. $Y=5-5\,e^{0.2t}$
6. $y=250e^{kt}$

9.5 APPLICATION TO DERIVE PHARMACOKINETICS EQUATIONS

1. After the intravenous injection of a drug to a patient, it distributing in the body and also eliminates in the body as first order kinetics is set into the differential $\frac{dX}{dt} = -KX$ where X is total amount of drug in the body of a patient in time t. Prove that the solution of the differential equation is $X = X_0e^{-kt}$

Solution:

$$\frac{dX}{dt} = -KX$$

Here $\frac{dX}{dt}$ can also written as X^1 = First order derivative

Then $X^1 = -KX$

Take Laplace Transform both side

$$L\{X^1\} = L\{-KX\}$$

$$L\{X^1\} = -k\,L\{X\}$$

$$\overline{X} - X_0 = -k\overline{X}$$

$$(S\overline{X} + K\overline{X}) = X$$

$$\overline{X} = \frac{X_0}{S+K}$$ S – Laplace operator

Take inverse Laplace transform both side

$$L^{-1}\{\overline{X}\} = X_0e^{-Kt}$$

$$X = X_0e^{-Kt}$$

X_0 – Amount of drug given to the patient when time is zero

2. In a two compartment model the amount of drug in each compartment is X_1 and X_2, the micro rate constants describing drug transfer between or out of the compartment (Ks) and a single X_0 is expressed by the differential equations

$$\frac{dX_1}{dt} = k_{12}X_2 - k_{21}X_1 - k_{10} \text{ and } \frac{dX_2}{dt} = k_{21}X_1 - k_{21}X_2$$

Show that $X_1 = \frac{K_{12}-a}{b-a}e^{-at} + \frac{K_{12}-b}{a-b}e^{-bt}$

$$X_1 = Ae^{-at} + Be^{-bt}$$

Solution:

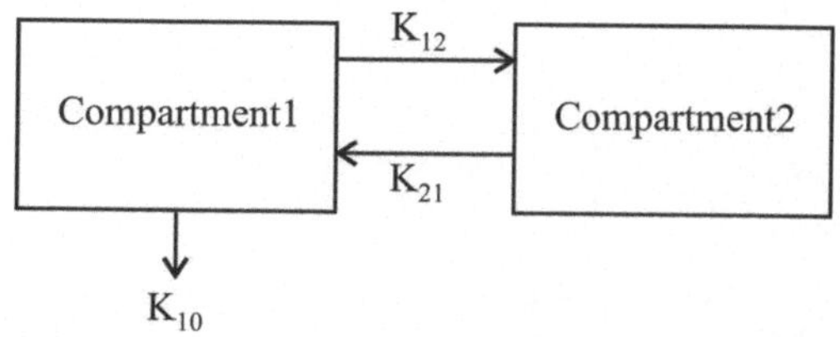

$$\frac{dX_1}{dt} = k_{12}X_2 - k_{21}X_1 - k_{01}$$

$$\frac{dX_2}{dt} = k_{21}X_1 - k_{12}X_2$$

Apply Laplace transform both side of the differential equations

$$L\left\{\frac{dX_1}{dt}\right\} = L\{k_{12}X_2\} - L\{k_{21}X_1 + k_{10}X_1\} \qquad .....(1)$$

$$L\left\{\frac{dX_2}{dt}\right\} = L\{k_{21}X_1\} - L\{k_{12}X_2\} \qquad .....(2)$$

$$s\overline{X}_1 - \overline{X}_1(0) = k_{12}\overline{X}_2 - (k_{21} + k_{10})\overline{X}_1$$

$$(s + k_{21} + k_{10})\overline{X}_1 - \overline{X}_1(0) = k_{12}\overline{X}_2$$

$$s\overline{X}_2 - \overline{X}_2(0) = k_{21}\overline{X}_1 - k_{12}\overline{X}_2$$

Because of normalization $\overline{X}_1 = (0) = 1$ in central compartment

$$(s + k_{21} + k_{10})\overline{X}_1 - 1 = k_{12}\overline{X}_2$$

$$(s + k_{21} + k_{10})\overline{X}_1 - k_{12}\overline{X}_2 = 1 \qquad .....(3)$$

$$-K_{21}\overline{X}_1 + (s + K_{12})\overline{X}_2 = 0 \qquad .....(4)$$

These two equations are in the system of linear equations which are solved by the method of Crammer's rule

$$a_1x + b_1Y = c_1$$

$a_2x + b_2Y = c_2$

$$\Delta = \begin{pmatrix} a_1 & b_1 \\ a_2 & b_2 \end{pmatrix} = a_1b_2 - a_2b_1$$

$$\Delta_1 = \begin{pmatrix} a_1 & c_1 \\ a_2 & c_2 \end{pmatrix} = a_1c_2 - a_2c_1$$

$$\Delta_2 = \begin{pmatrix} c_1 & b_1 \\ c_2 & b_2 \end{pmatrix} = c_1b_2 - c_2b_1$$

$$\Delta = \begin{pmatrix} s + k_{10} + k_{21} & -k_{12} \\ -k_{21} & s + k_{12} \end{pmatrix}$$

$$= (s + k_{10} + k_{21})(s + k_{12}) - (-k_{21} - k_{12})$$

$$= s^2 + (k_{10} + k_{12} + k_{21})s + k_{10}k_{12}$$

Take $a + b = (k_{10} + k_{12} + k_{21})$

$ab = k_{10}k_{12}$

$\Delta = s^2 + (a + b)s + ab$

This is a quadratic equation

$\Delta = (s + a)(s+ b)$

$$\Delta_1 = \begin{pmatrix} 1 & -k_{12} \\ 0 & s + k_{12} \end{pmatrix} = 1(s + k_{12}) - 0$$

$\Delta_1 = s + k_{12}$

$$\overline{X}_1 = \frac{s + k_{12}}{(s + a)(s + b)}$$

After finding the partial fraction for above rational function

$$\frac{(s + k_{12})}{(s + a)(s + b)} = \frac{A}{s + a} + \frac{B}{s + b}$$

$$\overline{X}_1 = \frac{k_{12} - a}{(b - a)(s + a)} + \frac{k_{12} - b}{(a - b)(s + b)}$$

Take Inverse Laplace Transform both side

$$X_1 = \frac{k_{12} - a}{b - a} e^{-at} + \frac{k_{12} - b}{b - a} e^{-bt}$$

$$X_1 = Ae^{-at} + Be^{-bt}$$

3. The differential equation

$\frac{d_u}{dt} = \frac{k_a k_e F x_0}{k_a - K}\left(e^{-kt} - e^{-k_a t}\right)$ represents Pharmacokinetics evaluation of urinary excretion data obtained after extra vascular administration of drug. Prove that

$$\overline{X}_u = \frac{k_a k_e F x_0}{k_a - K}\left[\frac{1}{k_a} + \frac{e^{-kt}}{k - k_a} - \frac{ke^{-k_a t}}{k_a (k - k_a)}\right]$$

Solution: The given equation is $\frac{dx_u}{dt} = \frac{k_a k_e F x_0}{k_a - K}\left(e^{-kt} - e^{-k_a t}\right)$

Take the Laplace transform both side of the equation, then

$$L\left\{\frac{dx_u}{dt}\right\} = \frac{k_a k_e F x_0}{k_a - K}\left(L\{e^{-kt}\} - l\{e^{-k_a t}\}\right)$$

$$s\,\overline{x}_u - X_u(0) = \frac{k_a k_e F x_0}{k_a - K}\left(\frac{1}{s + k} - \frac{1}{s + k_a}\right)$$

$$s\,\overline{x}_u - X_u(0) = \frac{k_a k_e F X_0}{k_a - K}\left(\frac{s + k_a - s - k}{(s + k)(s + k_a)}\right)$$

$$s\,\overline{x}_u = \frac{k_a k_e F X_0}{k_a - K}\left(\frac{k_a - k}{(s + k)(s + k_a)}\right)$$

$$s\,\overline{x}_u = k_a k_e F X_0\left(\frac{1}{(s + k)(s + k_a)}\right)$$

$$\overline{x}_u = k_a k_e F X_0\left(\frac{1}{s(s + k)(s + k_a)}\right)$$

When the equation is solved for x_u by applying partial fraction and taking inverse Laplace transformation, yield

$$x_u = k_a k_e F X_0\left(\frac{1}{k_a} + \frac{e^{-kt}}{k - k_a} + \frac{ke^{-k_a t}}{k_a (k - k_a)}\right)$$

INDEX

A

C

D

E

F

H

I

L

M

N

O

P

R

S

T

AUTHOR SUGGESTIONS

Pharmaceutical Mathematics is a tool to teach few subjects in Pharmacy course. In this regard herewith I am giving few of my suggestion With my 27 year experience of teaching for Pharmacy students. Since Mathematics is tool, in this connection I would like to suggest that, the mathematics subjects should not be taught as a course, but it should be divided into three parts and same has to be included and taught in the different subjects as suggested by the author.

SYLLABUS TO BE INCLUDED IN PHARMACEUTICS

Pharmaceutical Mathematics: **05 hrs**

Partial Fraction:

Introduction, Polynomial, Rational fractions, Proper and Improper fractions, Partial fraction, Resolution into Partial fraction, **Application of Partial Fraction to solve pharmaceutical problems**

Logarithms **05 hrs**

Introduction, Definition, Theorems on logarithms, Common logarithms, Characteristic and Mantissa, worked examples, **Application of Logarithm to Solve Pharmaceutical Problems.**

Analytical Geometry: **15 hrs**

Introduction: Signs of the Coordinates, Distance formula,

Straight Line : Slope or gradient of a straight line, Slope of a line joining two points, Point – slope form, General equation of a line,: **Application in Pharmacy**

SYLLABUS TO BE INCLUDED IN PHYSICAL PHARMACEUTICS

Function: Real Valued function, Classification real valued functions, **03 hrs**

Limits and continuity : Introduction, Limit of a function, Definition of limit of a function ($\in$ - δ definition),

$\lim_{x \to a} \frac{x^n - a^n}{x - a} = na^{n-1}$ (Without Proof)

Differentiation : Introductions, Derivative of a function, Derivative of a constant, Derivative of a product of a constant and a function , Derivative of the sum or difference of two functions, Derivative of the product of two functions (product formula), Derivative of the quotient of two functions (Quotient formula), Derivative of x^n *w.r.t.* x where n is any rational number , Derivative of e^x,, Derivative of $\log_e x$, Derivative of a^x , Differentiation of trigonometric functions (Without Proof), Differentiation of inverse trigonometric (Without Proof) , Function of a function or a composite function, Chain rule, Logarithmic differentiation, Differentiation of implicit functions, Successive Differentiation, Conditions for a function to be a maximum or a minimum at a point. Pharmaceutical Application **15 hrs**

Integration: Introduction, Definition, Standard formulae, Rules of integration , Method of substitution, Method of Partial fractions, Integration by parts, definite integrals, Application in Pharmaceutical derivation **07 hrs**

SYLLABUS TO BE INCLUDED IN BIOPHARMCEUTICS AND PHARMACOKINETICS

Differential Equations : Some basic definitions, Order and degree, Equations in separable form , Homogeneous equations, Linear Differential equations, Exact equations, **Application in solving Pharmacokinetic equations** **08 hrs**

Laplace Transform : Introduction, Definition, Properties of Laplace transform, Laplace Transforms of elementary functions, Inverse Laplace transforms, Laplace transform of derivatives, Application to Linear differential equations, **Application in solving Chemical kinetics and Pharmacokinetics equations** **05 hrs**

Matrices and Determinant **12 hrs**

Introduction, Recapitulation of types of matrices, Types of matrices, Operation on matrices, Transpose of a matrix, Matrix Multiplication, Determinants, Properties of determinants (Without Proof) , Minors and co Factors, Adjoint or adjugate of a square matrix , Singular and non-singular matrices, Solution of system of linear of equations using Cramer's rule, Characteristic equation and roots of a square , Application of Matrices in solving Pharmaceutical problems

9 789385 433788

Printed at Repro India Ltd.